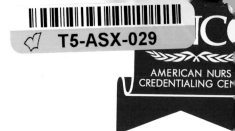

AMERICAN NURS
CREDENTIALING CEN

VOLUME 1

NURSING REVIEW AND RESOURCE MANUAL

Acute Care Nurse Practitioner

Published by American Nurses Credentialing Center
Authors: Pamela Smith, MSN, RN, ACNP-BC, CCRN
Tiffany Boysen, MSN, RN, ACNP-BC, CCRN
Julie Davey, MSN, RN, APRN-BC
Hope Moser, DNP, ANP, BC
Melanie Smith, MSN, RN, ACNP-BC

CONTINUING EDUCATION SOURCE
NURSING CERTIFICATION REVIEW MANUAL
CLINICAL PRACTICE RESOURCE

Library of Congress Cataloging-in-Publication Data

Acute care nurse practitioner : review and resource manual / by Pamela Smith ... [et al.].
   p. ; cm.
Includes bibliographical references and index.
ISBN 978-1-935213-46-8 (pbk.)
I. Smith, Pamela (Pamela Ann), 1955 May 11- II. American Nurses Credentialing Center.
[DNLM: 1. Critical Care–methods–Outlines. 2. Nursing Care–Outlines. WY 18.2]

616.02'8–dc23

                          2011047808

The American Nurses Credentialing Center (ANCC), a subsidiary of the American Nurses Association (ANA), provides individuals and organizations throughout the nursing profession with the resources they need to achieve practice excellence. ANCC's internationally renowned credentialing programs certify nurses in specialty practice areas; recognize healthcare organizations for promoting safe, positive work environments through the Magnet Recognition Program® and the Pathway to Excellence® Program; and accredit providers of continuing nursing education. In addition, ANCC's Institute for Credentialing Innovation provides leading-edge information and education services and products to support its core credentialing programs.

ISBN 13: 978-1-935213-46-8
© 2011 American Nurses Credentialing Center.
8515 Georgia Ave., Suite 400
Silver Spring, MD 20910

Acute Care Nurse Practitioner
Review and Resource Manual

JANUARY 2012

Please direct your comments and/or queries to: revmanuals@ana.org

The healthcare services delivery system is a volatile marketplace demanding superior knowledge, clinical skills, and competencies from all registered nurses. Nursing autonomy of practice and nurse career marketability and mobility in the new century hinge on affirming the profession's formative philosophy, which places a priority on a lifelong commitment to the principles of education and professional development. The knowledge base of nursing theory and practice is expanding, and while care has been taken to ensure the accuracy and timeliness of the information presented in the **Acute Care Nurse Practitioner Review and Resource Manual**, clinicians are advised to always verify the most current national guidelines and recommendations and to practice in accordance with professional standards of care used with regard to the unique circumstances that apply in each practice situation. In addition, every effort has been made in this text to ensure accuracy and, in particular, to confirm that drug selections and dosages are in accordance with current recommendations and practice, including the ongoing research, changes to government regulations, and the developments in product information provided by pharmaceutical manufacturers. However, it is the responsibility of each nurse practitioner to verify drug product information and to practice in accordance with professional standards of care. In addition, the editors wish to note that provision of information in this text does not imply an endorsement of any particular products, procedures or services.

Therefore, the authors, editors, American Nurses Association (ANA), American Nurses Association's Publishing (ANP), American Nurses Credentialing Center (ANCC), and the Institute for Credentialing Innovation cannot accept responsibility for errors or omissions, or for any consequences or liability, injury, and/or damages to persons or property from application of the information in this manual and make no warranty, express or implied, with respect to the contents of the **Acute Care Nurse Practitioner Review and Resource Manual**. Completion of this manual does not guarantee that the reader will pass the certification exam. The practice examination questions are not a requirement to take a certification examination. The practice examination questions cannot be used as an indicator of results on the actual certification.

Published by:
American Nurses Credentialing Center
The Institute for Credentialing Innovation
8515 Georgia Avenue, Suite 400
Silver Spring, MD 20910-3402
www.nursecredentialing.org

Introduction to the Continuing Education (CE) Contact Hour Application Process for *Acute Care Nurse Practitioner Review and Resource Manual*

Continuing education for this title is no longer available. The manual is up-to-date as a test resource, but does not grant any continuing education.

You can view a complete listing of CE offerings from the American Nurses Association online at **www.nursingworld.org**.

Acknowledgements

The authors would like to gratefully acknowledge the foundational work provided by the authors of these review manuals:

Elizabeth Blunt, PhD, MSN, FNP-BC
    Editor of *Family Nurse Practitioner Review and Resource Manual, 3rd Edition*
Sally Miller, PhD, ACNP-BC, GNP-BC, ANP-BC
    Author of *Adult Nurse Practitioner Review and Resource Manual, 3rd Edition*

The authors would also like to acknowledge the following contributors for their work on this manual:

Shirlee Drayton-Brooks, PhD, FNP-BC
Deborah Gilbert-Palmer, MSN, RN, CS, FNP
Elizabeth Petit de Mange, PhD, MSN, NP-C, RN

Contents

ACUTE CARE NURSE PRACTITIONER REVIEW AND RESOURCE MANUAL

Taking the Certification Examination

When you sign up to take a national certification exam, you will be instructed to go online and review the testing and renewal handbook (www.nursecredentialing.org/documents/certification/application/generaltestingandrenewalhandbook.aspx). Review it carefully and be sure to bookmark the site so you can refer to it frequently. It contains information on test content and sample questions. This is critical information; it will give you insight into the nature of the test. The agency will send you information about the test site; keep this in a safe place until needed.

GENERAL SUGGESTIONS FOR PREPARING FOR THE EXAM

Step One: Control Your Anxiety

Everyone experiences anxiety when faced with taking the certification exam.

- Remember, your program was designed to prepare you to take this exam.
- Your instructors took a similar exam, and have probably talked to students who took exams more recently, so they know how to help you prepare.
- Taking a review course or setting up your own study plan will help you feel more confident about taking the exam.

Step Two: Do Not Listen to Gossip About the Exam

A large volume of information exists about the tests based on reports from people who have taken the exams in the past. Because information from the testing facilities is limited, it is hard to ignore this gossip.

- Remember that gossip about the exam that you hear from others is not verifiable.
- Because this gossip is based on the imperfect memory of people in a stressful situation, it may not be very accurate.
- People tend to remember those items testing content with which they are less comfortable; for instance, those with a limited background in women's health may say that the exam was "all women's health." In fact, the exam blueprint ensures that the exam covers multiple content areas without overemphasizing any one.

Step Three: Set Reasonable Expectations for Yourself

- Do not expect to know everything.
- Do not try to know everything in great detail.
- You do not need a perfect score to pass the exam.
- The exam is designed for a beginner level—it is testing readiness for entry-level practice.
- Learn the general rules, not the exceptions.
- The most likely diagnoses will be on the exam, not questions on rare diseases or atypical cases.
- Think about the most likely presentation and most common therapy.

Step Four: Prepare Mentally and Physically

- While you are getting ready to take the exam, take good physical care of yourself.
- Get plenty of sleep and exercise, and eat well while preparing for the exam.
- These things are especially important while you are studying and immediately before you take the exam.

Step Five: Access Current Knowledge

General Content
You will be given a list of general topics that will be on the exam when you register to take the exam. In addition, examine the table of contents of this book and the test content outline, available at www.nursecredentialing.org/cert/TCOs.html.
- What content do you need to know?
- How well do you know these subjects?

Take a Review Course
- Taking a review course is an excellent way to assess your knowledge of the content that will be included in the exam.

- If you plan to take a review course, take it well before the exam so you will have plenty of time to master any areas of weakness the course uncovers.
- If you are prepared for the exam, you will not hear anything new in the course. You will be familiar with everything that is taught.
- If some topics in the review course are new to you, concentrate on these in your studies.
- People have a tendency to study what they know; it is rewarding to study something and feel a mastery of it! Unfortunately, this will not help you master unfamiliar content. Be sure to use a review course to identify your areas of strength and weakness, then concentrate on the weaknesses.

Depth of Knowledge

How much do you need to know about a subject?
- You cannot know everything about a topic.
- Remember that the depth of knowledge required to pass the exam is for entry-level performance.
- Study the information sent to you from the testing agency, what you were taught in school, what is covered in this text, and the general guidelines given in this chapter.
- Look at practice tests designed for the exam. Practice tests for other exams will not be helpful.
- Consult your class notes or clinical diagnosis and management textbook for the major points about a disease. Additional reference books can be found online at www.nursecredentialing.org/cert/refs.html.
- For example, with regard to medications, know the drug categories and the major medications in each. Assume all drugs in a category are generally alike, and then focus on the differences among common drugs. Know the most important indications, contraindications, and side effects. Emphasize safety. The questions usually do not require you to know the exact dosage of a drug.

Step Six: Institute a Systematic Study Plan

Develop Your Study Plan
- Write up a formal plan of study.
  - Include topics for study, timetable, resources, and methods of study that work for you.
  - Decide whether you want to organize a study group or work alone.
  - Schedule regular times to study.
  - Avoid cramming; it is counterproductive. Try to schedule your study periods in 1-hour increments.

- Identify resources to use for studying. To prepare for the examination, you should have the following materials on your shelf:
  - A good pathophysiology text.
  - This review book.
  - A physical assessment text.
  - Your class notes.
  - Other important sources, including: information from the testing facility, a clinical diagnosis textbook, favorite journal articles, notes from a review course, and practice tests.
  - Know the important national standards of care for major illnesses.
  - Consult the bibliography on the test blueprint. When studying less familiar material, it is helpful to study using the same references that the testing center uses.
- Study the body systems from head to toe.
- The exams emphasize health promotion, assessment, differential diagnosis, and plan of care for common problems.
- You will need to know facts and be able to interpret and analyze this information utilizing critical thinking.

Personalize Your Study Plan
- How do you learn best?
  - If you learn best by listening or talking, attend a review course or discuss topics with a colleague.
- Read everything the test facility sends you as soon as you receive it and several times during your preparation period. It will give you valuable information to help guide your study.
- Have a specific place with good lighting set aside for studying. Find a quiet place with no distractions. Assemble your study materials.

Implement Your Study Plan
You must have basic content knowledge. In addition, you must be able to use this information to think critically and make decisions based on facts.
- Refer to your study plan regularly.
- Stick to your schedule.
- Take breaks when you get tired.
- If you start procrastinating, get help from a friend or reorganize your study plan.
- It is not necessary to follow your plan rigidly. Adjust as you learn where you need to spend more time.
- Memorize the basics of the content areas you will be required to know.

Focus on General Material
- Most of what you need to know is basic material that does not require constant updating.
- You do not need to worry about the latest information being published as you are studying for the exam. Remember, it can take 6 to 12 months for new information to be incorporated into test questions.

Pace Your Studying

- Stop studying for the examination when you are starting to feel overwhelmed and look at what is bothering you. Then make changes.
- Break overwhelming tasks into smaller tasks that you know you can do.
- Stop and take breaks while studying.

Work With Others

- Talk with classmates about your preparation for the exam.
- Keep in touch with classmates, and help each other stick to your study plans.
- If your classmates become anxious, do not let their anxiety affect you. Walk away if you need to.
- Do not believe bad stories you hear about other people's experiences with previous exams.
- Remember, you know as much as anyone about what will be on the next exam!

Consider a Study Group

- Study groups can provide practice in analyzing cases, interpreting questions, and critical thinking.
  - You can discuss a topic and take turns presenting cases for the group to analyze.
  - Study groups can also provide moral support and help you continue studying.

Step Seven: Strategies Immediately Before the Exam

Final Preparation Suggestions

- Use practice exams when studying to get accustomed to the exam format and time restrictions.
  - Many books that are labeled as review books are simply a collection of examination questions.
  - If you have test anxiety, such practice tests may help alleviate the anxiety.
  - Practice tests can help you learn to judge the time it should take you to complete the exam.
  - Practice tests are useful for gaining experience in analyzing questions.
  - Books of questions may not uncover the gaps in your knowledge that a more systematic content review text will reveal.
  - If you feel that you don't know enough about a topic, refer to a text to learn more. After you feel that you have learned the topic, practice questions are a wonderful tool to help improve your test-taking skill.

- Know your test-taking style.
  - Do you rush through the exam without reading the questions thoroughly?
  - Do you get stuck and dwell on a question for a long time?
  - You should spend about 45 to 60 seconds per question and finish with time to review the questions you were not sure about.
  - Be sure to read the question completely, including all four answer choices. Choice "a" may be good, but "d" may be best.

The Night Before the Exam
- Be prepared to get to the exam on time.
  - Know the test site location and how long it takes to get there.
  - Take a "dry run" beforehand to make sure you know how to get to the testing site, if necessary.
  - Get a good night's sleep.
  - Eat sensibly.
  - Avoid alcohol the night before.
  - Assemble the required material—two forms of identification, admission card, pencil, and watch. Both IDs must match the name on the application, and one photo ID is preferred.
  - Know the exam room rules.
    - You will be given scratch paper, which will be collected at the end of the exam.
    - Nothing else is allowed in the exam room.
    - You will be required to put papers, backpacks, etc., in a corner of the room or in a locker.
    - No water or food will be allowed.
    - You will be allowed to walk to a water fountain and go to the bathroom one at a time.

The Day of the Exam
- Get there early. You must arrive to the test center at least 15 minutes before your scheduled appointment time. If you are late, you may not be admitted.
- Think positively. You have studied hard and are well-prepared.
- Remember your anxiety reduction strategies.

Specific Tips for Dealing With Anxiety

Test anxiety is a specific type of anxiety. Symptoms include upset stomach, sweaty palms, tachycardia, trouble concentrating, and a feeling of dread. But there are ways to cope with test anxiety.
- There is no substitute for being well-prepared.
- Practice relaxation techniques.
- Avoid alcohol, excess coffee, caffeine, and any new medications that might sedate you, dull your senses, or make you feel agitated.
- Take a few deep breaths and concentrate on the task at hand.

Focus on Specific Test-Taking Skills

To do well on the exam, you need good test-taking skills in addition to knowledge of the content and ability to use critical thinking.

All Certification Exams Are Multiple Choice

- Multiple-choice tests have specific rules for test construction.
- A multiple-choice question consists of three parts: the information (or stem), the question, and the four possible answers (one correct and three distracters).
- Careful analysis of each part is necessary. Read the entire question before answering.
- Practice your test-taking skills by analyzing the practice questions in this book and on the ANCC Web site.

Analyze the Information Given

- Do not assume you have more information than is given.
- Do not overanalyze.
- Remember, the writer of the question assumes this is all of the information needed to answer the question.
- If information is not given, it is not relevant and will not affect the answer.
- Do not make the question more complicated than it is.

What Kind of Question Is Asked?

- Are you supposed to recall a fact, apply facts to a situation, or understand and differentiate between options?
  - Read the question thinking about what the writer is asking.
  - Look for key words or phrases that lead you (see Figure 1–1). These help determine what kind of answer the question requires.

Figure 1–1. Examples of Key Words and Phrases

- avoid
- best
- except
- not
- initial

- first
- contributing to
- appropriate
- most
- significant

- likely
- of the following
- most consistent with

Read All of the Answers

- If you are absolutely certain that answer "a" is correct as you read it, mark it, but read the rest of the question so you do not trick yourself into missing a better answer.
- If you are absolutely sure answer "a" is wrong, cross it off or make a note on your scratch paper and continue reading the question.
- After reading the entire question, go back, analyze the question, and select the best answer.

- Do not jump ahead.
- If the question asks you for an assessment, the best answer will be an assessment. Do not be distracted by an intervention that sounds appropriate.
- If the question asks you for an intervention, do not answer with an assessment.
- When two answer choices sound very good, the best one is usually the least expensive, least invasive way to achieve the goal. For example, if your answer choices include a physical exam maneuver or imaging, the physical exam maneuver is probably the better choice provided it will give the information needed.
- If the answers include two options that are the opposite of each other, one of the two is probably the correct answer.
- When numeric answers cover a wide range, a number in the middle is more likely to be correct.
- Watch out for distracters that are correct but do not answer the question, combine true and false information, or contain a word or phrase that is similar to the correct answer.
- Err on the side of caution.

Only One Answer Can Be Correct

- When more than one suggested answer is correct, you must identify the one that best answers the question asked.
- If you cannot choose between two answers, you have a 50% chance of getting it right if you guess.

Avoid Changing Answers

- Change an answer only if you have a compelling reason, such as you remembered something additional, or you understand the question better after rereading it.
- People change to a wrong answer more often than to a right answer.

Time Yourself to Complete the Whole Exam

- Do not spend a large amount of time on one question.
- If you cannot answer a question quickly, mark it and continue the exam.
- If time is left at the end, return to the difficult questions.
- Make educated guesses by eliminating the obviously wrong answers and choosing a likely answer even if you are not certain.
- Trust your instinct.
- Answer every question. There is no penalty for a wrong answer.
- Occasionally a question will remind you of something that helps you with a question earlier in the test. Look back at that question to see if what you are remembering affects how you would answer that question.

ABOUT THE CERTIFICATION EXAMS

The American Nurses Credentialing Center Computerized Exam

The ANCC examination is given only as a computer exam, and each exam is different. The order of the questions is scrambled for every test, so even if two people are taking the same exam, the questions will be in a different order. The exam consists of 175 multiple-choice questions.

- 150 of the 175 questions are part of the test and how you answer will count toward your score; 25 are included to refine questions and will not be scored. You will not know which ones count, so treat all questions the same.
- You will need to know how to use a mouse, scroll by either clicking arrows on the scroll bar or using the up and down arrow keys, and perform other basic computer tasks.
- The exam does not require computer expertise.
- However, if you are not comfortable with using a computer, you should practice using a mouse and computer beforehand so you do not waste time on the mechanics of using the computer.

Know what to expect during the test.
- Each ANCC test question is independent of the other questions.
  - For each case study, there is only one question. This means that a correct answer on any question does not depend on the correct answer to any other question.
  - Each question has four possible answers. There are no questions asking for combinations of correct answers (such as "a and c") or multiple-multiples.
- You can skip a question and go back to it at the end of the exam.
- You cannot mark key words in the question or right or wrong answers. If you want to do this, use the scratch paper.
- You will get your results immediately, and a grade report will be provided upon leaving the testing site.

INTERNET RESOURCES:

- ANCC Web site: www.nursecredentialing.org
- ANA Web site: www.nursesbooks.org. Catalog of ANA nursing scope and standards publications and other titles that may be listed on your test content outline
- National Guideline Clearinghouse: www.ngc.gov

2

Professional Responsibility

Pamela Smith, MSN, RN, ACNP-BC, CCRN, and
Melanie Smith, MSN, RN, ACNP-BC

THE ACUTE CARE NURSE PRACTITIONER (ACNP)–PATIENT RELATIONSHIP

Establishing an Effective Professional Therapeutic Relationship

- Components of a therapeutic relationship
  - Mutual trust
    - Mutual trust is a shared belief between the patient and nurse practitioner that they can depend on each other to achieve a common purpose or goal.
  - Professional boundaries
    - The ACNP has access to private and personal patient information and may develop a long-term therapeutic relationship with a patient.
    - The atmosphere of intimacy in the ACNP–patient relationship and the need to touch the patient during the physical examination tends to accentuate the patient's vulnerability.
    - Boundaries must be established that acknowledge the appropriate use of patient information and intimacy to meet the patient's needs while providing care.

- Violations of the professional boundaries will alter the therapeutic relationship. The following are examples:
  - Sharing excessive personal information
  - Exhibiting sexually seductive behavior
- If the professional boundary is violated, the individual responsible must be removed from the relationship and other members of the healthcare team should attempt to restore the patient's integrity and trust.
- Confidentiality
  - The rule of confidentiality is the duty to not disclose information shared in an intimate and trusted manner.
- Cultural respect
  - Recognizing and respecting the cultural identification of patients is viewed as being essential to establishing a therapeutic relationship.
  - It is important to avoid making assumptions based solely on physical appearance or dress—many families have blended traditional beliefs and practices from multiple cultures.
  - The ACNP must individualize care based on an assessment of the cultural influences on both the perception of illness and reporting of symptoms.
  - Interactions that are complicated by cultural misunderstandings can result in incomplete or inaccurate assessments, misdiagnosis, inadvertent disrespect, and potentially suboptimal outcomes.
- Strategies for establishing therapeutic relationships
  - Use a conversational style when interacting with the patient.
  - Encourage the patient to actively participate in healthcare decisions.
  - Investigate cultural influences that will affect the healthcare course and treatment plan.
  - With noncommunicative patients, be aware of how the patient responds to the environment and what happens to them through:
    - Facial expressions
    - Body movements
    - Physiological parameters
    - What causes the patient discomfort and what alleviates it
  - Be an advocate for the patient's perspective and concerns to other members of the healthcare team or the family.
- Establishing rapport
  - Establishing rapport is an important foundation for the ACNP–patient relationship.
  - The patient must feel that he or she can trust in the competence of the ACNP and can confide in her or him.
  - The ability to listen, a natural curiosity, and empathy are qualities that help to establish rapport.
  - Listen to what the patient is saying and understand the emotional implications involved.
    - Allow the patient to use his or her own words.
    - Use a conversational style when interviewing.
    - Use a tone of voice and pace of speech appropriate to the topic being discussed.
- Planning for the patient and his or her family's psychosocial and spiritual needs
  - The ACNP should take a holistic approach to the patient and his or her family.
  - The holistic perspective examines the multiple dimensions of each person and his or her family:
    - Biological
    - Psychological

- · Social
- · Spiritual
- The relationship among these dimensions results in a whole that is greater than the sum of the parts.
- Another view of the holistic perspective includes the following:
  - · View the patient as an integral part of a larger social, physical, and energy environments.
  - · Assume that the mind, body, and spirit are closely related and one dimension should not be considered in isolation from the others.
  - · Focus on the meaning the patient assigns to health, illness experiences, and healthcare choices.
  - · View the patient's behaviors and responses as consistent with his or her life span patterns of response and choice.
- A functional assessment should be holistic and person-centered.
  - The functional assessment format includes the following:
    - · How the patient views his or her health and quality of life
    - · How the patient accomplishes self-care and household and job responsibilities
    - · The social, physical, financial, environmental, and spiritual factors that help or hinder the patient's overall functioning
    - · The strategies used by the patient and his or her family to cope with stresses and problems

Maintaining an Effective Professional Therapeutic Relationship

- Advanced directives
  - According to the American Nurses Association, it is the responsibility of the nursing profession to assist patients and families with informed decision-making about end-of-life choices.
  - Studies have shown that nurse practitioners are knowledgeable about advance care planning and should encourage patients to complete an advanced directive.
  - Methods to increase the use of advanced directives
    - · Direct patient contact
      - - Initiate the discussion when the patient is still healthy during:
        - · New patient visits
        - · Subsequent visits
        - · Yearly check-ups
      - - Educational methods
        - · Web sites
        - · Videos
        - · Pamphlets
  - Community involvement
    - · Support of existing programs
      - - Respecting choices
      - - Creating of educational seminars for the public
    - · The only way to identify the patient's wishes is by initiating the discussion about advanced care planning and revisiting the topic with the patient in an appropriate manner.

- Privacy and confidentiality
  - The Health Insurance Portability and Accountability Act (HIPAA) became law in 1996.
  - Legal requirements were finalized in 2002 by the U.S. Department of Health and Human Services.
  - The goal of HIPAA is to protect the privacy of a patient's identifiable health information.
    - Any information that can identify the patient
    - The patient's diagnosis or condition
    - The plan of care
    - The way the patient's care is paid for
  - A nurse practitioner must comply with HIPAA regulations if third-party reimbursement is accepted or he or she transmits health information in any form.
- Crisis situations and the therapeutic relationship
  - A crisis is a crucial situation or decisive point in a person's life.
    - May be an emotionally stressful event or traumatic change
    - Might be a point where a conflict reaches its highest point and must be resolved
  - The therapeutic relationship with the patient in crisis can serve as a stabilizing point.
    - Explore concerns with the patient.
    - The nurse practitioner can provide temporary relief and stability, and restore balance in the situation.
    - Be supportive and leave an opening for the patient to be heard.
      - Give legitimate and direct answers to the patient's questions or concerns.
      - Set limits and state positive options before negative ones.
    - Be conscious of nonverbal communication.
    - Show empathy and respect for the patient and the situation.
- Acting as a patient advocate regarding healthcare management
  - Advocacy can be described as a partnership between the nurse practitioner and a patient when the patient is confronting a health issue and they mutually agree upon the interpretation of the situation.
  - The relationship between the nurse practitioner and the patient is a practical one in which the professional has expertise to offer the patient who is experiencing an inherent ambiguity associated with his or her health concerns.
  - Advocacy has two levels:
    - Client-focused
      - Enhance patient autonomy
      - Assist patients in voicing their values
    - Systems-focused
      - Refers to influencing providers to improve existing services and to develop new ones
- Communicating therapeutically
  - Ethical practice requires honesty and integrity in all patient interactions.
  - Therapeutic communication starts with the nurse practitioner showing respect for the patient (and family members).
  - Communication comprises not only the verbal exchange between the nurse practitioner and the patient, but also nonverbal expressions such as tone of voice, body language, and facial expressions.
  - Communication techniques
    - Use the patient's name.
    - Show empathy.
    - Provide encouragement.

- Reorient the patient gently, as needed.
- Include the patient in decision-making whenever possible to promote collaborative care.
- Recognize limits and do not force the patient to express feelings or concerns until he or she is ready.
  - Respect the patient's right to silence and indicate an openness to talk.
- Promoting patient autonomy
  - The principle of respect of autonomy
    - The duty to respect others' personal liberty and individual values, beliefs, and choices
  - All persons have worth and dignity, and it is paramount that the nurse practitioner strive to preserve and protect these qualities.
  - Autonomy encompasses the ethical principle that patients have had or will develop the capacity to make decisions for and about themselves.
  - The nurse practitioner must advocate for and strive to protect the patient's health, safety, and rights.
  - Respect for autonomy is required because, given the natural course of health and the fragility of it, the capacity to remain autonomous may not remain fully intact.
- Collaborating
  - Collaboration between the nurse practitioner and the patient promotes improved clinical outcomes.
  - Patients are aware of collaborative relationships that are based on mutual respect and trust.
  - The benefits of collaboration include:
    - Improved quality of care
    - Increased patient satisfaction
    - Lower mortality rate
    - Improved patient outcomes
    - Increased sharing of responsibility
    - Reduced redundant care
    - Increased sharing of expertise

ACNP SCOPE OF PRACTICE

- The ACNP's focus is on providing curative, rehabilitative, palliative, and maintenance care.
  - Short-term goals
    - Stabilizing patient in or after acute or life-threatening illness
    - Minimizing or preventing complications
    - Attending to comorbidities
    - Promoting physical and psychological well-being
  - Long-term goals
    - Restoring the patient's maximum health potential
    - Providing palliative or end-of-life care
  - Practice environment
    - Any inpatient or outpatient setting that requires complex monitoring and high-intensity interventions with continuous nursing vigilance in the arena of high-acuity care

- Practice standards unique to the ACNP
  - Assessment of the dynamic health and illness status in the critically ill patient population
  - Need for continuous assessment and adjustment of the management plan because of the rapidly changing condition of the patient
  - Complexity of the required monitoring and therapeutics
  - Collaborative practice and interactive relationship between the ACNP and the heathcare institution
- The patient population of the ACNP includes acutely and critically ill patients with:
  - Episodic illness
  - Acute exacerbation of illness
  - Stable or progressive chronic illness
  - Terminal illness
- Scope and standards of acute care nurse practitioner practice
  - The scope of practice is influenced by five levels:
    - National (professional organizations)
    - State (government)
    - Healthcare institution
    - Service-related
    - Individual
  - The ACNP's scope of practice is broadly described in statements by professional nursing organizations and further defined by state governments and regulatory agencies as nurse practice acts or title-protection statutes.
  - Because ACNPs often provide services within healthcare facilities such as hospitals, subacute care facilities, nursing homes, and clinics, the scope of practice may be further defined by the policies of the institution.
  - *Domains and Competencies of Nurse Practitioner Practice* (2006)
    - National Organization of Nurse Practitioner Faculties (NONPF)
    - Describes entry-level competencies for graduates of master's and post-master's ACNP educational programs
  - *Scope and Standards of Practice of the Acute Care Nurse Practitioner* (2006)
    - American Association of Critical Care Nurses (AACCN)
    - Describes expert-level ACNP competencies
  - *Acute Care Nurse Practitioner Competencies* (2004)
    - National Panel for Acute Care Nurse Practitioner Competencies (NPACNPC)
    - Identifies entry-level knowledge and skills that should be achieved by the student at program completion and entry to ACNP practice
  - The federal government regulates nurse practitioners through statutes enacted by Congress, regulations, policies, and guidelines written by federal agencies.
    - Federal law covers:
      - Care of patients covered by Medicare
      - Care of patients covered by Medicaid
      - Care of hospitalized patients, in that the hospital's participation in the Medicare program is contingent on the hospital following certain regulations
      - Care of residents in nursing homes
      - In-office and hospital laboratories—Clinical Laboratories Improvement Act
      - Self-referral by healthcare providers—the Stark Acts
      - Prescription of controlled substances—Drug Enforcement Administration (DEA)

- Reporting of successful malpractice lawsuits against nurse practitioners to the National Practitioner Data Bank (NPDB)
- Confidentiality of information about patients under the Health Insurance Portability and Accountability Act (HIPAA)
- Discrimination in hiring and firing
- Facility access for the disabled
  - The ACNP national certification examination specifies the knowledge necessary to perform within the specialty scope of practice.
- Credentialing and privileging
  - Credentialing is providing the documentation necessary to be authorized by a regulatory body or institution to use a certain title and participate in certain activities.
    - May be mandatory or voluntary, depending on the individual state's regulations
  - Standards by which the advance practice nurse is monitored
    - Graduation from an accredited graduate-level nursing program
    - Attainment of national advanced practice nurse–level certification
    - State licensure, recognition as a registered nurse (RN) and advanced practice nurse, or both
    - Collaborative practice agreement with a physician if required by the state
    - Approval for prescriptive authority
    - Medicare and Medicaid provider numbers
    - National Provider Identifier (NPI) number
    - DEA number for prescribing controlled substances
    - Approval of hospital privileges
- Identifying situations outside the scope of practice
  - Be familiar with scope of practice guidelines for state(s) in which the nurse practitioner is licensed.
  - Refer to practice guidelines set forth by the NONPF, AACN, and National Panel for Acute Care Nurse Practitioners.
- Time management and establishing priorities
  - Time management is a concern for the ACNP because the accuracy and completeness of clinical thinking and decision-making may be affected by time limitations and pressures.
  - The novice ACNP may take longer to perform tasks and need more assistance with consultations and accessing resources than the experienced ACNP.
  - Actions to take to avoid thinking errors
    - Evaluate what data are critical in each patient's case.
    - Remain open to reevaluation of working diagnoses and treatments.
    - Listen to input from other providers.
    - Pay attention to the patient's concerns and descriptions of their problems to accurately set treatment priorities.
    - Critically think through the source of knowledge and how it relates to the individual patient's needs.
- Advocating for the nurse practitioner role
  - Advocacy can help move ideas into action.
  - Legislation is a way for an idea to become legal.
    - Promote change and improvement with physician collaborative agreements.

- Role delineation and consistency at the state and national level continues to evolve based on the efforts of ACNP leaders and professional organizations.
- Research guides the ACNP practice role and strengthens education strategies and mentoring to advance the advocacy role.
- Add the ACNP services to hospital or clinic brochures and directories.
- Patient education booklets provide a description of ACNP services.
- Distribute business cards to patients and their families.
- Join local, state, and national advanced practice nurse professional organizations.
- Collaboration with other healthcare providers
    - The basis of collaboration is that quality patient care will be achieved by including the contributions of all care providers.
        - It is the foundation of effective patient care.
        - It is the contribution of each member of the team that determines a successful patient outcome.
    - Attributes necessary for successful collaboration
        - Trust
            - Establishes a high-quality working relationship
            - Develops over time
        - Knowledge
            - Necessary for the development of trust
        - Shared responsibility
            - Joint decision-making for patient care and outcomes, practice issues within the organization
        - Mutual respect
            - Respect for the expertise of the team members; that is communicated to the patient
        - Communication
            - Ensures the sharing of patient information and knowledge
            - Does not question the approach to care in a critical fashion, but as method to enhance patient care
        - Cooperation and coordination
            - Promotes the use of skills of all team members, prevents duplication, and enhances productivity
        - Optimism
            - Promotes success when the involved parties support interdisciplinary collaboration
        - Consultation
            - The ACNP can create networks with other advanced practice nurses, physicians, and other colleagues by offering and receiving advice, information that will both improve patient care and enhance their own knowledge base.
            - Consultation allows the ACNP to positively influence patient outcomes beyond the direct patient encounter.
        - Patient-centered consultation
            - The consultant, at the request of the ACNP, assesses the patient and makes recommendations for the treatment plan.
            - The primary goal is to assist in management of the case.
        - Clinical resources
            - The ACNP, through collaboration, serving on hospital committees, membership in professional organizations, and participation in continuing education, can serve as a clinical resource for other members of the healthcare team.

ETHICAL AND LEGAL PRINCIPLES

- Ethical
  - "Ethics is a system of standards to motivate, determine, and justify actions directed to the pursuit of vital and fundamental goals" (Joel, 2009, p. 511).
  - Practice-based bioethics attempts to make human values the focus and the heathcare setting meaningful.
  - Ethical practice does not allow for violating a patient's individual rights.
  - Whenever two or more people are together, each individual has the right not to be subjected to aggression by the other.
  - "The rights agreement structures and defines human interaction and the pursuit of human values" (Joel, 2009, p. 512).
  - Principles and rules
    - Principles
      - Respect for autonomy
        - Duty to respect others' personal liberty, individual values, beliefs, and choices
      - Nonmaleficence
        - Duty not to inflict harm or evil
      - Beneficence
        - Duty to do good and prevent or remove harm
      - Formal justice
        - Duty to treat equals equally and those who are unequal unequally
    - Rules
      - Veracity
        - Duty to tell the truth and not to deceive others
      - Fidelity
        - Duty to honor commitments
      - Confidentiality
        - Duty not to disclose information shared in an intimate and trusted manner
      - Privacy
        - Duty to respect limited access to a person (Hamric, Spross, & Hanson, 2009)
- Legal
  - State licensure or recognition
    - Individual state nurse practice acts define the practice of nursing.
    - State laws overseeing advance practice nursing are divided into two forms:
      - Statutes, as defined by the nurse practice act, are regulated by the state legislature.
      - Rules and regulations are enforced by state agencies under the jurisdiction of the executive branch of state government.
      - Licensure, which provides standards for public safety, is delegated to the individual states by the federal Constitution.
  - Prescriptive authority
    - Requirements for advanced practice nurse prescribers
      - Graduation from an approved master's or doctoral-level advanced practice program
      - Licensure or recognition in good standing as an advanced practice nurse
      - National specialty certification
      - Recent pharmacotherapeutics course of at least 3 credit hours (45 contact hours)

- Evidence of a collaborative practice arrangement (in some states)
- Ongoing continuing education hours in pharmacotherapeutics to maintain prescribing status
- State prescribing and national DEA numbers (in some instances)
- Scope of practice
  - Elements of regulation for advanced practice nurses
    - Education
      - Master's
      - Post-master's
      - Doctoral
    - Accreditation of advanced practice nurse programs
    - National certification
      - Recertification
    - Licensure
      - Prescriptive authority
  - Credentialing
    - Graduation from an accredited graduate-level nursing program
    - Attainment of national advanced practice nurse-level certification
    - State licensure or recognition as an RN and advanced practice nurse
    - Collaborative practice agreement with a physician, if required by the state
    - Approval for prescriptive authority
    - Medicare and Medicaid provider numbers
    - NPI number
    - DEA number to prescribe controlled substances
    - Approval of hospital privileges
  - Specialty certification
    - National certification is used by state boards to ensure regulatory sufficiency.
    - ACNP certification is national in scope, and is a mandatory requirement for ACNPs to obtain and maintain credentialing in most states.
  - Collaborative practice agreements
    - Have replaced practice protocols
    - Are not required in all states
    - Are between ACNP and collaborating physician
    - Must be updated annually
    - Must have a current signature
    - Vary widely between acute care nursing specialties
  - Core competencies
    - Expert coaching and guidance of patients, families, and other care providers
    - Consultation
    - Research
    - Clinical, professional, and systems leadership
    - Collaboration
    - Ethical decision-making
    - ACNP core competencies
    - Direct clinical practice
      - Diagnosing and managing disease

- Demonstrate mastery of advanced pathophysiology, completion of a prioritized health history and both comprehensive and focused physical examinations, rapid assessment of unstable and complex health problems, implementation of diagnostic strategies and therapeutic interventions to stabilize healthcare problems, technical competence with procedures, modifications of the plan of care based on a client's changing condition and response to interventions, and collaboration with other healthcare providers to facilitate positive outcomes.
  - Promoting and protecting health and preventing disease
    - Provide anticipatory guidance and counseling to patients and their families.
- Standards of practice
  - ACNPs are held to both the standards of practice of the nursing profession and to the standards of the various advanced practice specialties.
  - Standards of practice describe the basic competency levels for safe and competent practice.
- Ethical dilemmas
  - "An ethical dilemma involves the need to choose from among two or more morally acceptable courses of action, when one choice prevents selecting the other, or the need to choose between equally unacceptable alternatives" (Hamric et al., 2009, p. 315)
  - Strategies for resolution of ethical conflict
    - Collaboration (best)
      - Step 1
        - Understand cognitive and emotional perspectives.
          - Perform nonjudgmental listening.
          - Deal with power imbalances.
          - Establish ground rules of mutual respect and shared decision-making.
      - Step 2
        - Engage all involved parties in active interaction and consensus-building.
          - Focus on interests instead of positions.
          - Acknowledge different perspectives.
          - Move toward identifying consensus positions.
      - Step 3
        - Make a decision and develop a plan.
          - Reframe
          - Identify shared interests, needs, and goals
          - Openly examine differences
    - Compromise
      - Used when:
        - Parties in conflict are committed to maintaining the relationship.
        - Parties each possess high moral certainty about opposing courses of action.
        - There is time before action is needed.
        - Each party relinquishes some control.
        - Trade-offs are made.
        - A compromise that preserves integrity can be achieved.

- Accommodation
  - Use when:
    - The issue is seen as minimally important.
    - Only one party is committed to preserving the relationship.
    - Time is limited.
    - Outcome is determined by one party because the other party relinquishes control.
    - It can be used as a negotiating tactic to decrease friction.
  - May not preserve integrity for all parties.
- Coercion
  - Occurs when time is short (emergency)
  - Reflects strong commitment to a particular position
  - One party takes an aggressive posture, so may be damaging to the relationship
  - Generates or encourages a power imbalance
- Avoidance
  - The moral issue is seen as unimportant or the situation is highly emotionally charged.
  - Time is short.
  - The conflict is not addressed or discussed, and no deliberate course of action is decided.
  - It may represent general conflict avoidance or abdicating moral accountability.
  - Repeated use can generate insensitivity to moral issues.
- Sample ethical decision-making framework
  - Gather information
    - Clinical indications
    - Patient preferences
    - Quality of life
    - Contextual factors
  - Identify the type of ethical problem.
    - Locus of authority: conflict involves who should make the decision
    - Ethical dilemma: see definition above
    - Moral distress: conflict in which the ethical course of action is perceived, but the agent feels unable to carry it out
  - Use ethical theories or approaches to analyze the problem
    - Utilitarian—focuses on the consequences of potential actions
    - Deontological—focuses on the duties of involved parties
  - Explore the practical alternatives
    - Ensure a wide range of alternatives are identified
    - Assess the feasibility of identified actions
  - Complete the action
    - Motivation to carry out the ethical action is essential
    - Not to act is a conscious choice with consequences
  - Evaluate the action
    - What went well and why?
    - To what other situations might this experience apply?
    - What do the patient, family, and other providers say about the course of action taken? (Hamric et al., 2009).

- Risk management
  - Negligence is the failure to act in a reasonable way as a healthcare clinician.
  - Negligence may lead to malpractice and legal action.
  - Four factors must be present for a malpractice suit to exist:
    - A duty of care must be owed to the injured party, either through direct office or hospital care or through phone or e-mail advice, and a patient–nurse relationship must be established.
    - The accepted standard of care must be breached.
    - The patient must have sustained an injury.
    - Causation must be demonstrated—the patient suffered an injury that was caused by the ACNP clinician.
  - National professional organizations set the standard of care.
  - ACNPs are often held to the medical standard of care as advanced practice nursing standards continue to be developed.
  - Risk management resources are available through professional advanced practice nursing organizations and public and private entities.
  - Liability insurance
    - A "claims-made" insurance policy covers claims against the ACNP only while the policy is in effect.
    - An "occurrence" policy covers the ACNP for alleged acts of negligence that occurred during the time that the policy was in effect (Hamric et al., 2009).
- Medical futility
  - Proposed therapy should not be performed because prevailing data show it will not improve the patient's condition
  - Remains ethically controversial
  - May be used by physicians to justify a decision not to pursue specific treatments requested or demanded by the patient, family, or both
  - No unanimity about statistical threshold for a treatment to be considered futile
  - Disputes may be avoided by optimal communication between physicians/ACNPs and patients or their surrogates.
    - Provide families with accurate, current, and frequent prognostic estimates; ensure the family's and patient's emotional needs are met.
    - Look at the problem from the family's perspective.
- Informed consent
  - Is both an ethical and a legal mandate that requires providers to obtain a competent patient's fully informed and voluntary consent before any medical or nursing treatment
  - The ACNP must describe the nature of the treatment and any consequences involved, the normal risks and hazards, any known side effects or complications that may occur, and any alternative treatments available to the patient.
  - Final informed consent consists of the patient's understanding of the information and the agreement to proceed.
  - Both the ACNP's information and the patient's agreement within the informed consent discussion must be documented in the patient's chart (Hamric et al., 2009).

EVIDENCE-BASED PRACTICE

- Evidence-based practice (EBP) is a scholarly and systematic problem-solving standard that results in the delivery of high-quality health care.
- To make the best clinical decisions using EBP, evidence from research is blended with practice-generated data, clinical expertise, and healthcare consumer values and preferences to achieve the best possible outcomes for individuals, groups, populations, and healthcare systems.
  - Research
    - The ACNP contributes to nursing knowledge by conducting or synthesizing research that discovers, examines, and evaluates knowledge, theories, criteria, and creative approaches to improve healthcare practice.
    - The ACNP should formally disseminate research findings through activities such as presentations, publications, consultation, and journal clubs (American Nurses Association, 2010b).
  - Standard of care
    - Nursing research and EBP contribute to the body of knowledge and enhance outcomes.
    - New knowledge is disseminated to decrease practice variations, improve outcomes, and create standards of excellence for care and policies.
    - Changes in practice should be based on current evidence.
- Research methods
  - Quantitative
    - Focuses on outcomes for patients that are measurable, generally using statistics
    - Dominant research method is the randomized controlled trial.
  - Qualitative
    - Based on the paradigms of phenomenology, grounded theory, ethnography, and others
    - Examines the experience of those receiving or delivering the nursing care, focusing on the meaning it holds for the individual
    - Commonly uses methods of interviews, case studies, focus groups, and ethnography (cultural anthropology)
- Integrating evidence into practice
  - Analyzing, synthesizing, and evaluating evidence
    - Use of clinical judgment
    - Read primary research reports and summaries of research findings.
    - Informally evaluate the soundness of the methods.
    - Adjust or fine-tune practice on the basis of credible findings
    - All forms of objective evidence should be used:
      - Quality improvement data
      - Data from internal databases
      - Expert opinion panels
      - Consensus statements
      - Data from benchmarking partners
      - Data from state and national databases
    - Systematically scan clinical journals relevant to one's specialty.

HEALTHCARE DELIVERY—COORDINATING PATIENT-FOCUSED CARE

Description

- One of the most important roles of the acute care nurse practitioner in healthcare delivery is to coordinate patient-focused care among healthcare providers across settings. Practitioners, therefore, must understand the policies and guidelines that define the standards and scope of their clinical practices, as well as the resources available to help deliver quality, cost-effective patient- and family-centered care within this legal framework. Skillful use of information technology and effective communication with patients, families, and members of the healthcare team are critical functions of the nurse practitioner in coordinating care. In the complex and ever-changing healthcare financing and care delivery settings, the nurse practitioner must be able to navigate the healthcare system on behalf of the patient.

Etiology

Healthcare policy encompasses the legislative and regulatory policies put into place by governments and governing bodies that affect the financing, organization, and delivery of health care. Policies range in scope from federal regulations ensuring the safety of prescription drugs and the quality of the air to state and local mandates describing the training guidelines and scope of practice of healthcare professionals.

- The first school of nursing was established in 1873; however, the first state law requiring licensure of practical nurses was not passed until 1938. Once this law was passed, uniformity and standardization in nursing education and qualifications for licensure quickly developed and evolved into the guidelines we have today for entry into professional practice.
- Current United States healthcare policy requires nurse practitioners (NPs) to:
  - Hold a graduate degree for entry level practice
  - Hold national board certification in a practice area of specialty, such as acute care or pediatrics
  - Be licensed or certified through their state board of nursing
  - Be licensed as an NP following completion of the educational and clinical components needed to earn a bachelor of science in nursing (BSN), followed by the graduate-level training required to receive a master's or doctoral degree
- Some programs award BSN degree to qualified nurse practitioner students holding bachelor's in non-nursing specialties as they "bridge" their education to the master's or doctoral degree in nursing as acute care NPs.
- Certification is a process by which a nongovernmental agency or association certifies that an individual licensed to practice a profession has met standards specified by that profession for specialty practice.
- Although the individual curriculum may vary across settings based on the student's subspecialty, certain pre-determined standards must be met by all who wish to qualify for licensure and sit for the board certification exam.

- A nurse practitioner's scope of practice is state-regulated, so the delivery of care and autonomy with which that care is provided, including prescriptive authority, varies widely in the United States. Some states require a collaborative agreement with a physician for practice, while other states allow for independent NP practice.
- The Joint Commission (formerly Joint Commission on Accreditation of Hospital Organizations or JCAHO) defines a licensed independent practitioner (LIP) as "any individual permitted by law and organization to provide care, treatment, and services without direction or supervision" (JCAHO, 2010).
- Hospitals and other healthcare institutions have internal policies that organize and govern their medical staffs and provide a framework for healthcare quality, called *medical staff bylaws*. Bylaws define medical staff structure, qualifications for appointment to staff, and the process for privileging and credentialing medical staff members for practice in that institution. They also define the duties related to each category of the medical staff and the process for terminating medical staff membership and privileges. Nurse practitioners are members of the medical staff.
- Ultimately, state law *and* hospital policies determine one's scope of practice, regardless of certification.
- Healthcare policy practice resources are numerous and widely available, both electronically and in print. Professional nursing organizations such as the American Nursing Association, the American Association of Nurse Practitioners, or American College of Nurse Practitioners; credentialing organizations such as American Nurses Credentialing Center (ANCC); state boards of nursing; hospital Web sites; government Web sites; and professional journals and position papers are all ways to remain current on healthcare policy and professional practice guidelines.

Incidence and Demographics

- Almost 350 colleges and universities have NP programs.
- In 2008, there were nearly 160,000 nurse practitioners with credentials in the United States; the majority were certified as adult or family NPs.
- NPs hold prescriptive privileges in all 50 states, with controlled substance privileges in 48.
- The average NP is female and 48 years old, and has been in practice 12.8 years as an NP.

Risk Factors

- Nurse practitioners are licensed and credentialed, so they are vulnerable to disciplinary and legal processes associated with violating practice standards. Although the number of lawsuits against healthcare providers continues to escalate, studies continue to validate the high quality of care and improved patient outcomes when nurse practitioners provide care. Despite a low overall incidence of malpractice claims against NPs compared with physicians, though, nurse practitioners are increasingly being named in malpractice suits, even when they appear to be minimally involved in the case.
- The most common sources of liability for NPs are
  - Failure to diagnose or a delay in diagnosis
  - Treatment errors
  - Medication errors

- A breach of confidentiality can also result in a malpractice claim. Nurse practitioners can be held liable for:
  - Discussing patient information where others can hear
  - Leaving patient records or computer screens with patient information in view of others
  - Releasing patient information without permission
  - As communication between interdisciplinary team members, patients, and families often falls to the nurse practitioner coordinating care delivery, confidentiality and protection of sensitive information must always remain a priority.
- Each state's Nurse Practitioner Practice Act provides general guidelines describing duties that can and cannot be performed. However, NPs must be aware of the education and experience needed to perform each specific job function and be able to defend their actions in court.
- Documentation is a crucial component of safe practice. It provides a record of patient care and the quality of care provided.
- Most experts recommend that nurse practitioners carry their own malpractice insurance policies, even if insurance is provided by their employers.

Prevention and Screening

Maintaining knowledge of health risks and common health problems specific to patients' age, gender, ethnicity, and family history is as important in the acute care setting as it is in the outpatient environment. Nurse practitioners are responsible for staying informed on current recommendations for health maintenance, chronic disease management, disease prevention, and risk factor modification, and incorporating these recommendations into the plan of care where appropriate. The nurse practitioner has a duty to follow up on potentially serious health concerns of a patient in his or her care until the issue has been resolved. Although not every issue identified merits an exhaustive inpatient workup, communication with outpatient providers and consultants about significant findings will ensure continuity of care.

Assessment

Patient care delivery is optimized not just through a comprehensive physical assessment, but by a thorough assessment of the patient's community resources, family support, personal and financial resources, belief system, and culture before to individualizing the plan of care.

Management

Expert management of patient care can be complicated, requiring not only clinical skill but expertise in navigating a complex healthcare system. Ongoing role development through research, collegial collaboration, and continuing education supports evidence-based practice and enhances professional development and management skills. Goals in managing patient care delivery include:

- Efficient use of financial, equipment, treatment, and supply resources
- Use of information technology for communication, continuity, and documentation of patient care
- Patient and family involvement when negotiating the goals of care
- Supporting patients recovering from illness or injury, often under the care of multiple providers and transitioning across a variety of healthcare settings, through ongoing discharge planning in conjunction with case management, social services, and other ancillary staff
- Keeping all healthcare providers informed and involved through expert professional communication

Special Considerations

The best care delivery and discharge plan is of no value if not individualized to each patient's unique medical, social, and financial circumstances. Noncompliance with the treatment plan is often a result of non-negotiation with the patient on realistic goals of care, or failure to assess barriers to achieving goals. Family, case management, and social services are all helpful resources for the nurse practitioner in supporting and coordinating a successful discharge plan.

As hospital practitioners, ACNPs are in a unique position to discuss and support end-of-life issues and palliative care.

When to Consult, Refer, or Hospitalize

Licensing, credentialing, and hospital bylaws and scope of practice legislation define the general role of the nurse practitioner, but one must always be aware of situational limitations on one's practice. NPs must be sensitive to the education and expertise needed to perform each specific job function and should defer care delivery to appropriate practitioners. Expert consultation for management of complex medical issues is always appropriate, as is transition to either a higher level of care or palliative and end-of-life care providers.

Follow-up

Expected Outcomes

Ideally, the ACNP's healthcare delivery plan is patient-centered, evidence-based, cost-effective, and carried out within the patient's expected length of stay. Post-hospital follow-up and continuity of care is enhanced by early discharge planning, clear discharge instructions, communication with providers in the outpatient setting or the next level of care, and careful documentation.

Complications

Patient noncompliance or social and financial circumstances that preclude a successful discharge leads to relapsing medical conditions and rehospitalization. Lack of continuity in care can be a result of poor documentation or faulty communication with members of the healthcare team and patient.

Healthcare Policy and Delivery of Care

- Federal regulation
  - The federal government regulates NP practice by way of statutes put in place by Congress and regulations, policies, and guidelines written by federal agencies.
  - Federal law may supersede state law; if the state and federal laws conflict, the federal law takes precedence.
  - When there is no federal law regarding an issue or if the state has been granted the responsibility to make a law, the state law will be followed.
  - Areas addressed by federal law that affect NP practice include:
    - Medicare
    - Medicaid
    - Nursing homes
      - Under federal regulation, the care of nursing home residents may be provided by a NP who is not an employee of the facility but who is working in collaboration with a physician.
    - In-office and hospital laboratories
    - Self-referral by healthcare providers
      - Regulated by Stark Acts (Ethics in Patient Referral of 1989, Omnibus Budget and Reconciliation Act of 1993, and Social Security Act)—not aimed at nurse practitioners; however, the NP may be involved if an inappropriate referral is made at the physician's request—the referrals would be imputed to the physician, not the NP
      - Prevents physicians from referring a patient to clinical laboratories or other designated health services where the physician may have a financial relationship
        - Unclear whether it is a Stark violation for NP to independently make a referral to an agency in which his or her employer has a financial relationship; these cases are independently reviewed
  - Prescription of controlled substances under the Drug Enforcement Agency (DEA)
    - The DEA licenses healthcare providers to prescribe controlled dangerous substances.
    - The DEA licenses NPs as mid-level providers.
    - The NP will be assigned a DEA number if:
      - There is no felony conviction.
      - The NP has a practice site.
      - The state law permits NPs to prescribe controlled substances.
        - Reporting to the National Practitioner Data Bank (NPDB)
          - The NPDB is a national repository of information on healthcare providers.
          - Under federal law, malpractice insurers must report damage awards paid on behalf of physicians, dentists, NPs, and other healthcare providers to the NPDB.
      - Patient confidentiality

- Federal law mandates that NPs and other healthcare providers to protect patient privacy and confidentiality.
- Through the Department of Health and Human Services, Congress required that rules be put in place under the Health Insurance Portability and Accountability Act (HIPAA) of 1996.
- Covered entities (health plans, healthcare clearinghouses, healthcare providers, hospitals, skilled nursing facilities, comprehensive outpatient rehabilitation facilities, home health agencies, hospice programs, nurse practitioners, certified nurse midwives, clinical nurse specialists, psychologists, clinical social workers, certified registered nurse anesthetists, physicians, physician assistants, "and any other person or organization who furnishes, bills, or is paid for health care in the normal course of business") must do the following:
  · Appoint a privacy officer.
  · Assess the office, hospital, or facility for potential breaches of patient privacy
  · Provide policies for handling and protecting of patient information.
  · Conduct training for staff.
  · Monitor office or facility for compliance with policies.
  · Have patients authorize in writing the release of their individually identifiable information for marketing purposes.
  · Notify patients in writing of their rights under the rules and make good faith efforts to have patients sign acknowledgements that they have received notice of these rights.
- An NP does not have to personally transmit health information in an electronic form for the above rules to apply.
  · If information is transmitted on the provider's behalf or that of the agency in which the provider is working, the rules apply.
- Basic requirements of the privacy rule are:
  · Providers and their staff may only convey the "minimum necessary information" about patients.
  · If information is to be released for marketing purposes, the patient must be told how the information will be used, to whom it will be disclosed, and the time frame in which it will be used.
  · The patient must release the information in writing.
- Information may be disclosed to oversight agencies (e.g., Center for Medicare and Medicaid Services [CMS]) without patient authorization.
- Psychotherapy notes have special rules:
  · Generally, the patient must authorize the release of information to disclose the notes for carrying out treatment, payment, or healthcare operations.
- Providers "must notify patients about how the personal medical information may be used and disclosed, and how individuals may access their own information."
  · Patients have no rights regarding three types of information:
    - Psychotherapy notes
    - Information gathered in anticipation of civil or criminal litigation
    - Some clinical laboratory information covered by the Clinical Laboratory Improvement Amendments
  · Providers must respect reasonable requests from patients who want to restrict the use of their information

- Discrimination in hiring and firing
  - Title VII of the Civil Rights Act of 1964 prohibits "discrimination based on race, color, or national origin" and applies to government employers and private employers with more than 15 employees.
  - The Age Discrimination Act of 1967 prohibits "discrimination based on age above 40 and applies to employer with more than 20 employees."
  - The Equal Pay Act of 1963 prohibits "wage discrimination between men and women" and applies to almost all employers.
- People with disabilities under the Americans with Disabilities Act
  - Title 1 of the Americans with Disabilities Act of 1990 prohibits "private employers from discriminating against qualified individuals in hiring, firing, advancement, compensation, job training, and conditions of employment" and applies to employers with more than 15 employees.
  - A disabled person is one who has a physical or mental impairment that substantially limits one or more major life activities.
- State regulations
  - Some states define scope of practice in statutes enacted by the state legislature.
  - Some states give the board of nursing the authority to define the scope of the NP.
  - State statutes describing NP practice fall into six categories regarding scope of practice:
    - Clearly defined by statute—most secure for the NP
    - Clearly defined by regulation
    - Vaguely defined by statute
    - Not defined
    - Defined by exception from a state law prohibiting practice of medicine without a license
    - Defined by the individual physician, who may delegate to an NP by law
  - State licensure as a registered nurse requires:
    - Graduation from an organized program of study
    - Certification by a national certifying agency required by some states
    - Master's degree required by many states
    - Prescriptive authority—requirements vary state to state
    - Continuing education—requirements vary state to state
- Healthcare financing
  - Reimbursement/billing
    - Fee-for-service Medicare
      - Payment for specific type of service under a fee schedule
      - Fees based on:
        - *Current Procedural Terminology* (CPT) and *International Classification of Diseases*, 9th revision (ICD-9)
        - Geographic area
        - Office and training expenses of the provider
      - Under a fee-for-service system, the more services an NP performs, the more revenue he or she will generate.
      - An NP who wishes to provide service to a Medicare patient with a fee-for-service reimbursement plan must have a Medicare number.
        - National Provider Identifier (NPI) number

- "Incident to" services
  - Legal definition:
    - "Services furnished as an integral, although incidental, part of the physician's personal professional services in the course of diagnosis or treatment of an injury or illness"
  - Incidental to a physician's professional service
  - Used for Medicare
    - Services of non-physicians must be provided in a physician's office under a physician's direct personal supervision (physician must be in the office suite)
    - Non-physician must be an employee of a physician, physician group, or have an independent contractual agreement with the group
- Capitated Medicare
  - Fee paid by a managed care organization (MCO) to a healthcare provider, per patient, per month, for the care of an MCO member
  - NPs and physicians are paid a set fee per patient per month for all services agreed to.
  - An NP desiring to provide care for a Medicare patient enrolled in a MCO applies to the MCO for admission to the organization's provider panel.
  - Individuals covered by Medicare may choose between traditional fee-for-service and managed care.
- Medicaid
  - A federal program administered by the states
  - Mothers and children qualify based on poverty
  - Adults who are disabled for 1 year or less may qualify on the basis of poverty.
  - Some patients are enrolled in MCOs like Medicare.
  - To serve a Medicaid patient not enrolled in an MCO, the NP must apply and be accepted as a Medicaid provider by the state Medicaid agency.
  - To serve a patient enrolled in an MCO, the NP must apply and be admitted to the provider panel of the MCO in which the patient is enrolled.
  - States may apply to the federal government for Medicaid waivers.
    - Gives the state permission from CMS to administer Medicaid in ways that differ from federal laws and regulations
- Indemnity insurer
  - An insurance company that pays for the medical care of the insured but does not deliver health care
  - Pays healthcare providers on per-visit, per-procedure basis
  - To be reimbursed, NP submits billing form to insurance company
  - Fee schedules negotiated between provider and payer
- Managed care organization
  - An insurer that provides both healthcare services and payment for services.
  - Umbrella term that includes:
    - Health maintenance organizations
      - Prepaid, comprehensive system of health benefits that combines the financing and delivery of health services to subscribers
    - Other types of health plans
  - NP may be granted admission to provider panels
    - Designated primary care provider (PCP)
    - Contract for providing care, credentialing, directory listing, and reimbursement

- PCP has full responsibility for the patient's primary care, such as:
  - Complying with the MCOs quality, utilization, and patient satisfaction standards
  - Coordinating care with specialists, hospitals, and long-term-care facilities
  - Providing referrals for specialty care
  - Being cost-effective care
  - Providing 24-hour access to care
  - PCPs are reimbursed on a fee-for-service basis
- Group model MCO
  - Employer–employee arrangement
  - Example: Kaiser Permanente
  - Pays provider a set salary for taking care of patients
- Practice model MCO
  - Contract with independent providers, group practices, or practice associations for a "product line" of services
- Both models allow the option of choosing an NP for the PCP
- Not all MCOs currently contract with NPs
- Provider credentialing
  - MCOs credential providers
    - Collect educational, license, malpractice, employment, and certification data on each provider.
- Self-pay patients
  - May pay in cash, with credit cards, or by credit extension
  - Coding
    - All reimbursable services have Current Procedural Terminology (CPT) codes.
      - Most common in primary care is Evaluation and Management (E&M) Services
    - Requires providers to bill on the basis of the extent and complexity of history-taking, physical examination, and medical decision-making
  - CPT is a coding system developed by the American Medical Association and is used by third-party payers when claims are submitted.
  - All CPT codes have corresponding Medicare fees.
    - For current codes, use the CPT for the year being billed
      - Office visits are billed according to the complexity of the visit
        - There are five levels of office visits
        - As the level of visit becomes more complex, the more components are required.
          - History taking, examination, and medical decision-making are the key components in determining code selection.
          - Other components to be considered include counseling, coordination of care, and the nature of the presenting problem.
      - A billable visit is face-to-face contact with the nurse practitioner.
      - In the office setting, the nurse practitioner must distinguish between a new and established patient.
        - A new patient has not received professional services within the past 3 years from a provider in the same specialty in the same practice.
        - Telephone communication is considered a professional service.
      - A practice will bill using a variety of E & M codes because patient encounters vary in the amount of attention required.
      - Failure to bill for all services rendered can result in lower revenues for the practice.
      - All medical diagnoses will have an ICD-9 code.

- Reviewing data
- All medical diagnoses have ICD-9 codes.
- Concepts in healthcare policy
  - Access and use
    - Accessibility
    - Use of services
  - Episodes
    - Of illness; visits/procedures related to a particular illness, disease, or condition
  - Equity/inequity
    - Equity in health
      - Absence of systematic differences in one or more aspects of health status across socially, demographically, or geographically defined groups
    - Inequity in health
      - Presence of systematic differences in one or more aspects of health status across socially, demographically, or geographically defined groups
  - Health services components
    - Structure
      - The design of health services that influences the way in which they are delivered.
        - Types of personnel and staff
        - Organization of work
        - Range of services offered
        - The way the eligible population is determined
    - Processes of health care
      - The behavior or performance of the healthcare system or facility
      - Clinical care
        - Problem recognition
        - Diagnostic process
        - Recommendation of treatment and management
        - Follow-up
    - Outcomes
      - Aspects of health that result from interventions provided by a health system, the facilities, and its personnel
  - Prevention
    - Interventions that interrupt the framework of causality leading to one or more aspects of ill health
    - Primary
      - Interruption of causality before a physiological or psychological abnormality is identified
    - Secondary
      - Interruption of causality when a physiological or psychological abnormality is present but before the signs/symptoms manifest themselves
    - Tertiary
      - Intervention after a sign or symptom is present and to reduce progression or persistence of the disease state

Promotion of Quality Health Care

- Quality improvement (QI) processes
  - The NP should be competent in a variety of specific techniques, tools, and methodologies used to evaluate process performance and outcome.
    - Use of charts
      - Statistical control charts
      - Cause-and-effect diagrams
      - Scatter diagrams
    - Analytic data tools
      - Statistical software
    - Ability to interpret data in reports
    - Continuous quality improvement (CQI)/total quality management (TQM)
      - Ensure the delivery of care that is appropriate, safe, competent, and timely
      - Maximize favorable patient outcomes
      - Guided by use of established indicators of best practice
        - National guidelines for care
        - Indicators that may be developed internally in the institution or externally by expert panels who use existing evidence to specify which indicators are the most reasonable and targets for outcome achievement
- Numerous frameworks for improving performance
  - All quality improvement frameworks have common features
    - The focus of a QI effort must be measurable
    - Once measured, analysis is applied in a systematic way to improve and/or transform the healthcare delivery
    - Root cause analysis
      - Approach to identifying underlying causes of problems and process failures in the healthcare system
      - Useful for examining adverse events and patient safety issues
        - Sentinel events
          - Any unanticipated event in a healthcare setting resulting in death or serious physical or psychological injury to a patient or patients, not related to the natural course of the patient's illness
            - Tracked by The Joint Commission to ensure events are analyzed and appropriate changes made
            - Examples:
            - Medication error
            - Delayed treatment
            - Wrong surgery site
            - Suicide
            - Fall
            - Restraints
- Safety initiatives
  - The Joint Commission
    - National Patient Safety Goals

- Assisted accredited institutions to address specific concerns in regards to patient safety
- Updated annually
- Development and updating performed by a panel of patient safety experts who have hands-on experience in patient safety issues in a variety of healthcare environments
  - Nurses
  - Physicians
  - Pharmacists
  - Risk managers
  - Clinical engineers
- Accreditation
  - Obtained by many levels of the healthcare system
    - Hospitals
    - Physician's offices
    - Nursing homes
    - Office-based surgery centers
    - Behavioral treatment centers
    - Providers of home care services
- Benefits of accreditation
  - Helps organize and benefit patient safety measures
  - Strengthens community confidence in the quality, safety, and patient care of the organization
- Core measures
  - Part of a program established by The Joint Commission in 1997 that required hospitals to contract with selected performance measurement vendor systems to collect and submit data used in the accreditation process
  - Reportable evidence-based practices and outcomes in high-risk, high-volume populations
  - Used by CMS; mandates that hospitals report performance data for specified diagnoses
- Institute for Healthcare Improvement (IHI)
  - Offers resources and teaching tools to help healthcare professionals develop effective improvement efforts and enhance clinical outcomes in a variety of areas
  - Wide range of topics may be accessed via the Web site (www.ihi.org)
  - Examples of programs
    - Improvement map
      - Helps hospitals improve in nine core areas
        - Adverse drug events
        - Catheter-associated urinary tract infections
        - Central-line-associated blood stream infections
        - Injuries from falls and immobility
        - Obstetrical adverse events
        - Pressure ulcers
        - Surgical site infections
        - Venous thromboembolism
        - Ventilator-associated pneumonia
    - IHI Global Trigger Tool for measuring adverse events
      - Identifies adverse events and measures the rate of occurrence over time

REFERENCES

American Academy of Nurse Practitioners. (2011). *Nurse practitioner facts.* Retrieved from http://www.aanp.org/NR/rdonlyres/B899F71D-C6EE-4EE6-B3EE-466506DFED60/5145/AANPNPFactslogo72011.pdf

American College of Nurse Practitioners. (n.d.). *Numbers of nurse practitioners.* Retrieved from http://acnpweb.org/i4a/hpages/index.cfm

American Nurses Association. (2010a). *Nursing's social policy statement: The essence of the profession.* Silver Spring, MD: Author.

American Nurses Association. (2010b). *Scope and standards of practice.* Silver Spring, MD: Author.

Bell, L. (Ed.). (2006). *American Association of Critical Care Nurses scope and standards of practice for the acute care nurse practitioner.* Retrieved from http://www.aacn.org/WD/Practice/Docs/128102-ACNP_Scope_and_Standards

Barkley, T. W., & Myers, C. M. (Eds.). (2008). *Practice guidelines for acute care nurse practitioners* (2nd ed.). St. Louis, MO: Saunders Elsevier.

Bernat, J. L. (2005). Medical futility: Definition, determination, and disputes in critical care. *Neurocritical Care, 2*(2), 198–205.

Buppert, C. (2008). *Nurse practitioner's business practice and legal guide.* Boston: Jones & Bartlett.

Fowler, M. (2010). *Guide to the code of ethics for nurses, interpretation and application.* Silver Spring, MD: American Nurses Association.

Hamric, A., Spross, J., & Hanson, C. (2009). *Advanced practice nursing: An integrative approach.* St. Louis, MO: Saunders Elsevier.

Joel, L. (2009). *Advanced practice nursing, essentials for role development.* Philadelphia: F. A. Davis.

Joint Commission on Accreditation of Hospital Organizations. (2010). *Comprehensive accreditation manual for hospitals: The official handbook (CAMH).* Retrieved from www.jcrinc.com/Joint-Commission-Requirements/Hospitals/#MS

Klein, T. (2007). Scope of practice and the nurse practitioner: Regulation, competency, expansion, and evolution. *Topics in Advanced Practice Nursing eJournal.* Retrieved from www.medscape.org/viewarticle/506277

Marks, D., Murray, M., Evans, B., & Estacio, E. (2011). *Health psychology: Theory-research-practice.* Los Angeles: Sage Publications.

Melnick, D. E, Dillon, G. F., & Swanson, D. B. (2002). *Medical licensing examinations in the United States: Critical issues in dental education.* Retrieved from http://www.jdentaled.org/cgi/reprint/66/5/595.pdf

Polit, D., & Tatano Beck, C. (2009). *Essentials of nursing research: Appraising evidence for nursing practice.* Philadelphia: Wolters Kluwer Health/Lippincott Williams & Wilkins.

Starfield, B. (2001). Basic concepts in population health and health care. *Epidemiology and Community Health, 55,* 452–454.

Thomas, J., Finch, L., Schoenhofer, S., & Green, A. (2005). The caring relationships created by nurse practitioners and the ones nursed: implications for practice. *Topics in Advanced Practice Nursing eJournal, 4*(4). Retrieved from www.medscape.com/viewarticle/496420

U.S. Department of Health & Human Services. (n.d.). *Historical highlights.* Retrieved from http://www.hhs.gov/about/hhshist.html

Wikipedia. (n.d.). *Nurse practitioner.* Retrieved from http://en.m.wikipedia.org/wiki/Nurse_practitioner

Wright, W. L. (2005). *Malpractice prevention: Everything the NP needs to know.* Retrieved from http://www.conferenceprogram.com/np/presentations/2E-Wright-Malpractice-Prevention

3

General Assessment and Management

Pamela Smith, MSN, RN, ACNP-BC, CCRN;
Julie Davey, MSN, RN, ANP-BC, ACNP-BC;
and Melanie Smith, MSN, RN, ACNP-BC

ASSESSMENT OF THE AT-RISK PATIENT

- Several patient populations will have high-risk patients and need focused screening during history and physical assessment.
  - Elderly
    - Functional assessment—evaluate:
      - Mobility, hearing, vision
      - Ability to carry out activities of daily living safely
      - Changes in cognition
        - Nutrition
          - Thorough dietary history
          - Weight loss or gain
          - Ability to go the grocery store
          - Dentition
        - Financial stability
    - Social support/caregiver issues
    - Presence of anxiety/depression
  - Homeless
    - Living conditions
    - Length of homelessness

- Presence of untreated illness
  - Mental illness/depression
  - Malnutrition
  - Dentition
- Patients with chronic illness
  - Screening
    - Cardiovascular disease
      - Abdominal aortic aneurysm
        - One-time ultrasound for men 65 to 75 years of age
        - No routine screening for women
      - Aspirin use
        - Used by men age 45 to 79 years when potential benefit of decreased risk of myocardial infarction outweighs risk of gastrointestinal bleeding
        - Used by women age 55 to 79 years when potential benefit of decreased risk of ischemic stroke outweighs risk of gastrointestinal bleeding
        - Insufficient evidence for use in patients age 80 or older
        - Not recommended for stroke prevention in women younger than 55 years of age and myocardial prevention in men younger than 45 years of age.
    - Hypertension
      - Blood pressure screening for adults over 18 years of age
    - Diabetes
      - Screen for type 2 diabetes in asymptomatic adults with blood pressure (treated or untreated) > 135/80 mm Hg
    - Hyperlipidemia
      - Screen men age 35 and older
      - Screen men 20 to 35 for lipid disorders if at increased risk for coronary artery disease
      - Screen women aged 45 and older for lipid disorders if at increased risk of coronary artery disease
      - Screen younger women 20 to 45 if history is strong for coronary artery disease
      - No recommendation for or against routine screening for lipid disorders in men 20 to 35 or in women 20 and older who are not at risk for coronary artery disease
    - Osteoporosis
      - Screen periodically in women > 65 years or > 60 if at risk
    - Cancer
      - Breast cancer—mammography
        - Women > 40 years of age every 1 to 2 years
      - Colorectal cancer
        - Screen adults > 50
        - Occult blood yearly
        - Sigmoidoscopy every 5 years *or* colonoscopy every 10 years
      - Pap smear
        - Within 3 years of onset of sexual activity or 21 to 65 years of age
- Obesity/malnutrition
  - Assess for physical inactivity
  - Screen for diet and exercise

- Tobacco and substance abuse
  - Smoking cessation counseling/screening
  - Alcohol use and screening
  - National Institute of Drug Abuse (NIDA)
    - Modified Alcohol, Smoking, and Substance Involvement Screening Test
      - Web-based interactive tool
      - Generates score that suggests level of intervention needed
  - Fast Alcohol Screening Test (FAST)
    - Similar to CAGE test
    - Four-question test
    - Used in emergency department and clinics
  - CAGE
    - Four-question test that evaluates alcohol problems over a lifetime
  - Occupational risk and exposure
    - ChemSTEER—Chemical Screening Tool for Exposures and Environmental Releases
      - Estimates occupational inhalation and dermal exposure to chemicals during industrial and commercial manufacturing
    - Exposure to ionizing radiation
  - Environmental risk and exposure
    - Secondhand tobacco smoke
    - Pesticides
    - Lead
    - Mercury
- Screening tools for risk assessment
  - Health risk assessment tools
    - Several forms exist
    - Evaluate a variety of factors
      - Lifestyle
      - Biometric and laboratory results
      - Compliance with recommended preventive screenings
      - Existing chronic illness
      - Future disease risk
      - Workplace productivity
  - Subjective Global Assessment (SGA)
    - Method of evaluating malnutrition
    - Used at the bedside
    - Classifies patients into one of three categories
      - SGA grade A—well-nourished
      - SGA grade B—moderately or suspected malnutrition
      - SGA grade C—severely malnourished
  - Surgical patients
    - Cardiac risk stratification for non-cardiac surgery
      - Presence of coronary artery disease, congestive heart failure, cerebrovascular disease, or chronic kidney disease due to atherosclerosis
      - Presence of diabetes—cardiovascular disease equivalent that increases risk of cardiac complications

- Major abdominal, thoracic, and vascular surgeries—higher risk of post-operative complications
- Revised Cardiac Risk Index
  - Tool used to assess and communicate cardiac risk
  - Incorporated in some perioperative management guidelines
- Non-invasive ischemia test (stress test) for high revised cardiac risk index, congestive heart failure, or angina symptoms
- Risk stratification for cardiac surgery
  - Society of Thoracic Surgeons (STS) online risk calculator
  - EuroSCORE—European System for Cardiac Operative Risk Evaluation
    - Both used in coronary artery bypass and valvular surgery
  - Both provide objective way of stratifying risk

Development of Differential Diagnoses

- The development of differential diagnoses is derived from the data collected from the history and physical examination.
- Data from the chief complaint, history of present illness, past medical history, family history, and review of symptoms are particularly helpful.
  - Identify abnormal findings.
  - Localize the finding anatomically.
    - Localized symptoms may lead directly to the problem: a sore, inflamed throat, for example.
    - More generalized symptoms may make it more difficult to pinpoint the source; for example, chest pain may be cardiac, gastrointestinal, or musculoskeletal.
  - Interpret the findings in terms of what is probable based on signs and symptoms.
  - Form a hypothesis (or hypotheses) about the nature of the problem.
  - Consult the clinical literature for evidence-based decision-making.
- Steps in clinical decision-making
  - Select the most specific and critical findings to form the diagnostic hypothesis.
  - Match the findings with all conditions associated with them.
  - Eliminate diagnostic possibilities that fail to explain the findings.
  - Weigh the competing possibilities and choose the most likely diagnosis from among the conditions that might be responsible for the patient's findings.
  - Pay special attention to possible explanations that may be life-threatening and treatable; for example:
    - Meningococcal meningitis
    - Acute myocardial infarction
    - Aortic dissection
    - Bacterial endocarditis
    - Pulmonary embolism
    - Subdural hematoma
  - Always include the worst-case scenario in the list of differential diagnoses.
- Order additional testing to confirm or rule out the tentative diagnosis (diagnoses).
- Once a working diagnosis is confirmed, discuss the treatment plan with the patient.
- Manage the data.

- Separate clusters of observations and analyze one cluster at a time.
  - By body system
  - By associated symptoms

Clinical Management & Health Promotion

- Assisting individuals obtain optimum states of health.
- Evidence-based practice
  - Apply evidence to the development, implementation, and evaluation of effective programs in the healthcare field.
  - The practice of health promotion has a direct link with the research that supports its effectiveness.
- Disease and age-related risk factors
  - Cardiovascular disease (hypertension, coronary artery disease, heart failure, stroke) is the leading cause of death in the United States.
    - Primary prevention includes lifestyle modifications such as exercise, healthy nutrition, tobacco cessation, stress reduction, and modification of all risk factors such as hypertension, hyperlipidemia, and diabetes mellitus.
  - Osteoporosis
    - Preventing fractures involves maintenance of bone density by:
      - Maintaining endocrine control of bone density (selective estrogen receptor modifiers, bisphosphonates, calcitonin)
      - Adequate intake of calcium and vitamin D
      - Weight-bearing activities
    - Higher risk for falls and injuries
      - Prevention includes maintaining strength of the lower extremities, balance training, environmental modifications, and review of medications as a potential contributing factor.
  - Diabetes mellitus type 2
    - Development most often occurs between ages 50 and 60.
    - Prevention includes lifestyle modifications such as exercise, healthy nutrition, and maintaining a healthy weight.
  - Osteoarthritis is the most common disease affecting older adults.
    - Excessive weight increases the risk.
    - Prevention and reduction in symptoms includes proper exercise (conditioning), proper training for activities, and the use of assistive gait devices when necessary.
  - Polypharmacy
    - Older adults are at higher risk for multiple medication use and drug interactions.
    - Healthcare providers must be aware of polypharmacy and review medications frequently.
    - Encourage patients to use only one pharmacy so medications from multiple providers can be monitored and evaluated.

Patient Education

- Self-care strategies
  - The successful management of many disease processes and chronic health conditions requires the compliance of the patient and their families.
  - Compliance requires education.
  - Before education, an assessment of the patient's needs, beliefs, goals, judgment standards, and comprehension of skills must be undertaken.
  - Development of positive behaviors is the goal.
- Considerations for adult learners
  - Create a climate for collaboration.
  - Determine the adult learner's preferred method of learning—how he or she learns the best.
  - The learner brings personal experiences to the educational session.
  - Social roles play a part in readiness to learn.
  - Immediate application of knowledge will increase the potential for behavioral change.
- Determining learning needs
  - Assess the patient's and family's motivation to learn.
  - Assess the existing knowledge base for the topic at hand.
  - Determine past experiences with this type of health-related issue.
  - Identify by what method the patient learns best.
  - Ask how culture might play a role in his or her willingness to adapt new behaviors.
  - Assess the patient's literacy level.
  - Identify what educational materials are available on the topic at hand.
  - Determine what motivates the patient to change behavior.
  - Identify any barriers to learning.
  - Ask how the education and behavioral change will be evaluated.
- Coaching through behavioral changes
  - Assists in improving self-management of chronic illness
  - Assessment of and attention to the emotional status of the patient is important to success.
  - Appropriate use of educational materials should be individualized.
  - Development of a trusting and caring relationship between the learner(s) and educator is imperative for success.
  - Develop a collaborative set of goals with the learner.
  - The use of open-ended questions allows the learner to focus on his or her needs and concerns.
  - Affirming the learner's strengths instills confidence.
  - The use of reflective listening demonstrates the educator's interest.

EVALUATING THE PLAN OF CARE

Description

Once the complex tasks of assessment, diagnosis, and care planning have been completed by the acute care nurse practitioner (ACNP), an essential clinical management piece remains: evaluation of the patient's progress and response to interventions. This includes evaluation of the patient's and family's response to teaching interventions. Evaluation of the patient, as well as the plan of care, is an ongoing process that guides modification of the treatment plan and optimization of expected patient outcomes.

Etiology

- The basis for the standard of professional practice by the ACNP as a care provider is best described using the nursing process as framework. The ACNP:
  - Performs **assessments** that collect and incorporate data from a variety of sources to support clinical decision-making
  - Determines accurate **diagnoses** as a basis for interventions
  - **Identifies** appropriate and measurable patient-specific **outcomes**
  - Develops an interdisciplinary, cost-effective **care plan** designed to reach those outcomes
  - Implements the plan of care through **advanced nursing interventions**
  - **Evaluates** patients' responses to interventions and progress toward anticipated goals
- The ACNP incorporates advanced practice competencies, critical thinking, continuing education, and the use of relevant theory and research into this framework and provides evidence-based care planning and advanced nursing care to acutely and critically ill patients.

Incidence and Demographics

- In 2008, there were nearly 160,000 credentialed nurse practitioners (NPs) in the United States; most were certified as adult or family NPs, with 5.6% holding certification as ACNPs.
- A 2008 national survey specific to ACNP practice found that the overwhelming majority of practitioners are White females with an average age of 42, hold master's degrees in nursing as one of their highest degrees, and practice in inpatient hospital settings.
- A recent review of 69 studies published between 1990 and 2008, analyzing outcomes of the care provided by advanced nursing practitioners, found similar or better patient outcomes in numerous clinical areas compared to care provided by physicians. The review also found that advanced practice nurses consistently provided safe, effective, quality care.

Risk Factors

- Planning care for the patient with chronic, acute, and critical illness should include an evaluation for risk factors that could lead to complications while undergoing treatment. Interventions should be modified accordingly.

- The ACNP should consider, when possible, the need to screen patients for potential undetected health problems based on data collected in the history and physical exam, the presence of risk factors, or pertinent findings from lab or test results. Complications of coronary artery disease, cerebrovascular disease, or diabetes often present acutely when patients are critically ill. Disease-specific interventions for prophylaxis and enhancement of risk reduction must be implemented whenever possible.
- The acutely ill patient is at risk for exacerbation of previously stable chronic health problems as well, despite continuation of home treatment regimens. Modifications to treatment for chronic health problems should be incorporated into the plan of care when indicated.
- It is necessary to perform ongoing assessments of the patient's risk for or development of adverse responses to complex medical treatment and hospitalizations and plan or modify interventions accordingly. Those risks can be:
  - **Physiological**, including complications from invasive tests and procedures, exacerbation of chronic health problems, and the side effects of:
    - Medications
    - Prolonged immobility
    - Fluid and electrolyte shifts
    - Impaired nutrition
  - **Psychological** risks associated with separation from family and significant others, sleep deprivation, effects of psychoactive medications, impaired communication in the presence of invasive tubes, environmental factors such as lack of privacy, and the stress of coping with life-threatening diagnoses and illness.
  - **Healthcare system risks,** which are a challenging part of providing care to complex patients with multiple providers and include lack of care coordination and continuity of care, polypharmacy, and suboptimal communication between team members and with patient and family members as common barriers to achieving success in meeting expected outcomes in a timely, cost-effective manner.
- The ACNP must consider that care ultimately may be provided at a variety of acute and outpatient care settings, and that the focus of care at times may be on palliative treatment. Creating a sustainable care plan requires comprehensive initial planning and ongoing modifications to the plan after evaluating each patient's unique and dynamic response to illness and treatment.
- Factors such as the patient's financial resources and support system, his or her ability or willingness to respond to education or comply with treatment, and recognition that interventions may need to be carried out across the continuum of care also play a role in care plan modification. Ensuring a successful outcome requires the ACNP to take a leadership role in communicating changes in the patient's clinical status and goals of care to all members of the multidisciplinary team, and to provide clear and thorough documentation of the care plan and the care provided.
- Nurse practitioners are licensed and credentialed, and are therefore at risk for the disciplinary and legal processes associated with violating practice standards. The most common sources of liability for NPs are:
  - Failure to diagnose or a delay in diagnosis
  - Treatment errors
  - Medication errors

- A breach of confidentiality can result in a malpractice claim. Because communication among interdisciplinary team members, patients, and families often falls to the nurse practitioner coordinating care delivery, confidentiality and protection of sensitive information must always remain a priority.
- Clear, confidential documentation is a crucial component of safe practice in care planning and plan modification by the ACNP. Documentation should be available to all healthcare team members and provides a record of the care plan and the team members accountable for the care provided.

Prevention and Screening

- Maintaining knowledge of health risks and common health problems specific to patients' age, gender, ethnicity, and family history is as important in the acute care setting as it is in the outpatient arena. Nurse practitioners are responsible for staying informed on current recommendations for health maintenance, chronic disease management, risk factor modification, and disease prevention. These recommendations should be incorporated into the plan of care when appropriate.
- Nurse practitioners have a duty to follow up on any potentially serious health concerns for patients in their care until such issues have resolved. Although not every issue identified merits a comprehensive inpatient workup, significant findings must be communicated to outpatient providers and consultants to ensure continuity of care.
- Knowledge of quality indicators that reflect the provision of safe, cost-effective, evidence-based care is essential. Thromboembolic events, gastritis, hospital-acquired infections, or the development of decubitus ulcers are often preventable. Whether planning initial acute care interventions, modifying the care plan based on ongoing evaluation of the patient's response to treatment, or transitioning the patient to a different care setting, prophylaxis against common complications of acute care should be incorporated into the ACNP's care plan.

Assessment

- Planning for patient care delivery and outcomes is optimized not just through a comprehensive physical assessment, but by a thorough assessment of the patient's community resources, family support, personal and financial resources, belief system, and culture, before individualizing the plan for physical care and patient/family teaching.
- Modification of the plan of care is based on continual assessment of the patient's changing condition in response to interventions.

Management

- Patients' responses to illness and treatment are dynamic and clinical pictures can change rapidly. Patients may progress as expected or more quickly than expected in response to intervention. Conversely, patients can deteriorate due to the complexity of ongoing illness and hospitalization, despite the most thoughtful, comprehensive care plan. Therefore, the management plan must be dynamic as well.

- As a patient's condition changes, or fails to change, the ACNP must evaluate interventions and identified outcomes, and be prepared to modify the plan of care. Outcomes should be individualized and continuously modified based on:
  - The patient's clinical status and mutually agreed-upon goals of treatment
  - The ethics, financial implications, and costs of providing ongoing care
  - Potential risks and benefits of interventions and treatment
  - The quality of care that can be provided
  - Resources that are available to the patient across healthcare settings
  - The patient's demonstrated compliance or noncompliance with therapy
  - The patient's and family's beliefs regarding planned interventions and therapy
- Successful outcomes are enhanced and strengthened when interventions are evidence-based, shaped by multidisciplinary and patient/family input, and sustainable across a variety of healthcare settings.
- When the patient's goals are not compatible with those of their providers because of financial, psychosocial, and–at times–ethical considerations, interventions and outcomes must be modified accordingly to reflect mutually agreed-upon treatments and endpoints of care.

Nonpharmacologic Treatment
- Information technology, medical equipment, and monitoring devices are important tools in care planning. Such modalities can help to assess, diagnose, treat, evaluate, and modify treatment, both historically and in real time.
- Medical and information technology can be a vehicle for clinical assessment, information management, documentation, or communication with members of the healthcare team, or used for staff and patient education. They aid critical thinking and evaluation of patients' response to treatment; provide efficiency in modifying care plans; and facilitate provision of quality, coordinated, evidence-based care.

Pharmacologic Treatment
- The ACNP often plays a key role in prescribing and modifying pharmacological interventions for the acutely or critically ill patient. It is important that interventions are based on scientific evidence, consistent with the desired outcomes of care, and prescribed and manageable within the nurse practitioner's scope of practice, particularly when managing pain.
- Medication management in the setting of polypharmacy can be complex and challenging when patients are critically ill. The ACNP must consider the costs of therapy, the goals of care, the sustainability of treatment, and the risk or benefit to the patient before initiating new pharmacologic interventions.
- Collaboration, careful documentation, and communication with all members of the healthcare team, particularly physicians, pharmacists, and the bedside nurse, aid in delivery of safe, effective, and timely implementation of pharmacological interventions.
- When medications are modified day by day, and at times minute by minute, patients are at risk for adverse drug reactions, synergistic side effects, medication errors, the burden of multiple medication costs, and noncompliance with prescribed regimens. The ACNP must be vigilant in ensuring the plan of care for pharmacologic treatment is continually reassessed and modified for safety, quality, appropriateness, and cost-effectiveness.

Special Considerations

Patient Teaching

- Planning and providing for patient and family education plays a vital role in achieving successful patient outcomes. Education should be incorporated into the ACNP's care plan and the response to teaching should guide plan modification. Teaching helps patients and families:
  - Understand disease processes and the complications that develop when treating complex, chronic, and acute illnesses.
  - Understand treatment options and the goals of planned interventions and therapies.
  - Make informed treatment and discharge planning decisions.
  - Enhance compliance with medication regimens and follow-up.
  - Enhance compliance with nonpharmacologic therapies.
- Teaching by the ACNP may be carried out informally in response to a situational knowledge deficit demonstrated by a patient or family member, or in a formal setting with an individualized teaching plan. Teaching may be delegated to qualified individuals.
- Patients may learn best in classroom settings, with personalized instruction, or both. Appropriate electronic resources or written material may be suitable for teaching as well. The ACNP must perform an educational assessment and determine the teaching method most appropriate to the patient's age, educational level, and preferred learning style.
- Like all aspects of care planning, support for patient's and family's educational needs should be individualized. Whether participating in family care conferences in the hospital, setting aside time for answering questions from patients and family members, or providing electronic resources that supplement formal or informal teaching, the nurse practitioner often has a leadership role in communicating with patients and families, determining knowledge deficits, and planning appropriate educational interventions.

Cost-Effectiveness

- In today's healthcare environment, healthcare dollars must be spent wisely, whether a patient is insured, uninsured, or underinsured. Care of the patient experiencing acute or critical illness often entails a rapid escalation toward complex interventions and technologically driven treatments. Whether prescribing medication or planning for transition to the next level of care, interventions should be carried out ethically, but with a concern for the patient's disease processes, financial resources, ability and willingness to comply with ongoing treatment, and goals of care.
- Although quantifying the financial benefit of care provided by the ACNP and the best strategies for third-party reimbursement of NP care continues to be difficult, outcome studies consistently demonstrate the benefits of care provided by nurse practitioners versus physicians in terms of quality and cost-effectiveness.
- The ACNP, no matter the practice setting, always must consider the financial impact of care when planning interventions and treatments, and incorporate cost-effectiveness and quality benefits into the changing plan of care.

When to Consult, Refer, or Hospitalize

- Licensing, credentialing, hospital bylaws, and scope of practice legislation define the general role of the nurse practitioner. Nevertheless, the ACNP must always be aware of situational limitations on practice. Having the education and expertise needed to perform each specific job function must be balanced with referring care, when appropriate, to specialized practitioners. Expert consultation for management of complex medical issues is always appropriate, as is a transition to either a higher level of care or palliative and end-of-life care providers. It is important, if possible, to define the threshold for such referrals when designing the plan of care.

Follow-up

Expected Outcomes
- The ACNP ideally designs a healthcare delivery plan that is patient-centered, collaborative, coordinated, evidence-based, and cost-effective. Achievement of successful outcomes is driven by continuous patient evaluation and modification of the care plan-based on the patient's response or lack of response to interventions.
- Continuity of care as the patient transitions across care settings is supported by ongoing discharge planning, clear discharge instructions, communication with providers in the outpatient setting or at the next level of care, and careful documentation.

Complications
- Multiple factors can derail the most thorough care plan. Failure to set mutually agreed-upon goals of care with patients and families can lead to patient noncompliance, unwanted financial burdens for the patient, and ethical challenges for the healthcare team. Failure to consider social and financial circumstances that preclude a successful discharge leads to relapsing medical conditions and rehospitalizations. Lack of continuity in care can be a result of poor documentation or communication with members of the healthcare team and the patient.
- The ACNP should be prepared for the challenges associated with planning care for complex acutely ill patients who can have dynamic and highly individualized responses to illness. Interdisciplinary collaboration and communication, and using resources necessary to plan evidence-based interventions, are key factors in avoiding setbacks and preventable complications in delivery of care.

REFERENCES

American Academy of Nurse Practitioners. (2011). *Nurse practitioner facts.* Retrieved from http://www.aanp.org/NR/rdonlyres/B899F71D-C6EE-4EE6-B3EE-466506DFED60/5145/AANPNPFactslogo72011.pdf

American Association of Critical Care Nurses. (2006). *Scope and standards of practice for the acute care nurse practitioner.* Retrieved from http://www.aacn.org/WD/Practice/Docs/128102-ACNP_Scope_and_Standards.pdf

American College of Nurse Practitioners. (2011). *APRNs achieve comparable or better outcomes than physicians, review suggests.* Retrieved from http://www.acnpweb.org/i4a/pages/index.cfm?pageid=1

American College of Nurse Practitioners. (2011). *Numbers of nurse practitioners.* Retrieved from http://www.acnpweb.org/i4a/pages/index.cfm?pageid=3353.

Barkley, T. W., & Myers, C. M. (Eds.). (2008). *Practice guidelines for acute care nurse practitioners* (2nd ed.). St. Louis, MO: Saunders Elsevier.

Bickley, L., & Szilagyi, P. (Eds). (2009). *Bates' guide to physical examination.* Philadelphia: Lippincott Williams & Wilkins/Wolters Kluwer.

Cohagen, A., & Brenner, B. (Eds.) (2011). *Alcohol and substance abuse evaluation.* Retrieved from http://emedicine.medscape.com/article/805084-overview

Fauci, A., Braunwald, E., Kasper, D., Hauser, S., Longo, D., Jameson, J., & Loscalzo, J. (2008). *Harrison's principles of internal medicine.* New York: McGraw Hill.

Hahn, J., Kushel, M., Bangsber, D., Riley, E., & Moss, A. (2006). Brief report: The aging of the homeless population: Fourteen-year trends. *Journal of General Internal Medicine, 21*(7), 775–778.

Linder, H., Menzies, D., Kelly, J., Taylor, S., & Shearer, M. (2003). Coaching for behaviour change in chronic disease: A review of the literature and the implications for coaching as a self-management intervention. *Australian Journal of Primary Health, 9*(3), 177–185.

Logan, P. (1999). *Principles of practice for the acute care nurse practitioner: Part A.* Stamford, CT: Appleton & Lange.

Makhija, S., & Baker, J. (2008). The subjective global assessment: A review of its use in clinical practice. *Nutrition in Clinical Practice, 23*(4), 405–409.

National Institute on Drug Abuse. (2008). *Screening for tobacco, alcohol and other drug use.* Retrieved from http://www.nida.nih.gov/nidamed/screening

United States Environmental Protection Agency. (2004). *Exposure assessment tools and models.* Retrieved from http://www.epa.gov/opptintr/exposure/pubs/chemsteer.htm

Williams, A. (2008). *Health promotion and wellness for older persons.* Missoula: Montana Geriatric Education Center.

Zajarias, A., & Cribier, A. (2009). Outcomes and safety of percutaneous aortic valve replacement. *Journal of the American College of Cardiology, 53*(20), 1829–1836.

4

Cardiovascular Disorders

Julie Davey, MSN, RN, ANP-BC, ACNP-BC

ACUTE CORONARY SYNDROMES AND CORONARY ARTERY DISEASE

Description

- Coronary artery disease (CAD) is defined as the atherosclerotic process of plaque accumulation within the walls of the coronary arteries. Acute coronary syndrome (ACS) is a broad term that encompasses unstable angina, non-ST-elevation myocardial infarction (NSTEMI), and ST-elevation myocardial infarction (STEMI).

Etiology, Incidence, and Demographics

- CAD is the number-one cause of death among men and women in the United States.
- 16 million Americans have CAD.
- 600,000 deaths per year occur secondary to CAD.
- Prevalence increases with age.
- CAD is more common in men before age 70. After age 70, gender distribution is equal.

Risk Factors

- Positive family history (first-degree relatives and early onset increase risk)
- Male gender
- Dyslipidemia (the higher the low-density lipoprotein [LDL], the greater the risk)
- Hypertension
- Diabetes mellitus
- Physical inactivity, obesity, or both
- Tobacco abuse

Prevention and Screening

- Modify risk factors, including hypertensive control, hyperlipidemia control, weight loss, and smoking cessation
- Anti-platelets
- Beta-blockers
- Routine exercise regimen
- Screening tests, such as ECG and stress testing, as appropriate based on symptomatology and risk factors

Assessment

- Angina pectoris (ischemic chest pain) described as a substernal, tight/pressure sensation
- Discomfort may radiate to the jaw, neck, left arm
- Lasts 5 to 20 minutes
- Brought on by exertion, stress, exposure to cold weather, or ingestion of a large meal
- Relieved by rest, sublingual nitroglycerin
- Associated symptoms may include dyspnea, nausea, diaphoresis
- Area of physical examination is rarely specific or sensitive

Differential Diagnosis

- Aortic dissection
- Pulmonary embolism
- Tension pneumothorax
- Pericarditis
- Esophageal spasm
- Peptic ulcer disease
- Gastroesophageal reflux disease

Diagnostic Studies

- Cardiac isoenzymes (CPK, CK-MB, Troponin): enzymes elevated with NSTEMI and STEMI
- Electrocardiogram: may demonstrate non-specific changes, ST depression, T-wave inversion; ST elevation only with STEMI
- Other labs, including CBC (assess for anemia or infectious process as contributing factors to ischemia), lipid panel, and glucose level to screen for risk factors
- Stress testing for patients with angina to assess for ischemia
- Echocardiogram to assess left ventricular function and presence of valvular heart disease as cause of presenting symptomatology
- Coronary angiography to assess for presence of CAD and provide intervention such as angioplasty and/or stent placement, when appropriate

Management

- Aspirin: inhibits platelet aggregation by blocking production of thromboxane A2
  - Dosage for CAD: enteric-coated ASA 81 to 325 mg p.o. q.d.
  - Dosage for ACS: 81 to 325 mg chewed upon presentation to increase absorption and onset.
  - Contraindications: documented drug allergy, active bleeding
- Nitrates: systemic and coronary vasodilator, reduces preload
  - SL NTG 0.4 mg Q 5 minutes for chest pain relief × 3 doses
  - IV NTG for refractory CP, titrate to relief (monitor for hypotension)
  - Contraindications: hypotension, critical aortic stenosis, recent use of phosphodiasterase type 5 inhibitor medications for erectile dysfunction
- Anticoagulation
  - Unfractionated heparin: IV heparin bolus followed by gtt, titrate to PTT 1.5 to 2 × normal
  - Low molecular weight heparin: SC dosing
    - Advantages: better bioavailability, less protein binding, no monitoring
    - Disadvantages: longer T1/2, caution in renal patients
  - Contraindications: active bleeding
- Beta-adrenergic-blocking agents: reduce oxygen demand by inhibiting catecholamine effects on heart rate and contractility
  - Decrease mortality, infarct size, and rate of reinfarction
  - Should be given to patients with history of myocardial infarction (MI), angina pectoris, and within the first 24 hours post-MI unless contraindicated
  - Contraindications: significant bronchospastic lung disease, bradyarrhythmias, decompensated heart failure
- Morphine: improves myocardial oxygen demand by reducing preload
  - Decreases sympathetic drive and is recommended analgesic and anxiolitic
  - Usual dose 2 to 4 mg IV p.r.n. pain
  - Potential side effects: hypotension, respiratory depression, nausea or vomiting
  - Antiplatelets
- Clopidogrel (Plavix): inhibits ADP-mediated platelet aggregation
  - Dosage: clopidegrel 75 mg p.o. q.d.; may give loading dose (300 to 600 mg) in acute situations to accelerate onset
  - If ASA contraindicated, clopidegrel is first line

- Prasugrel (Effient): inhibits ADP-mediated platelet aggregation
  - May be used as an alternative to clopidegrel
- Glycoprotein IIb/IIIa antagonists: final common pathway for platelet aggregation by blocking IIb/IIIa receptors on platelet surface
  - Use in combination with ASA and UFH in high risk ACS patients.
  - Contraindications: active bleeding, thrombocytopenia, uncontrolled hypertension, or cerebrovascular accident or surgery in the last 30 days
- Calcium channel blockers
  - Third-line agent in patients with persistent chest pain despite adequate doses of nitrates and beta-adrenergic blockers
  - Very useful in vasospastic or Prinzmentals angina
  - Contraindications: non-dihydroperidines in patients with systolic heart failure and conduction system abnormalities
- Reperfusion strategies for STEMI
- Thrombolytics (see next page)
  - Indicated for ST elevation > 0.1 mv in two or more contiguous leads
  - Time to therapy < 12 hours
  - Age < 75 years
  - Advantages: wide availability and faster administration
- Percutaneous coronary intervention (angioplasty/stent placement)
  - Goal: balloon inflation within 90 min of arrival
  - Advantages: lower incidence of recurrent ischemia, reinfarction, and death

When to Consult, Refer, or Hospitalize

- All patients with ACS require hospitalization.
- Obtain cardiology consultation to determine treatment plan and perform procedures such as cardiac catheterization.

Follow-up

- Careful management of comorbid conditions
- Patient and family education on the underlying disease process and warning signs of future events
- Discuss risk factor modification:
  - Lipid management
  - Blood pressure control
  - Blood glucose control
  - Maintenance of body mass index (BMI) 18–25
  - Tobacco cessation
- Discuss importance of medication compliance in detail

CONTRAINDICATIONS TO THROMBOLYTIC THERAPY

Absolute

- Previous intracranial bleed
- Stroke less than 3 months previously
- Closed head or facial trauma within 3 months
- Suspected aortic dissection
- Ischemic stroke within 3 months (except in ischemic stroke within 3 hours' time)
- Active bleeding diathesis
- Uncontrolled high blood pressure (> 180 systolic or > 100 diastolic)
- Known structural cerebral vascular lesion

Relative

- Current anticoagulant use
- Invasive or surgical procedure in previous 2 weeks
- Prolonged cardiopulmonary resuscitation (CPR)—defined as more than 10 minutes
- Known bleeding diathesis
- Pregnancy
- Hemorrhagic or diabetic retinopathies
- Active peptic ulcer
- Controlled severe hypertension

DYSLIPIDEMIA

Description

- Dyslipidemia is term used to describe any variety of lipid abnormalities, including low-density lipoproteins (LDL), high-density lipoproteins (HDL), and triglycerides (TGL), that deviate from normal ranges and increase risk of cardiovascular disease. Ranges of normal for total cholesterol and lipoproteins are defined by the National Cholesterol Education Program.

Etiology, Incidence, and Demographics

- More common in males
- Affects > 120 million Americans
  - Familial or genetic syndromes
    - Familial hypercholesterolemia
    - Familial defective apolipoprotein B-100

- Familial hypertriglyceridemia
- Familial combined hyperlipidemia
- Endocrine causes
  - Thyroid disease
  - Cushing's syndrome
  - Hepatic disease
- Other contributors
  - Underlying malignancy
  - Pancreatitis

Risk Factors

- Cigarette smoking
- High-fat, high-cholesterol diet
- Sedentary lifestyle
- Family history or genetic predisposition
- Excess alcohol use

Prevention and Screening

- National Cholesterol Education Program (NCEP)
  - Recommends that all adults over age 20 have cholesterol screening every 5 years
  - More frequent screening if risk factors for vascular disease are present
- United States Preventive Services Task Force
  - Recommended: routine screening to begin at age 35 for men and age 45 for women
  - Screening earlier if risk factors for heart disease present

Assessment

- Rarely produces signs and symptoms. If present, physical exam or inquiry findings may include:
  - Xanthomas
  - Xanthalesmas
  - Corneal arcus
- Earlobe crease
  - Plaques (on fundoscopic exam)
- Symptoms of underlying predisposing disease
  - Weight gain
  - Cold intolerance
  - Constipation
  - Edema
  - Central obesity
  - Purple striae
  - Fat-wasting
  - Hepatomegaly

Differential Diagnosis

- Transient increase in lipid profiles because of acute illness or drug therapy
- Thiazide diuretics
- Acute pancreatitis
- Hepatitis
- Renal disease

Diagnostic Studies

- Fractionated lipid profile, to include:
  - Total cholesterol
    - LDL
    - HDL
  - Triglycerides
  - Apolipoprotein
    - As indicated to assess for transient or endocrine causes
  - Liver function tests
    - Amylase and lipase
  - Basic metabolic panel
  - Renal function tests
    - Urinalysis
    - TSH
    - As indicated to evaluate comorbid risk factors for heart disease
  - Electrocardiogram
  - Fasting glucose

Management

- Therapy includes lifestyle modifications, pharmacologic therapy, or both.
- Goals of therapy:
  - High-risk:
    - CAD or PAD
    - Diabetes mellitus
    - 2 or more risk factors and a 10-year risk of MI > 20% (based on Framingham criteria)
    - LDL < 100 mg/dL
  - Very high-risk:
    - Recent MI
    - CAD and diabetes mellitus or severe or poorly controlled risk factors
    - LDL < 70 mg/dL
  - Moderately high risk:
    - 2 or more risk factors and a 10%–20% risk of having an MI within 10 years
    - LDL < 130 mg/dL
    - Option of lowering LDL < 100 mg/dL

- Moderate to lower risk:
  - Moderate: 2 or more risk factors and a < 10% risk of MI in 10 years
  - Goal < 130
  - Low: 0–1 risk factor
  - Goal < 160
- Decision to implement drug therapy based on the presence of other risk factors for cardiovascular disease

Nonpharmacologic Treatment
- Increase exercise
- Smoking cessation
- Low-cholesterol, low-fat diet
- Weight loss for obese patients

Pharmacologic Treatment
- HMG-CoA reductase inhibitors (statins)
  - Drug of choice for all patients with diagnosed CAD or CAD risk-equivalent (peripheral arterial disease, diabetes mellitus, abdominal aortic aneurysm)
  - Should be dosed in the evening
  - May produce muscle symptoms or rhabdomyolysis
  - Monitor liver function tests
  - Contraindicated in:
    - Pregnancy
    - Liver disease
- Niacin
  - Therapeutic effect upon LDL, HDL, and triglycerides
  - Contraindicated in diabetes mellitus and gout
  - May produce vasomotor flushing; pretreat with ASA 30 to 60 minutes before taking
  - May produce GI side effects; start with low dose, titrate upward slowly
  - Monitor with liver function tests
- Fibric acid derivatives
  - Greatest impact on HDL
  - Generally well-tolerated
  - < 10% LDL reduction
  - Bile acid sequestrants
  - Safe for use with other lipid-lowering agents
  - Safe in pregnancy
  - Will interfere with absorption of other drugs and fat-soluble vitamins—take separately from other medicines
  - May produce GI side effects
- Cholesterol absorption inhibitors
  - Site of action localized to cholesterol-absorbing sections of intestine
  - Used primarily to enhance the efficacy of HMG-CoA reductase inhibitors by approximately 15%
  - Minimal side effect profile

When to Consult, Refer, or Hospitalize

- Consult lipid specialist for patients not achieving goal on multiple medications.
- Consult appropriate specialist if underlying cause for hyperlipidemia is present (e.g., endocrinology for Cushing's syndrome).

Follow-up

- Adherence to low-fat, low-cholesterol diet
- Exercise regimen
- Tobacco cessation
- Side effects of medications as appropriate
- Routine screening of lipids, especially if on pharmacologic therapy

HYPERTENSION

Description

- Hypertension (HTN) is persistent elevation of either systolic or diastolic blood pressure measured at least three times on two separate occasions.

Table 4–1. Classification of Hypertension

BP Classification	Systolic BP (mmHg)	Diastolic BP (mmHg)
Normal	< 120	< 80
Pre-hypertension	120–139	80–89
Stage 1 hypertension	140–159	90–99
Stage 2 hypertension	≥ 160	≥ 100

*Based on the average of two or more readings taken at each of two or more visits after an initial screening. Adapted from National Heart, Lung, and Blood Institute, 2003, *Seventh report of the Joint National Committee on prevention, detection, evaluation, and treatment of high blood pressure (JNC-7) (NIH Publication no. 5233)*, Bethesda, MD: National Institutes of Health.

- Primary or essential hypertension: no identifiable cause (95% of cases)
- Secondary hypertension: identifiable etiology present (5% of cases)

Etiology, Incidence, and Demographics

- Affects 58 million Americans
- The most common primary diagnosis in the United States
- Prevalence increases with age
- Higher prevalence in men until the fifth to sixth decade; by age 65, women have a higher prevalence
- Higher incidence among Blacks
- Primary or essential hypertension—theories of causation include:
  - Impaired renin-angiotensin cascade
  - Sympathetic nervous system hyperactivity
  - Defect in natriuresis (sodium excretion)
  - Elevated intracellular calcium (excess arterial constriction)
- Secondary hypertension—potential identifiable causes include:
  - Renal disease
    · Medical renal disease (disease of the parenchyma resulting in excess renin release)
    · Renal vascular disease (renal vasculature perceives fall in pressure, responds with water-conserving compensatory mechanisms)
  - Vascular disease
    · Renal artery stenosis
    · Coarctation of the aorta
  - Sleep apnea
  - Endocrine disease
    · Cushing's syndrome
    · Hyperaldosteronism
    · Pheochromocytoma
    · Hyperthyroidism
  - Pregnancy
  - Drug effects
    · Oral contraceptives
    · Corticosteroids
    · Nonsteroidal antiinflammatory drugs (NSAIDs)
    · Sympathomimetics (decongestants, rescue asthma inhalers)

Risk Factors

- Obesity and sedentary lifestyle
- Increased sodium intake
- Diet high in fat
- Excessive alcohol intake
- Family history

Prevention and Screening

- Screening is recommended for all adults at each clinical visit.

Assessment

- Frequently referred to as the "silent killer"
  - Does not typically exhibit signs and symptoms until target organ damage has occurred
  - Headache may be present but is a nonspecific finding—if present, usually located in occipital region
- Manifestations of target organ damage
  - Cardiovascular: left ventricular hypertrophy, diastolic dysfunction, heart failure
  - Cerebrovascular: transient ischemic attack, cerebrovascular accident
  - Renal: decreased renal function, chronic kidney disease
  - Retinopathy: hemorrhages, exudates, papilledema
- Signs and symptoms of underlying etiology may be present in secondary HTN (see Table 4–2)

Table 4–2. Symptoms of Underlying Disease in Secondary Hypertension

Pheochromocytoma	Primary Aldosteronism	Hyperthyroidism	Renal Disease
Flushing	Cramps	Tremor	Oliguria
Palpitations	Parasthesias	Anxiety	Hematuria
Pallor	Muscle weakness	Palpitation	
Tremor		Hair loss	
Pounding headache		Heat intolerance	
Angina		Fine sweat	
Diaphoresis			

Differential Diagnosis

"White-coat" hypertension is said to occur when patients exhibit elevated blood pressure in a clinical setting but not in other settings. It is typically secondary to anxiety.

Diagnostic Studies

- As indicated to assess for causes of secondary hypertension, comorbid risk factors for cardiac disease, or target organ damage:
  - Chest x-ray
  - Lipid profile
  - Blood chemistries, including serum glucose
  - Renal function tests (BUN/Cr)
  - Screening panels for various endocrine disorders: TSH, urine catecholamines and VMA, serum cortisol, serum aldosterone
  - Evaluate for target organ damage: electrocardiogram, echocardiogram, urinalysis

Management

Nonpharmacologic Treatment

- Lifestyle modifications:
  - DASH (Dietary Approaches to Stop Hypertension): diet high in fruits, vegetables, nuts, whole grains; low in red meat, sodium, saturated fats
  - Weight reduction
  - Dietary sodium reduction
  - At least 30 minutes of physical aerobic activity daily
  - Moderate alcohol consumption—no more than two drinks per day for men and one drink per day for women and lightweight individuals

Note. The decision to implement lifestyle modifications alone or in combination with pharmacologic therapy depends upon the presence or absence of comorbidities such as chronic kidney disease, diabetes mellitus, or other compelling indications.

Compelling Indications

- Heart failure
- Post–myocardial infarction
- High coronary artery disease risk
- Recurrent CVA prevention

Treatment Algorithm (Pharmacologic Therapy)

- Institute lifestyle modifications for all patients with BP ≥ 140/90 mm Hg and persons with diabetes mellitus or chronic kidney disease with BP ≥ 130/80 mm Hg.
- Drug therapy is initiated in those with stage 1 or greater hypertension, on the basis of the presence or absence of compelling indications:
- Patients without compelling indications
  - Stage 1 hypertension: thiazide diuretics, may consider angiotensin-converting enzyme (ACE) inhibitor, angiotensin II receptor blocker (ARB), beta-adrenergic antagonist, calcium channel antagonist, or a combination of agents
  - Stage 2 hypertension: two-drug combination to include a thiazide diuretic and one of the other agents described above
- Patients with compelling indications:
  - Choice of agents dictated by the compelling indication; specific agents determined by provider

Special Considerations

- Thiazide diuretics are typically used as first-line treatment.
- Beta-blockers, ACE inhibitors, ARB, and CCB can be used as monotherapy or in combination with other antihypertensive classes.
- CCB and thiazide diuretics work well in the Black population.

When to Consult, Refer, or Hospitalize

- See Hypertensive Crisis below.

Follow-up

- Dietary restrictions (limiting Na and ETOH intake)
- Exercise regimen (30 to 45 minutes on most or all days of the week)
- Overall risk factor modification
- Medication side effects as appropriate
- BP self-monitoring (instruct patient to rest for 5 minutes before taking BP and no caffeine or nicotine 30 minutes before taking BP)
  - If monitoring BP at home, instruct on proper technique: arm supported at heart level (4th ICS), appropriate size cuff (bladder of cuff should encircle at least 80% of upper arm), place cuff 1 cm above the antecubital fossa

Hypertensive Crises

- The terms *hypertensive urgency* and *hypertensive emergency* are used to describe these crises.
- *Hypertensive urgencies* are situations where blood pressure must be lowered within a few hours.
  - Asymptomatic severe HTN (BP often > 220/125 mm Hg)
  - Rarely require emergency therapy
  - Typically treated with oral medications
  - Goal is to decrease to 20% to 25% below initial MAP or DBP ≤ 100–110 mm HG
  - Commonly used agents: alpha-adrenergic stimulant (e.g., clonidine), ACEI, CCB
    Note. The most important rule is to avoid overly rapid reduction in BP because this may lead to ischemia.
- *Hypertensive emergencies* are situations that require rapid reduction in blood pressure within 1 hour to avoid morbidity or mortality.
  - DBP often > 130 mm Hg
  - Evidence of acute target organ damage is present:
    - Hypertensive encephalopathy (AMS, headache, irritability, papilledema)
    - Hypertensive nephropathy (hematuria, proteinuria, progressive kidney dysfunction)
    - Intracranial hemorrhage
    - Acute coronary syndrome
    - Aortic dissection
    - Preeclampsia, eclampsia
- Goal is to reduce MAP by 10% to 15% in first 30 to 60 minutes (or to DBP of 110 mmHG), reduce MAP by 25% of initial MAP over first few hours
- Intensive care management and arterial line placement in most cases
- Parenteral medication required
  - Commonly used agents: nitoprusside, nitroglycerin, labetalol, hydralazine

HEART FAILURE (HF)

Description

- Heart failure (HF) is syndrome characterized by insufficient cardiac output to meet the metabolic demands of the body, because of either decreased contractility (systolic failure) or decreased ventricular filling (diastolic failure).

Etiology, Incidence, and Demographics

- Approximately 5 million cases in the United States
- 500,000 new cases diagnosed each year
- 990,000 hospitalizations each year secondary to HF
- Equal gender distribution
- Twice as common in patients who are hypertensive patients than in patients who are normotensive; 25% more common in the Black population
- Age—occurs in 10% of persons over 70 years of age
- Medication noncompliance often a contributing factor

Classifications

- Systolic heart failure: occurs secondary to poor left ventricular function
  - Causes
- Ischemic heart disease
- Valvular heart disease
- Dilated cardiomyopathy
- Alcohol abuse
- Diabetes mellitus
- Diastolic heat failure: occurs secondary to diastolic dysfunction (poor relaxation and ventricular filling)
- Causes
  - Hypertension
  - Hypertrophic cardiomyopathy

Risk Factors

- Presence of any of above conditions can lead to development of acute or chronic heart failure

Prevention and Screening

- Assessment for and prevention of ischemic heart disease
- Control of comorbid conditions, including hypertension, hyperlipidemia, diabetes mellitus
- Healthy lifestyle habits, including normalization of weight (maintenance of BMI of 18 to 25), exercise, healthy diet
- Tobacco and alcohol cessation

Assessment

- Dyspnea
- Anxiety
- Chest discomfort or heaviness
- Pallor
- S3/S4 gallop
- Frothy sputum
- Typically no symptoms of systemic fluid overload
- Easily fatigued
- Paroxysmal nocturnal dyspnea
- Orthopnea
- Anorexia
- Bibasilar rales
- Abdominal fullness
- Jugular venous distention
- Lower extremity edema
- Hepatosplenomegaly
- Displaced point of maximal impulse

Differential Diagnosis

- Acute coronary syndrome
- Pulmonary embolus
- Cirrhosis
- Chronic obstructive pulmonary disease (COPD)
- Nephrotic syndrome
- Myxedema

Diagnostic Studies

- Chest x-ray demonstrates fluid in all fields (Kerley's lines)
- ECG may demonstrate underlying cardiac event, ischemia, or arrhythmias; left ventricular hypertrophy; atrial enlargement
- Pulse oximetry or arterial blood gas demonstrates hypoxemia
- Echocardiogram determines systolic vs. diastolic dysfunction; also identifies if valvular abnormality is present

- Liver function tests may indicate chronic elevated liver pressure—increased GGT, alkaline phosphatase
- Serum electrolytes in any variety of abnormal patterns—BUN/Cr typically demonstrates pre-renal insufficiency
- Complete blood count may demonstrate anemia of chronic disease

Management

Treat underlying cause as appropriate
- Myocardial ischemia
- Valvular disease
- Uncontrolled hypertension
- Drug-induced myocardial depression

Nonpharmacologic Treatment
- 2 to 2.5 g sodium restriction—greater restrictions are difficult to attain and have no appreciable benefit
- Gradual, tailored exercise program for stable patients

Pharmacologic Treatment
- Diuretic therapy required for symptom control in moderate and severe heart failure
  - Loop diuretics generally required because of comorbid renal insufficiency
  - May add metolazone to refractory patients because of its activity at lower glomerular filtration rates
  - May produce hypokalemia, hyponatremia, and metabolic alkalosis
- ACE inhibitors
  - Renin-angiotensin-aldosterone system activated early in failure and contributes to progression of disease
- First-line treatment
  - Indicated for all patients with ejection fraction < 40% to reduce progression to symptomatic failure and can improve left ventricular function over time
  - Use cautiously in patients with serum creatinine > 3 mg/dL
  - Most common side effect is cough
- Angiotensin II receptor antagonist
  - Also inhibits renin-angiotensin-aldosterone cascade
  - Does not provide other ACE inhibitor effects such as increase in bradykinin, prostaglandins, and nitric oxide
  - May be used in ACE inhibitor–intolerant patients
- Beta-adrenergic antagonists
  - Block progressive, chronic, epinephrine, and sympathetic nervous system stimulation to the myocardium
  - Have been shown to produce 10% increase in cardiac output in 3 to 6 months of treatment
  - First-line therapy in compensated heart failure
- Aldosterone antagonists
  - Used as a neurohormonal antagonist; mediates major effects of the renin-angiotensin-aldosterone system as well as sodium retention
  - Consider for patients with symptoms and exacerbation despite maintenance therapy with drug classes described previously

- Cardiac glycosides (digoxin)
  - Role limited to those with systolic dysfunction unresponsive to other treatments
  - No mortality benefit
- Vasodilators
  - Third-line pharmacologic agent
  - Decreases preload via venodilation while increasing myocardial oxygenation
- Biventricular pacing
  - Used for patients with systolic heart failure
  - Enhances degree of contraction and reduces mitral regurgitation in those patients with chronic and severe symptoms
  - Typically includes implantable defibrillator component
  - Variety of criteria must be met for this intervention

When to Consult, Refer, or Hospitalize

- Admit
  - Decompensated patients
  - Acutely symptomatic
  - Severe volume overload
  - Heart failure refractory to maximum outpatient treatment
- Consult
  - Consult cardiology for newly diagnosed patients to determine underlying etiology and outline treatment course

Follow-up

- Educate patient and family on disease process and motivate them to take active role in management
- Stress compliance with medication
- Track daily weights and report weight gain of more than 2 lbs in 2 days
- Low sodium diet
- Exercise training program
- Report new or recurrent symptoms promptly to avoid hospitalization if possible

VALVULAR DISEASE

Description

- Valvular disease involves abnormality of one or more of the cardiac valves.

Note. All valvular abnormalities are typically asymptomatic until they become severe.

MITRAL REGURGITATION

Description

Mitral regurgitation (MR) is the failure of the mitral valve to close completely, thereby allowing blood to flow into the left atrium during systole.

Etiology, Incidence, and Demographics

- Rheumatic heart disease
- Ischemic heart disease
- MVP
- Congenital abnormalities
- Ruptured chordae tendineae
- Papillary muscle dysfunction
- Infective endocarditis
- Blunt chest trauma

Risk Factors

- Any of the conditions listed above place a patient at risk for the development of MR.

Prevention and Screening

- Prevention of rheumatic fever
- Prevention of ischemic heart disease with risk factor modification
- Echocardiogram for screening if suspected

Assessment

- Acute MR
  - Dyspnea on exertion (DOE)
  - Fatigue
  - Peripheral edema
  - Cough with clear sputum production
  - Pansystolic murmur
- Chronic MR
  - Symptoms develop with severe disease
  - Exertional dyspnea
  - Fatigue
  - Pansystolic murmur
  - Hyperdynamic left ventricle (LV) impulse
  - Brisk carotid upstroke

Differential Diagnosis

- Aortic stenosis
- Tricuspid regurgitation
- Hypertrophic obstructive cardiomyopathy
- Atrial septal defect
- Ventricular septal defect

Diagnostic Studies

- ECG: Left atrial enlargement is common in chronic MR; LVH may also be present.
- Chest x-ray: increased left ventricular and left atrial size
- Echocardiogram is diagnostic and can quantify the degree of MR and detect any other structural abnormalities.

Management

- Consider anticoagulation to prevent systemic emboli (depends on degree of severity and presence of comorbidities)
- Low-sodium diet and diuretics for symptom control
- Afterload reduction with ACE-I
- Surgery for acute MR or severe chronic MR
- Surgery also indicated in asymptomatic patients with declining LV function or marked LV dilation

When to Consult, Refer, or Hospitalize

- Hospitalization required for management of complications such as heart failure or pulmonary edema
- Refer to cardiology or cardiothoracic surgery for patients with severe symptoms despite medical management, severe or worsening valvular disease, or decreased left ventricular function to determine need for surgical intervention

Follow-up

- Educate patient and family on disease process
- Educate on the importance of reporting symptoms—may indicate worsening of the disease and need for surgical intervention
- Low-sodium diet
- Hypertensive control

MITRAL STENOSIS (MS)

Description

- Mitral stenosis (MS) is the narrowing of the mitral valve, resulting in obstructed flow from the left atrium to the left ventricle.

Etiology, Incidence, and Demographics

- Typically occurs secondary to rheumatic heart disease
- Atrial myxoma
- Vegetation or thromboembolus
- Severe calcification of the mitral annulus
- Usually asymptomatic for 10 to 20 years

Risk Factors

- Any of the above conditions place people at risk for the development of MS.

Prevention and Screening

- Prevention of rheumatic fever
- Echocardiogram for screening if suspected

Assessment

- Symptoms of severe MS:
  - Dyspnea, orthopnea, PND
  - Fatigue
  - Palpitations
  - Hemoptysis
  - Angina
- PE findings:
  - Loud S1
  - Opening snap
  - Diastolic rumble
  - Palpable thrill

Differential Diagnosis

- Austin-Flint murmur
- Triscuspid stenosis

Diagnostic Studies

- ECG: left atrial enlargement, right axis deviation, right ventricular hypertrophy
- Chest x-ray: prominent pulmonary vasculature with chronic pulmonary hypertension
- Echocardiogram: diagnostic; determines extent of valvular disease and LV size and function
- TEE: assesses for vegetation, congenital disease, or aortic root abscesses

Management

- Anticoagulation for patients who have experienced previous thromboemboli
- Medical therapy directed at slowing progression of pulmonary HTN, reducing HF symptoms, and slowing the development of endocarditis
- Severe MS requires surgery.

When to Consult, Refer, or Hospitalize

- Required for management of complications such as heart failure or pulmonary edema
- Refer to cardiology or cardiothoracic surgery: patients with severe symptoms despite medical management, severe or worsening valvular disease, or decreased left ventricular function, to determine need for surgical intervention

Patient Education

- Educate patient and family on disease process
- Educate on importance of reporting symptoms—may indicate worsening of the disease and need for surgical intervention

MITRAL VALVE PROLAPSE

Description

- Mitral valve prolapse (MVP) is the prolapse of the valve leaflets during systole.

Etiology, Incidence, and Demographics

- Connective tissue disorders (e.g., Marfan syndrome)
- Rheumatic endocarditis
- Rupture of the chordae tendineae
- More common in females age 20 to 40
- More common in thin patients

Risk Factors

- Connective tissue disease
- Family history
- Female gender

Prevention and Screening

- Prevention of rheumatic fever
- Echocardiogram for screening if suspected

Assessment

- Frequently asymptomatic
- Nonspecific chest pain
- Anxiety
- Palpitations
- Fatigue
- Dyspnea
- Dysrhythmia

- Characteristic mid-systolic clicks—only typically have benign disease
- Late systolic murmur—typically more significant disease with associated MR
- In advanced states, finding consistent with decompensated HF

Differential Diagnosis

- Mitral regurgitation
- Aortic stenosis
- Infective endocarditis
- Tricuspid regurgitation

Diagnostic Studies

- Diagnosis often clinical
- Echocardiogram for confirmation
- ECG may show changes consistent with left atrial enlargement or ventricular hypertrophy in advanced states

Management

- Majority of patients require no treatment
- Beta-adrenergic blockade when supraventricular dysrhythmia present

When to Consult, Refer, or Hospitalize

- Rarely required
- May be required for management of complications such as heart failure or pulmonary edema
- Refer to cardiology or cardiothoracic surgery: patients with severe symptoms despite medical management, severe or worsening valvular disease, or decreased left ventricular function, to determine need for surgical intervention.

Patient Education

- Educate patient and family on disease process
- Educate on the importance of reporting symptoms—may indicate worsening of the disease and need for surgical intervention

AORTIC STENOSIS

- Aortic stenosis (AS) is a condition characterized by stiffening of the aortic valve, offering increased resistance to left ventricular outflow. Aortic stenosis is the most common surgical valve lesion in developed countries.

Etiology, Incidence, and Demographics

- Progressive calcification of the aortic valve
- Less commonly follows rheumatic heart disease
- Occurs in 25% of patients > 65 years of age
- Occurs in 35% of patients > 70 years of age
- 10% to 20% of patients affected will develop hemodynamically significant stenosis
- Three to four times more common in males

Risk Factors

- Tobacco use
- Male gender
- Hypertension

Prevention and Screening

- Control hypertension
- Tobacco cessation
- Echocardiogram for screening if suspected

Assessment

- Frequently asymptomatic
- Harsh systolic murmur at second intercostal space, right sternal border
- Palpable thrill at the right sternal border
- Auscultation of murmur precedes clinical symptoms
- Murmur transmits to carotid artery
- Diminished or absent A2
- Delayed carotid upstroke
- Symptoms of left ventricular failure with progressive disease
- Angina pectoris common as disease progresses
- Exertional syncope if severe
- Associated coronary artery disease in 50% of patients

Differential Diagnosis

- Mitral regurgitation
- Supravalvular obstruction
- Outflow obstruction

Diagnostic Studies

- ECG may suggest left ventricular hypertrophy
- Chest x-ray (later diseases)
- Enlarged cardiac shadow
- Calcification of aortic valve
- Dilation and calcification of ascending aorta
- Echocardiogram to assess valve thickness, function, and gradient
- Cardiac catheterization for definitive diagnosis; valve area < 0.8 cm^2 suggests severe stenosis

Management

- Surgery indicated for all symptomatic patients
- Surgical mortality 10% in the > 75-year-old population
- Ross procedure
- Patient's pulmonary valve transplanted to aortic position
- Bioprosthesis valve placed in pulmonary position
- Bioprostheses do not deteriorate as quickly on pulmonary side
- Excellent long-term outcomes without anticoagulation
- Balloon valvuloplasty provides only very short-term results—greatest utility to stabilize high-risk patients before surgery

When to Consult, Refer, or Hospitalize

- May be required for management of complications such as heart failure, pulmonary edema, angina, or syncope
- Refer to cardiology or cardiothoracic surgery patients with severe symptoms despite medical management, severe or worsening valvular disease, or decreased left ventricular function to determine need for surgical intervention

Follow-up

- Educate patient and family on disease process
- Educate on importance of reporting symptoms because this may indicate worsening of disease and need for surgical intervention

AORTIC REGURGITATION

Description

- Aortic regurgitation (AR) is incomplete closure of the aortic valve, allowing blood to flow into the left ventricle during ventricular systole.

Etiology, Incidence, and Demographics

- Structural disease (unicuspid, bicuspid valves)
- Inflammatory (rheumatic fever, syphilis, rheumatoid arthritis)
- Disruptive (trauma, dissection)
- Hypertension

Risk Factors

- Any of the conditions listed above place patients at risk for the development of AR.

Prevention and Screening

- Control hypertension
- Prevention of rheumatic fever and syphilis
- Echocardiogram to screen if suspected

Assessment

- Symptoms of severe, chronic AR
  - Dyspnea
  - Fatigue
  - Paroxysmal nocturnal dyspnea
  - Angina pectoris or atypical chest pain
- Symptoms of acute AR
  - Dyspnea
  - Pulmonary edema
  - Orthopnea
  - PND
- Physical exam findings with chronic AR
  - Widened pulse pressure
  - Low diastolic pressure
  - Water-hammer pulse
  - Hyperdynamic, prominent, laterally displaced point of maximum impulse (PMI)
  - Soft, high-pitched, decrescendo diastolic murmur

- PE findings with acute AR
  - Pulmonary edema
  - Crackles
  - Increased tactile fremitus
  - Pulse pressure usually normal
  - Diastolic murmur soft with minimal intensity

Differential Diagnosis

- Pulmonic regurgitation
- Ventricular septal defect

Diagnostic Studies

- ECG: LVH with chronic AR, sinus tachycardia with acute AR
- Chest x-ray: "boot-shaped" cardiac silhouette, prominent aortic knob
- Echocardiogram as diagnostic to determine severity and left ventricular function

Management

- Surgery is indicated for acute AR.
- For chronic AR
  - Vasodilators
    - Nifedipine
      - For patients with severe AR and LV dilation who are asymptomatic, can decrease disease progression and time to surgery by 1 to 2 years
    - ACE-I may be used.
    - Advise against strenuous activity.

When to Consult, Refer, or Hospitalize

- May be required for management of complications such as heart failure, pulmonary edema, angina, or syncope
- Refer to cardiology or cardiothoracic surgery patients with severe symptoms despite medical management, severe or worsening valvular disease, or decreased left ventricular function to determine need for surgical intervention

Follow-up

- Educate patient and family on disease process
- Educate on importance of reporting symptoms because this may indicate worsening of disease and need for surgical intervention

PERIPHERAL VASCULAR DISEASE

Description

- Peripheral vascular disease (PVD) involves disorders of the peripheral arteries and vein, including:
  - Peripheral arterial disease (PAD): insufficient blood flow to the lower extremities, most often secondary to atherosclerotic process
  - Chronic venous insufficiency (CVI): occurs secondary to high venous pressures in the lower extremities

Etiology, Incidence, and Demographics

- Approximately one in five adults is affected by PVD.
- PAD occurs secondary to an atherosclerotic process.
- CVI is often a result of previous DVT, obesity, prolonged standing, or pregnancy.

Risk Factors

- PAD
  - Hypertension
  - Hyperlipidemia
  - Diabetes mellitus
  - Tobacco abuse
  - Other atherosclerotic disease processes (e.g., CAD, carotid stenosis, cerebral vascular disease)
- CVI
  - History of deep vein thrombosis
  - History of lower extremity trauma
  - Obesity

Prevention and Screening

- PAD
  - Modify risk factors, including smoking cessation, achievement of excellent hypertension, hyperlipidemia, and diabetes mellitus control.
  - Screening includes Ankle Brachial Index (ABI) testing. This test compares systolic pressures in the brachial artery with systolic pressures in the dorsalis pedis and posterior tibial arteries. The results are expressed in a ratio. An ABI of 0.9 or greater is normal. An ABI of 0.75 to 0.5 is consistent with claudication. An ABI below 0.5 is consistent with rest pain or gangrene.
  - USPST does not recommend screening for PAD.
  - According to the PAD Coalition and screening, we should follow the ACC/AHA Guidelines for Management of Patients with PAD, according to which the following patients should be screened:
    - Age < 50 with diabetes and one other atherosclerotic risk factor (hypertension, dyslipidemia, tobacco abuse)

- Age 50 to 69 and history of diabetes or tobacco abuse
- Age 70 years and older
- Leg symptoms with exertion (claudication) or ischemic rest pain
- Abnormal lower extremity pulse examination
- CVI
  - Early, aggressive management of DVT to minimize valvular damage
  - Thrombolysis or thrombectomy of acute DVT may also prevent CVI.

Assessment

- PAD
  - Intermittent claudication
  - Diminished hair growth on lower extremities
  - Diminished pulses and cool extremities
  - Erectile dysfunction in men with iliac disease
  - 5 Ps
    - Pain
    - Pallor
    - Pulse (diminished or absent)
    - Paresthesias
    - Poikilothermia
- CVI
  - Dependent edema
  - Shiny taut skin
  - Hyperpigmented (brownish) skin
  - Venous varicosities and ulcerations
  - Thick and fibrous subcutaneous tissue

Differential Diagnosis

- PAD
  - Sciatica
  - Acute peripheral arterial occlusion
  - Peripheral neuropathy
  - Buerger's disease
- CVI
  - Lower extremity edema secondary to cardiac, renal, or hepatic etiology
  - Lymphedema
  - Medication induced

Diagnostic Studies

- PAD
  - ABI
  - Arterial Doppler
  - CT angiography (CTA) and magnetic resonance angiography (MRA)
  - Peripheral angiography
- CVI
  - Venous Doppler
  - Venography

Management

- PAD
  - Risk factor modification
  - Walking regimen
  - Oral phosphodiesterase inhibitors (e.g., cilostazol 100 mg twice daily)
  - Antiplatelets (e.g., aspirin daily)
  - Endovascular techniques, such as angioplasty with or without stent placement
  - Surgical intervention, such as bypass
  - Fibrinolytic therapy for acute arterial thrombus
  - Embolectomy
- CVI
  - Assess for other causes of edema (e.g., cardiac, renal, hepatic, medication-induced)
  - Decrease sodium intake
  - Elevate extremities
  - Graduated compression stockings
  - Weight reduction
  - Meticulous skin care
  - Pneumonic compression devices

When to Consult, Refer, or Hospitalize

- Admit
  - Acute arterial thrombus
  - CVI with development of nonhealing ulceration or infected ulceration
- Refer to vascular specialist for severe PAD requiring possible intervention.
- Refer to wound care specialist for nonhealing ulcerations.

Follow-up

- Educate regarding risk factor modification for both PAD and CVI.
- Follow routinely on an outpatient basis.

DEEP VEIN THROMBOSIS

Description
- Deep vein thrombosis is acute thrombus formation in a deep leg or pelvic vein. The thrombus may detach and travel to the pulmonary vasculature, causing a pulmonary embolus.

Etiology, Incidence, and Demographics

- Stasis secondary to immobilization—bed rest, para- or quadriplegia
- Venous wall injury
- Hypercoagulable states
- Polycythemia vera
- Essential thrombocytosis
- Blood malignancies
- Estrogen usage
- More common in women than men
- 800,000 new cases annually
- Occurs in 3% of patients following major surgical procedures
- Incidence of venous thromboembolism (VTE), which includes DVT and PE, among hospitalized patients is 20% of low-risk patients and 80% of critical care and high-risk patients

Risk Factors

- Immobility
- Estrogen use, particularly in smokers and women over 30 years of age
- Underlying malignancies that predispose a person to clot formation
- Surgical procedures without thrombus prophylaxis

Prevention and Screening

- Early ambulation postoperatively and after major medical illnesses
- Awareness of high-risk patients and screen as appropriate

Assessment

- May be asymptomatic
- Dull, generalized ache in the affected leg
- Discomfort exacerbated by walking
- Slight, generalized edema of affected calf or leg
- Distention of superficial collaterals
- Palpable cords

Differential Diagnosis

- Fluid retention
- Trauma
- Lymphedema
- Cellulitis
- Musculoskeletal strain

Diagnostic Studies

- Venous duplex Doppler ultrasonography is diagnostic study of choice
- Ascending venography when diagnosis is uncertain

Management

- Prophylaxis and management in high-risk situation
- Postoperative subcutaneous heparin, unfractionated or low molecular weight
- Thromboembolic stockings or pneumatic compression devices
- Encourage ambulation
- Elevate legs with knees slightly flexed
- Adjusted-dose heparin to PTT 1.5 to 2.0 times normal for prophylaxis of hip and pelvic procedures
- Heparinization for first 7 to 10 days (unfractionated or low molecular weight)
- Oral anticoagulation with warfarin for a minimum of 3 months

When to Consult, Refer, or Hospitalize

- May require hospitalization for initiation of anticoagulation if patient is clinically unstable or has multiple comorbidities

Follow-up

- If patient on oral contraceptives, discuss alternative contraceptive methods, especially if patient uses tobacco
- Discuss need for anticoagulation with warfarin to achieve goal INR of 2.0–3.0
- Discuss frequent monitoring of INR needed with warfarin, reporting signs of bleeding, and dietary modifications
- Educate on use of graduated compression stockings

PULMONARY HYPERTENSION

Description

- Pulmonary hypertension involves elevated pressures in the pulmonary vasculature.

Etiology, Incidence, and Demographics

- Increased pulmonary vascular resistance
  - Occlusion of the pulmonary vasculature (pulmonary emboli)
  - Vasoconstriction (hypoxemia)
  - Decreased vasculature (chronic obstructive pulmonary disease)
- Increased pulmonary pressures
  - Left ventricular hypertrophy
  - Valvular heart disease (mitral stenosis, aortic stenosis)
- Increased pulmonary blood flow (left-to-right intracardiac shunt)
- Increased blood viscosity (polycythemia)
- Primary pulmonary hypertension; most common in young females
  - Often has a genetic link (autosomal dominant pattern)
- Incidence related to incidence of the underlying cause
- Primary pulmonary hypertension (PPH) is uncommon; affects 1 to 2 persons per 1 million people worldwide

Risk Factors

- Valvular heart disease
- Left ventricular hypertrophy
- Pulmonary embolism
- Polycythemia

Prevention and Screening

- Control hypertension to avoid development of LVH
- No routine screening
- Avoid tobacco

Assessment

- Subjective
  - Dyspnea
  - Chest pain—dull, substernal
  - Fatigue
  - Syncope
- Objective
  - Split S2
  - Peripheral edema if right ventricular failure is present
  - Signs/symptoms of right ventricular failure

Diagnostic Studies

- ECG: right axis deviation
- Chest x-ray: increased pulmonary artery size, changes associated with COPD if present
- Echocardiogram: shows elevated pulmonary artery pressures and valvular heart disease or left ventricular hypertrophy if present
- Cardiac catheterization (right) confirms diagnosis
- CT angiogram may show evidence of pulmonary emboli if present
- CBC: increased hemoglobin and hematocrit (polycythemia) if hypoxemia present and chronic

Differential Diagnosis

- Cor pulmonale
- Heart failure
- Restrictive lung disease
- Obstructive lung disease
- Obstructive sleep apnea

Management

- Treatment of the underlying disorder/cause
- Supplemental oxygen
- Anticoagulation in patients with pulmonary emboli
- For severe polycythemia, consider phlebotomy
- Vasodilator therapy

When to Consult, Refer, or Hospitalize

- Admit
  - To initiate vasodilator therapy
  - For diuresis with close monitoring
- Consult
  - Pulmonology to determine treatment course

Follow-up

- Educate patient and family on disease process
- Moderate activity (avoid strenuous activity)
- Medication side effects as appropriate
- Low-sodium diet

CARDIAC RHYTHM DISTURBANCES

Description

- All cardiac rhythms other than normal sinus rhythm are disturbances.

Atrial Fibrillation

- ECG characteristics: Disorganized atrial activity characterized by atrial rate in excess of 300 beats per minute with variable ventricular conduction; no discernible P waves, narrow QRS complex

Etiology, Incidence, and Demographics

- Wide variety of cardiac and extracardiac conditions can precipitate transient or permanent atrial fibrillation
  - Rheumatic heart disease
  - Cardiomyopathy
  - Atrial septal defect
  - Hypertension
  - Mitral valve prolapse
  - Trauma
  - Heart failure
  - Hyperthyroidism
  - Sick sinus syndrome
  - Alcohol withdrawal or intoxication
  - Drug toxicity (beta-adrenergic antagonists)
- May be idiopathic
  - Most common dysrhythmia
  - More common in males
  - Affects 2% to 4% of the population

Risk Factors

- Preexisting disease processes identified in Etiology and Demographics
- History of paroxysmal atrial fibrillation

Assessment

- May be asymptomatic
- Palpitations
- Angina
- Fatigue
- Dyspnea
- Syncope
- Tachycardia
- Irregular pulse
- Other findings consistent with causative disease

Differential Diagnosis

- Atrial flutter
- Atrial tachycardia
- Supraventricular tachycardia (SVT)

Management

- Treat underlying disorders as appropriate.
- Ultimate goal is conversion to normal sinus rhythm
- If onset of dysrhythmia is unknown, anticoagulate with warfarin for 3 to 4 weeks before conversion attempted
- Conversion may be electrical with synchronous cardioversion of 100 to 200 joules.
- Chemical cardioversion with a class IC antidysrhythmics
- Propafenone
- Flecainide
- Other antidysrhythmic options
- Sotalol
- Ibutilide
- Amiodarone
- Dronederone
- In patients who fail to convert, rate control is treatment goal
- Beta-adrenergic antagonists
- Calcium channel blockers (non-dihydroperidines)
- Digoxin
    - In chronic patients
    - Those with no comorbid disease, including structural heart disease, under age 60 may be anticoagulated with ASA 325 mg daily.
    - All other patients should be anticoagulated with warfarin with a goal INR of 2.0 to 3.0.

When to Consult, Refer, or Hospitalize

- Admit patients with atrial fibrillation with RVR who are symptomatic, hemodynamically unstable, or both.
- Consult cardiology and electrophysiology to determine treatment course.

NARROW COMPLEX SUPRAVENTRICULAR TACHYCARDIA

Description

- Narrow complex supraventricular tachycardia presents with ECG characteristics: regular rhythm, P wave difficult to distinguish, QRS complex narrow, and rate of 160 to 250 bpm.

Etiology

- Anxiety
- Stimulants
- Digitalis toxicity

Risk Factors

- See above

Assessment

- Palpitations
- Dizziness, syncope
- Hypotension

Differential Diagnosis

- AV node reentry tachycardia

Management

- Vagal maneuvers
  - Carotid massage
  - Valsalva maneuver
- Adenosine
- Beta-blockers (e.g., metoprolol)
- Non-dihydroperidine calcium channel blockers (e.g., diltiazem, verapamil)

When to Consult, Refer, or Hospitalize

- Admit patients who are symptomatic, hemodynamically unstable, or both.
- Consult cardiology and electrophysiology to determine treatment course if recurrent event.

VENTRICULAR TACHYCARDIA

Description

- Ventricular tachycardia presents with ECG characteristics: P waves not discernable, QRS complex wide and regular, rate of 100 to 250 bpm.

Etiology

- Irritability of myocardium with ventricles assuming control of cardiac rhythm

Risk Factors

- Myocardial ischemia
- Electrolyte imbalance
- Cardiomyopathy
- Myocarditis

Assessment

- Palpitations
- Dizziness or syncope
- Chest pain
- Hypotension, hemodynamic instability
- Weak or absent pulse

Differential Diagnosis

- Supraventricular tachycardia with aberrancy
- Severe hyperkalemia (sine wave)
- Torsades de pointes

Management

- Initiate ACLS protocol
- Unstable VT or pulseless VT
  - Direct current cardioversion (100, 200, or 360 joules with biphasic defibrillator; monophasic defibrillators begin with 100 joules)
- Follow ACLS guidelines.

When to Consult, Refer, or Hospitalize

- All patients require hospitalization.
- Consult cardiology and electrophysiology to determine the need for additional testing and possible ICD implantation.

VENTRICULAR FIBRILLATION

Description

- Indications of ventricular fibrillation are ECG characteristics: no P waves, no QRS complex, and chaotic rhythm produced by fibrillation of the ventricles.

Etiology

- Irritability of myocardium with ventricles assuming control of the cardiac rhythm

Risk Factors

- Ischemia
- Electrolyte imbalance
- Acidosis

Assessment

- Syncope
- Pulselessness
- Apnea
- Cyanosis

Differential Diagnosis

- Ventricular tachycardia
- *Torsades de pointes*

Management

- ACLS protocol
- Same as for pulseless VT

When to Consult, Refer, or Hospitalize

- All patients require hospitalization.
- Consult cardiology and electrophysiology to determine the need for additional testing and possible ICD implantation

ASYSTOLE

Description

- A patient with asystole has these ECG characteristics: no P waves, No QRS complexes, and "flat line" on telemetry.

Etiology

- There is no ventricular contraction and, therefore, no cardiac output.

Risk Factors

- Ischemia
- Drug overdose
- Electrolyte imbalance

Assessment (cardiopulmonary arrest)

- Syncope
- Pulselessness
- Apnea

Differential Diagnosis

- None

Management

- ACLS protocol
- Medications
- Epinephrine
- Atropine

When to Consult, Refer, or Hospitalize

- All patients with asystole require hospital admission.
- Consult cardiology and electrophysiology to determine the need for additional testing.

COMPLETE HEART BLOCK (THIRD-DEGREE ATRIOVENTRICULAR BLOCK)

Description

- ECG characteristics of a patient with complete heart block (third-degree atrioventricular block) are: complete disassociation between the atria and ventricles. Atrial rate is typically normal (60 to 100 bpm); ventricular rate is slow (40 to 60 bpm).

Etiology

- Acute myocardial infarction is the most common cause.
- Digoxin toxicity
- Degeneration of the conduction system

Risk Factors

- Myocardial ischemia
- Digoxin use

Assessment

- Dizziness
- Syncope
- If ventricular rate is adequate, may be asymptomatic

Differential Diagnosis

- Second-degree AVB (Mobitz I)
- Second-degree AVB (Mobitz II)

Management

- Atropine
- Consider epinephrine
- Transcutaneous or transvenous pacing
- Treatment of underlying cause
- May require permanent pacemaker implantation

When to Consult, Refer, or Hospitalize

- All patients require hospitalization.
- Consult cardiology and electrophysiology to determine need for additional testing and possible permanent pacemaker implantation.

Patient Education

- Patient education for all arrhythmias is based on the specific arrhythmia, underlying cause, and procedures required.

PERICARDITIS

Description

- Pericarditis is acute, painful inflammation of the pericardium. Pericarditis can be mild, self-limiting, and treatable on an outpatient basis, or a life-threatening condition requiring hospitalization. An accurate history is essential to making a diagnosis of pericarditis.

Etiology, Incidence, and Demographics

- Virus (most common)
- Bacteria
- Postmyocardial infarction
- Renal failure
- Tuberculosis
- Neoplastic
- Collagen disease
- Drug-induced
- Trauma

Risk Factors

- Recent upper respiratory virus
- Bacterial infection
- Recent myocardial infarction
- Renal failure
- Trauma
- Malignancy
- Connective tissue disease

Prevention and Screening

- None

Assessment

- Localized retrosternal or precordial chest pain (rarely may radiate)
- Pain increased by deep inspiration, coughing, swallowing, or recumbency
- Pain relieved by sitting forward
- Shortness of breath secondary to pain with inspiration
- Pericardial friction rub characteristically present (absence does not preclude diagnosis)
- Pleural friction rub may also be present
- Fever may be present, depending on underlying cause
- Various physical findings consistent with underlying cause

Differential Diagnosis

- Acute coronary syndrome
- Costochondral pain
- Dyspepsia
- Pleuritis
- Pneumothorax

Diagnostic Studies

- CBC: leukocytosis
- ECG: ST segment elevation in all leads
- Depression of PR segment highly indicative
- ESR elevation
- Blood culture if bacterial cause suspected
- Echocardiogram to assess for presence of pericardial fluid; may be normal

Management

- NSAIDs are mainstay of treatment.
  - ASA
  - Indomethacin
  - Corticosteroids are indicated only when there is total failure of high-dose NSAIDs over several weeks and with relapsing pericarditis; these agents can increase viral replication.
  - When indicated, dexamethasone 4 mg IV may relieve pain in a few hours.
  - Prednisone 60 mg daily decreased by 10 mg q3 to 5d until a dose of 15 mg is reached, then 15 mg for 5 days; alternate with 10 mg for 5 days, then alternate with 5 mg for 5 days, then d/c.
  - Antibiotics in cases of bacterial infection
  - Other treatments as indicated by underlying cause (e.g., dialysis)

When to Consult, Refer, or Hospitalize

- Admit
  - If bacterial infection involved, may require IV antibiotics
  - For acute kidney injury with need for hemodialysis
- Consult
  - Nephrology consultation for patients requiring hemodialysis

Patient Education

- Educate patient and family on the underlying disease process.
- Discuss treatment regimen and need to report persistent symptoms that do not resolve.

CARDIAC TAMPONADE

Description

- Cardiac tamponade is the accumulation of fluid or blood in the pericardial space, resulting in a life-threatening decrease in cardiac output.

Etiology, Incidence, and Demographics

- Blunt or penetrating trauma to the chest
- Postoperative cardiac catheterization or cardiac surgery
- Pericarditis
- Acute coronary syndrome
- Neoplasms resulting in pericardial effusion
- Infections (viral, bacterial, fungal)
- Ruptured aortic aneurysm with bleeding into pericardial space
- Chronic kidney disease

Risk Factors

- Presence of conditions listed above

Prevention and Screening

- Close monitoring of patients with above conditions to detect pericardial effusions early before the problem becomes severe enough to result in tamponade

Assessment

- Subjective
  - Dyspnea
  - Chest pain
- Objective
  - Beck's Triad
    - Jugular venous distension
    - Narrowing pulse pressure
    - Distant heart sounds
  - Pulsus paradoxus—greater than 10 mm Hg decrease in SBP during inspiration
  - Oliguria
  - Cool, pale, diaphoretic skin
  - Altered mental status (confusion, anxiety)
  - Hypotension
  - Tachycardia

Differential Diagnosis

- Cardiogenic shock
- Tension pneumothorax
- Right ventricular failure

Diagnostic Studies

- Echocardiogram: confirms diagnosis (presence of pericardial effusion large enough to impede normal ventricular filling and contraction)
- Chest x-ray: may demonstrate widened mediastinum
- ECG: may show electrical alterans (alternating large and small QRS complexes)
- Hemodynamic monitoring: equalization of pressures: mean RA, RV diastolic, pulmonary artery occusion pressure (PAOP), and LV diastolic

Management

- Temporary support of hemodynamics with intravascular volume expansion (250–500 cc NS) and ionotropic agents (dobutamine, dopamine)
- Oxygen
- Pericardiocentesis
- Possible pericardial window (an opening in the pericardium that allows fluid to drain into the pleural space)

When to Consult, Refer, or Hospitalize

- All patients with cardiac tamponade require hospitalization.
- Consult cardiothoracic surgery for possible pericardiocentesis or pericardial window.

Patient Education and Follow-up

- Provide education on the diagnosis and underlying cause once identified.
- Prepare patient and family for emergent procedures.
- Discuss the underlying etiology and need for additional treatment accordingly.

CARDIOMYOPATHY

Description

- Cardiomyopathy is a group of entities primarily affecting the myocardium and classified by their anatomic appearance and pathophysiology.

Etiology, Incidence, and Demographics

- Approximately 1 in 5,439
  - 0.02% of the U.S. population
  - Deaths from cardiomyopathy: 27,260 deaths per year; 35,000 hospitalizations for cardiomyopathy per year

DILATED CARDIOMYOPATHY

Description

- In dilated cardiomyopathy, the hallmark is cardiac enlargement.
- All four chambers are usually dilated.
- Myocyte degeneration and hypertrophy, and myofibrillary atrophy, occur.
- Interstitial fibrosis may occur.
- Ventricular enlargement progresses.

Etiology

- Most often idiopathic
- Toxins (e.g., ETOH, chemotherapeutic agents)
- Metabolic abnormalities
- Infectious
- Inflammatory
- Tachycardia

Risk Factors

- Alcohol or illicit drug abuse
- Chronic tachyarrhythmias

Prevention and Screening

- Avoid or discontinue alcohol and drug use.
- Echocardiogram if there is clinical suspicion

Assessment

- Dyspnea
- Chronic fatigue
- Fluid overload
- Palpitations
- Anginal type CP
- Crackles
- JVD
- Laterally displaced PMI
- S3
- Signs of RHF
- PVCs

Diagnostic Studies

- ECG: may demonstrate ST-T wave changes or conduction abnormalities
- Chest x-ray: cardiomegaly, pulmonary congestion
- Echocardiogram: left ventricular dysfunction and dilation
- Labs: routine screening and to assess for underlying etiology (see above)
  - Chemistry
  - CBC
  - LFTs
  - TFT

Differential Diagnosis

- Hypertrophic obstructive cardiomyopathy
- Restrictive cardiomyopathy

Management

- Determine and treat the underlying cause.
- Treat decompensated HF (see heart failure section).
- Daily weights
- Low-sodium Na diet
- Long-term:
  - Diuretics, ACE I, and beta-blockers (improve long-term survival)
- Both long-term and acute management are the same as for HF.
- If life-threatening arrhythmias present, will need ICD, long-term antiarrhythmic therapy, or both
- ICD for patients with EF of 35% to prevent sudden cardiac death

HYPERTROPHIC CARDIOMYOPATHY

Description

- The hallmark of hypertrophic cardiomyopathy is unexplained hypertrophy of the muscle and thickening of the intraventricular septum.
- Hypertrophy may become severe enough to encroach on the LV cavity.
- Movement of the mitral valve may be restricted.
- Myocytes form in a disorganized pattern throughout the LV.
- Can be obstructive or nonobstructive

Etiology, Incidence, and Demographics

- Chronic HTN
- Hereditary
- Most common genetically transmitted cardiac disease
- Autosomal dominant trait

Risk Factors

- Hypertension, especially chronic and poorly controlled
- Family history

Prevention and Screening

- Control hypertension.
- Screen with echocardiogram if family history of HCM

Assessment

- Dyspnea
- Chest pain
- Syncope
- Palpitations
- Hyperdynamic apical impulse
- Brisk carotid upstroke
- Bisferiens pulse may be present
- S4
- Harsh crescendo–decrescendo systolic murmur

Differential Diagnosis

- Hypertensive heart disease
- Restrictive cardiomyopathy
- Aortic stenosis

Diagnostic Studies

- ECG: LVH, possible septal Q waves
- Chest x-ray: usually unremarkable unless pulmonary edema present
- Echocardiogram: LVH, if outflow tract obstruction present, the mitral valve will have an anterior systolic motion
- Labs: routine as stated above in DCM section

Management

- Control blood pressure
  - Beta-blockers
  - CCB may also be used
- Myocardial septal excision has been successful in some severely symptomatic individuals.
- Dual-chamber pacing
- Septal ablation
- Possible ICD to prevent sudden cardiac death

RESTRICTIVE CARDIOMYOPATHY

Description

- The hallmark of restrictive cardiomyopahty is diastolic dysfunction.
- Stiff ventricular walls
- Systolic function preserved
- Myocardial fibrosis, hypertrophy, and thickening
- Increased cardiac pressures
- Venous and systemic congestion occur.
- Decreased stroke volume and cardiac output

Etiology

- Noninfiltrative
- Infiltrative
- Hemochromatosis
- Malignancy
- Radiation injury

Risk Factors

- See Etiology

Prevention and Screening

- None
- Echocardiogram if suspected

Assessment

- Dyspnea
- Fatigue
- Systemic congestion
- Increased jugular venous pressures
- Possible systolic murmur
- Symptoms of right heart failure

Differential Diagnosis

- Constrictive pericarditis
- Hypertrophic obstructive cardiomyopathy
- Hypertensive heart disease

Diagnostic Studies

- ECG: ST-T wave changes, conduction abnormalities, low voltage
- Chest x-ray: cardiomegaly
- Echocardiogram: normal or mildly reduced left ventricular systolic function, small or normal left ventricular size, diastolic dysfunction
- Labs: routine as outlined above in DCM section
- Biopsy as indicated, especially if amyloidosis suspected

Management

- Treat underlying cause
- Diuretics, sodium restriction
- Beta-blockers, CCB, and ACE-I often used but have shown no benefit

When to Consult, Refer, or Hospitalize

- For all cardiomyopathies:
  - Admit
    · Decompensated heart failure
    · Failed outpatient therapy
  - Consult
    · Consult cardiology for all patients with new cardiomyopathies to determine underlying cause and recommended treatment course

Follow-up

- Educate patient and family on the underlying disease process.
- Sodium restriction, lifestyle modifications
- Daily weights; report 2-lb weight gain in 2 days
- Alcohol, drug, and tobacco cessation
- Importance of medication compliance

ANEURYSM

Description

- An aneurysm is an abnormal dilation of the arterial wall, resulting in bulging of the intima.

Etiology, Incidence, and Demographics

- Aneurysms are a result of a degenerative process of the arterial wall. Age, as well as the atherosclerotic process, play a role. Decreased elastin in the arterial wall leads to a dilated, weakened vessel wall.
- Male > female
- Types of aneurysms:
  - Fusiform: uniform dilation of the entire segment of an artery (most common type)
  - Saccular: outpouching or bulging of one side of the arterial wall (typically found in the distal abdominal aorta, proximal to the origin of the renal arteries)
  - Dissecting: rupture or tear in the weakened arterial wall; blood forced between the layers of arterial wall and creates "false lumen"

Risk Factors

- Increasing age
- Male gender
- Family history of aneurysm
- Hypertension
- Tobacco abuse
- Coronary artery disease
- Peripheral vascular disease

Prevention and Screening

- USPSTF recommends screening for AAA by Doppler in men aged 65 to 75 who have a history of smoking

Assessment

- Most are asymptomatic and found incidentally during imaging studies for other problems.
- Abdominal pain
- Sensation of pulsation in the abdomen
- Back pain; dull ache or ripping or tearing with rupture or dissection
- Pulsating abdominal mass
- Abdominal bruit
- Patient with ruptured aneurysm may present hemodynamically as unstable and be in shock

Differential Diagnosis

- Ruptured disc
- Urinary tract infection
- Renal obstruction
- Peptic ulcer perforation
- Abdominal neoplasm

Diagnostic Studies

- Ultrasound for screening
- CT scan provides better images and is test of choice for suspected rupture or dissection
- Chest x-ray may show widened mediastinum with thoracic aortic aneurysm rupture or dissection
- Hemoglobin and hematocrit, type and cross, chemistry, PT, INR, PTT for patients with dissection

Management

- Stabilize hemodynamically and obtain vascular surgery consultation for suspected rupture or dissection.
- For aneurysms < 5 cm in low-risk patients, follow by ultrasound or CT at 6- to 12-month intervals.
- Hypertension control is of utmost importance.

When to Consult, Refer, or Hospitalize

- Admit
  - Suspected or confirmed rupture or dissection
- Consult
  - Patients with aneurysms measuring 4 cm or larger—refer to a vascular specialist for further evaluation
  - Consult vascular surgery for all patients with aortic dissection.

Follow-up

- Discuss risk factor modification (e.g., lifestyle changes) and risk of rupture.
- Discuss the need for routine follow-up and repeat imaging studies to monitor growth pattern.
- Instruct the patient to seek immediate medical attention for any symptoms consisting of sudden-onset severe back or abdominal pain.
- If surgery is indicated, discuss the procedure, risks, and benefits with the patient and family.

ENDOCARDITIS

Description

- Endocarditis is systemic infection beginning with colonization of an infective organism on the valve, progressing to produce signs and symptoms consistent with bacteremia.

Etiology, Incidence, and Demographics

- *Viridans streptococci* (most common)
- *S. aureus* (second-most common)
- Enterococci
- Gram-negative organisms
- Fungi

Risk Factors

- Preexisting murmur
- Congenital lesions
- Rheumatic heart disease
- Transient bacteremia
- Injection drug use
- Prosthetic valve

Assessment

- Fever
- Arthralgias
- Dyspnea
- New or changing murmur (not in all cases)
- Splinter hemorrhages: linear, subungual hemorrhages on nail beds
- Osler's nodes: painful cutaneous nodules on pads of fingers and toes
- Janeway lesions: painless hemorrhagic macules on palms or soles of feet
- Roth spots: exudative lesions in retina

Differential Diagnosis

- Other causes of constitutional illness
- Valvular abnormalities without endocarditis (e.g., MVP, AS)

Diagnostic Studies

- Blood cultures: 3 sets at least 1 hour apart
- Echocardiogram: transespohageal is most sensitive for detection of vegetation.
- CBC: leukocytosis
- Chest x-ray—may demonstrate cardiac abnormality
- Duke criteria—80% accuracy (see below for criteria)
- Two major criteria *or*
  - One major criterion and three minor criteria *or*
  - Five minor criteria

Table 4–3. Duke Criteria for Endocarditis

Major Criteria	Minor Criteria
Two positive blood cultures for typical microorganism	Predisposing condition
Endocardial involvement documented via echocardiography	Fever > 100° F (37.7° C) Embolic disease Immunologic manifestations Positive blood cultures not meeting major criteria Positive echocardiogram not meeting major criteria

Adapted from "New criteria for diagnosis of infective endocarditis: Utilization of specific echocardiographic findings," by D. T. Durak, A. S. Lukes, & D. K. Bright, 1994, *American Journal of Medicine*, 96(3), 220–222.

Management

- Active infection requires antibiotic treatment appropriate to organism
  - Penicillin G for *Viridans streptococci*
  - Penicillin G + aminoglycoside for enterococci
  - Narrow spectrum beta lactamase-resistant choice for staphylococci
  - Vancomycin for MRSA
- Variety of regimens available for prophylaxis treatment
  - Amoxicillin 2 g, 1 hour before procedure
  - Clindamycin, cephalexin, or macrolide alternatives for penicillin-allergic
  - Add aminoglycoside for high-risk patients who have GI or GU procedures; vancomycin for those who are allergic to penicillin

When to Consult, Refer, or Hospitalize

- All patients with infective endocarditis require hospitalization and IV antibiotics.
- Cardiology/cardiovascular surgery if severe valvular heart disease present

Patient Education

- Educate patient and family on the underlying disease process.
- Discontinue IV drug use.
- Discuss the need for SBE prophylaxis in the future.

REFERENCES

Anderson, J. L., Adams, C. D., Antman, E. M., Bridges, C. R., Califf, R. M., Casey, Jr., D. E., et al. (2007). ACC/AHA 2007 guidelines for the management of patients with unstable angina and non-ST-segment elevation myocardial infarction: Executive summary. A report of the American College of Cardiology/American Heart Association Task Force on Practice Guidelines (Writing Committee to Revise the 2002 the Guidelines for the Management of Patients with Unstable Angina and Non-ST-Segment Elevation Myocardial Infarction). *Circulation: Journal of the American Heart Association, 116,* 803–877.

Antman, E. M., Hand, M., Armstrong, P. W., Bates, E. R., Green, L. A., Halasyamani, L. K,. et al. (2008). 2007 focused update of the ACC/AHA 2004 guidelines for the management of patients with ST-elevation myocardial infarction: A report of the American College of Cardiology/American Heart Association Task Force on Practice Guidelines (2007 Writing Group to Review New Evidence and Update the 2004 Guidelines for the Management of Patients With S-T Elevation Myocardial Infarction). *Journal of the American College of Cardiology, 51,* 210–247.

Barkley, T. W., & Myers, C. (2008). *Practice guidelines for acute care nurse practitioners.* Philadelphia: W. B. Saunders.

Bongard, F., Sue, D., & Vintch, J. (2008). *Current diagnosis and treatment: Critical care* (3rd ed.). New York: Lange/McGraw Hill.

Buttaro, T., Trybulski, J., Bailey, P., & Sandberg-Cook, J. (2008). *Primary care* (3rd ed.). St. Louis, MO: Mosby.

Fauci, A. S., Braunwalk, E., Kasper, D. L., Hauser, S. L., Longo, D. L., Jameson, J. L., et al. (2008). *Harrison's principles of internal medicine* (17th ed.). Philadelphia: McGraw Hill.

Fiebach, N. H., Barker, L. R., Burton, J. R., & Zieves, P. D. (2007). *Principles of ambulatory medicine* (7th ed.). Philadelphia: Lippincott, Williams, & Wilkins.

Fraker, T. D., Fihn, S. D., & 2002 Chronic Stable Angina Writing Committee. (2007). 2007 chronic angina focused update of the ACC/AHA 2002 guidelines for the management of patients with chronic stable angina: A report of the American College of Cardiology/American Heart Association Task Force on Practice Guidelines Writing Group to Develop the Focused Update of the 2002 Guidelines for the Management of Patients with Chronic Stable Angina. *Journal of the American College of Cardiology, 50,* 2264–2274.

Fuster, V., Ryden, L. E., Cannom, D. S., Crijns, H. J., Curtis, A. B., Ellenbogen, K. A., et al. (2006). ACC/AHA/ESC 2006 guidelines for the management of patients with atrial fibrillation: A report of the American College of Cardiology/American Heart Association Task Force on Practice Guidelines and the European Society of Cardiology Committee for Practice Guidelines (Writing Committee to Revise the 2001 Guidelines for the Management of Patients With Atrial Fibrillation). *Journal of the American College of Cardiology, 48,* e149–246.

Joint National Committee on Prevention, Detection, Evaluation, and Treatment of High Blood Pressure (JNC). (2004). *7th report of the JNC.* Bethesda, MD: National Institutes of Health.

Marino, P. T. (2007). *The ICU book* (3rd ed.). Philadelphia: Lippincott, Williams, & Wilkins.

McPhee, S., & Papadakis, M. (2010). *Current medical diagnosis and treatment* (49th ed.). New York: Lange/McGraw Hill.

National Cholesterol Education Panel. (2002). *Third report of the expert panel on detection, evaluation, and treatment of high blood cholesterol in adults (Adult Treatment Panel III).* Bethesda, MD: National Institutes of Health.

Parrillo, J., & Dellinger, R. (Eds.). (2008). *Critical care medicine: Principles of diagnosis and management in the adult* (3rd ed.). St. Louis, MO: Mosby.

5

Pulmonary Disorders

Julie Davey, MSN, RN, ANP-BC, ACNP-BC

CHRONIC OBSTRUCTIVE PULMONARY DISEASE (EMPHYSEMA AND CHRONIC BRONCHITIS)

Description

- Chronic obstructive pulmonary disease (COPD) is:
- A term used collectively to describe chronic bronchitis and emphysema—two diseases with different features, epidemiology, and treatment modalities, but that both result in a chronic obstruction to exhalation airflow.
- *Chronic bronchitis* is characterized by excessive secretion of bronchial mucus and is manifested by productive cough for 3 months or more in at least 2 consecutive years in the absence of any other disease that may account for the symptom.
- *Emphysema* denotes abnormal, permanent enlargement of air spaces distal to the terminal bronchiole.

Etiology, Incidence, and Demographics

- Cigarette smoking is the cause in 80% of cases.
- Prolonged exposure to industrial pollutants
- Alpha-1 proteinase deficiency causes pure emphysema in young patients.
- 14 million diagnosed cases annually—estimated 14 million additional undiagnosed cases

Risk Factors

- Cigarette smoking
- Prolonged exposure to industrial or environmental dusts or fumes
- Atopy
- History of bronchoconstriction in response to nonspecific stimuli

Prevention and Screening

- Tobacco cessation or avoidance
- Avoiding exposure to environmental pollutants

Assessment

Chronic Bronchitis
- Intermittent mild or moderate dyspnea
- Onset of symptoms > age 35
- Copious purulent sputum production
- Stocky, obese habitus
- Barrel chest
- Increased hematocrit
- Hypercapnia, hypoxemia by arterial blood gas

Emphysema
- Progressive, constant dyspnea
- Onset of symptoms > age 50
- Mild sputum (clear)
- Thin, wasted habitus
- Normal hematocrit
- Increased total lung capacity
- Hyperresonance to percussion

Differential Diagnosis
- Acute bronchitis
- Asthma
- Bronchiectasis
- Cystic fibrosis

Diagnostic Studies

- Chest x-ray
  - Chronic bronchitis: "dirty lungs," nonspecific peribronchial and perivascular markings
  - Emphysema: hyperinflation, bulla, blebs
- Pulmonary function tests: consistent with obstructive disease as described in Asthma section
- Complete blood count (CBC)
  - Chronic bronchitis: increased hematocrit
  - Emphysema: normal hematocrit
- Electrocardiogram (ECG) may show evidence of right ventricular hypertrophy

Management

- Four components of COPD management
  - Assess and monitor disease.
  - Reduce risk factors; smoking cessation is single most important treatment modality.
  - Manage stable COPD.
  - Manage exacerbations.

Antibiotic Therapy
- Indicated for acute exacerbation of COPD because of the high risk of secondary bacterial infection
- Acute exacerbation of COPD is defined as any change from baseline cough, dyspnea, or sputum.
- Indicated for any condition causing an acute worsening of pulmonary status in a patient with COPD
- Common medications
  - Trimethoprim/sulfamethoxazole DS b.i.d. for 7 to 10 days
  - Broad-spectrum beta lactamase-sensitive or -resistant penicillin 500 mg b.i.d. for 7 to 10 days
  - Doxycycline 100 mg b.i.d. for 7 to 10 days
  - Fluroquinolones
- Oxygen therapy can halt progression of disease in patients with resting hypoxemia

Table 5-1. Staging and Pharmacologic Management of COPD

Stage	0	I	II	III	IV
Definition	At risk	Mild COPD	Moderate COPD	Severe COPD	Very severe COPD
	Lung function is normal.	FEV_1/FVC < 70% predicted	FEV_1/FVC < 70% predicted	FEV_1/FVC < 70% predicted	FEV_1/FVC < 70% predicted
		FEV_1 > 80%	50% < FEV_1 < 80%	30% < FEV_1 < 50%	FEV_1 < 30% or < 50% *plus* chronic respiratory failure
	Chronic cough and sputum production	Symptoms may be present or absent.	Symptoms may be present or absent.	Symptoms may be present or absent.	Symptoms may be present or absent.
Treatment		Short-acting bronchodilator PRN (anticolinergics or beta agonists)	Same as for stage I	Same as for stage II	Same as for stage III
			Regular treatment with one or more long-acting bronchodilators	Add inhaled glucocorticosteroids for repeat exacerbations.	Add long-term oxygen.
			Pulmonary rehabilitation	Pulmonary rehabilitation	Consider surgical referral

Adapted from "Global Strategy for the Diagnosis, Management, and Prevention of Chronic Obstructive Pulmonary Disease: GOLD Executive Summary," by K. F. Rabe, S. Hurd, A. Anzueto, P. J. Barnes, S. A. Buist, P. Calverly et al., (2007), *American Journal of Respiratory and Critical Care Medicine, 176,* 532–555.

When to Consult, Refer, or Hospitalize

- Admit
  - Severe or worsening symptoms that do not respond to outpatient therapy
  - Altered mental status, lethargy, or respiratory muscle fatigue
  - Persistent or worsening hypoxemia despite use of oxygen
  - Worsening or severe acidosis
  - Presence of high risk comorbid conditions
- Refer or consult
  - Frequent exacerbations despite optimal treatment (2 or more per year)
  - Need for long-term oxygen therapy
  - Severe or rapidly progressive disease

Follow-up

- Educate the patient and family on the underlying disease process.
- Smoking cessation
- Report worsening symptoms.
- Report signs and symptoms of infection.
- Discuss the need for and initiate referral to pulmonary rehabilitation.
- Annual influenza vaccination
- Pneumococcal vaccination every 5 years
- Small, frequent meals to avoid abdominal distention, which may impair diaphragmatic function

ASTHMA

Description

- Asthma is a complex disorder characterized by variable and recurring symptoms, airflow obstruction, bronchial hyperresponsiveness, and an underlying inflammation. Airflow obstruction is widespread but variable, and is often reversible, either spontaneously or with treatment.

Etiology, Incidence, and Demographics

- Affects 17 million Americans
- Primary complaint for 10 million office visits annually

Allergic Triggers

- Pollen
- Feathers
- Pet dander
- Dust mites
- Cockroach excrement
- Molds
- Food additives

Nonallergic Triggers

- Exercise
- Drug-induced
- ASA and NSAIDs
- Beta-adrenergic antagonists
- Occupational factors
- Gastroesophageal reflux disease (GERD)

Risk Factors

- Hygiene hypothesis: Certain infections early in life, exposure to other children, less-frequent use of antibiotics, and "country living" are all associated with a lower incidence of asthma.
- Genetic predisposition
- Atopy

Prevention and Screening

- Avoid environmental triggers
- Smoking cessation or avoidance

Assessment

- Episodic wheezing
- Chest tightness
- Dyspnea
- Chronic dry cough
- Symptoms worsen in aftermath or presence of:
  - Exercise
  - Emotional stress
  - Viral upper respiratory infection
  - Irritants
  - Changes in weather
  - Inhalant allergens

- Dermatitis
- Nasal polyps
- Tachypnea
- Tachycardia
- Use of accessory muscles
- Nasal flaring
- Hyperresonance to percussion

Classification of Asthma

Asthma is classified according to frequency and severity of symptoms, as shown in Table 5–2.

Table 5–2. Asthma Classification

Classification	Severity of Symptoms	Nightime Symptoms	FEV
Mild intermittent	Symptoms < 2 times per week, otherwise asymptomatic	Symptoms ≤ 2 times per month	> 80%
Mild persistent	Symptoms > 2 times per week, < 1 time/day	Symptoms ≥ 2 times per month	> 80%, variability from 20 to 30%
Moderate persistent	Daily symptoms daily use of a beta$_2$ agonist	Symptoms ≥ 1 time per week	60% to 80%
Severe persistent	Continual symptoms, limited physical activity	Frequent symptoms	< 60%

Adapted from *Current Medical Diagnosis and Treatment* by S. McPhee & M. Papadakis, 2011, New York: McGraw-Hill.

Differential Diagnosis

- Airway obstruction
- Aspiration
- Anaphylaxis
- Chronic obstructive pulmonary disease (COPD)
- Adverse drug reaction
  - Angiotensin-converting enzyme (ACE) inhibitors
  - Beta-adrenergic antagonists
- Pulmonary embolism

Diagnostic Studies

Pulmonary function tests demonstrate obstruction to airflow (see Definitions of Pulmonary Function Tests, Table 5–3)
- Forced vital capacity (FVC) decrease
- Forced expiratory volume (FVC_1) decrease
- FEV_1/FVC ratio < 75%
- Measures of airflow should be assessed before and after administration to assess for significant reversibility after bronchodilator therapy: > 12% and 200 mL in FEV_1 or > 15% and 200 mL in FVC
- Peak expiratory flow < 200 mL indicates severe obstruction
- Bronchial provocation testing causes decrease in FEV_1 by 20%.
- CBC may reveal eosinophilia > 3% during acute episodes
- Mild hypoxia and hypocapnia by arterial blood gas—significant hypoxemia and hypercapnia indicate fatigue of accessory muscles and critically ill patient
- Chest x-ray normal—hyperinflation not a common feature

Stepwise Approach for Managing Asthma in Persons > 12 Years Old
- All forms of asthma require patient education on environmental control, proper use of inhalers, management of comorbidities, and when to seek emergency care.
- Steps 2 to 4—consider subcutaneous allergen immunotherapy in those with allergic asthma

Step 1
- No daily medication needed
- Rescue therapy with short-acting beta-adrenergic agonists as needed for acute episodes

Table 5-3. Definitions of Pulmonary Function Tests

Test	Definition
Spirometry	
FVC	Forced vital capacity—volume of gas that can be forcefully expelled from lungs after maximal inspiration
FEV_1	Forced expiratory volume in 1 second—volume of gas expelled in first second of FVC (most commonly used to determine asthma status)
FEF_{25-75}	Forced expiratory flow from 25%–75% of the FVC—maximal airflow rate
PEFR	Peak expiratory flow rate—maximal airflow rate achieved in FVC maneuver
MVV	Maximum voluntary ventilation—maximum volume of gas that can be breathed in 1 minute (measured in 15 seconds and multiplied by 4)
Lung Volumes	
TLC	Total lung capacity Volume of gas in lungs after a maximal inspiration
RV	Residual volume—volume of gas remaining in lungs after maximal expiration
ERV	Expiratory reserve volume—volume of gas representing difference between functional residual capacity and residual volume
FRC	Functional residual capacity—volume of gas in lungs at end of normal tidal expiration
SVC	Slowed vital capacity—volume of gas that can be exhaled slowly after maximal inspiration

Adapted from "Heart." in Tierney, L.M. Jr., McPhee, S.J., & Papadakis, M. A. (Eds.), *Current Medical Diagnosis and Treatment* (p. 269), by M. S. Chesnutt & T. J. Prendergrast (2007) New York: Lange Medical Books/McGraw-Hill.

Step 2
- Requires one daily medication
- Preferred treatment is a low-dose inhaled steroid
- Alternative treatments include
  - Inhaled antimediator
  - Leukotriene receptor antagonist
  - Sustained-release theophylline
- Rescue therapy with short-acting beta-adrenergic agonist for breakthrough symptoms

Step 3
- Preferred therapy
  - Daily maintenance therapy including either addition of long-acting beta adrenergic agonist to low-dose inhaled steroid *or*
  - Single use of medium-dose inhaled steroid
- Alternative treatments include
  - Low-dose inhaled corticosteroid with either leukotriene receptor antagonist, theophylline, or Zileuton
- Rescue therapy with short-acting beta-adrenergic agonist for breakthrough symptoms

Step 4
- Preferred treatment
  - Daily medications include medium-dose inhaled steroid and long-acting beta-adrenergic agonist
- Alternative treatments include
  - Medium-dose inhaled corticosteroid with either leukotriene receptor antagonist, theophylline, or Zileuton
- Rescue therapy with short-acting beta-adrenergic agonist for breakthrough symptoms

Step 5
- Preferred treatment
  - High-dose inhaled corticosteroids and long-acting beta-adrenergic agonist *and*
  - Consider omalizumab for patients with allergies

Step 6
- Preferred treatment
  - High-dose inhaled corticosteroid with long-acting beta-adrenergic agonist and oral corticosteroid *and*
  - Consider omalizumab for patients with allergies

When to Consult, Refer, or Hospitalize

- Admit
  - Progressive dyspnea
  - Hypoxemia
  - Signs of systemic infection
  - Consider admission for patients with FEV_1 < 70% of predicted
  - FEV_1 < 50% predicted

- Refer or consult
  - Complicating comorbid conditions (multiple environmental allergies, rhinosinusitis, etc.)
  - Inability to meet goal after 3 to 6 months of treatment
  - Suboptimal response to therapy
  - Patients requiring high-dose inhaled corticosteroids
  - Patients requiring two or more courses of oral prednisone in the last year

Follow-up

- Educate the patient and family on the underlying disease process.
- Discuss environmental control measures.
- Instruct on the use of medications and delivery devices.
- Emphasize the importance of using long-term control medications.
- Discuss when to use quick-relief medications.
- Discuss early recognition and treatment of exacerbations.
- Discuss the importance of influenza and pneumococcal vaccinations.

BRONCHITIS (ACUTE BRONCHITIS)

Description

- Bronchitis is an acute respiratory infection in which cough, regardless of phlegm production, is the predominant feature and has persisted for < 3 weeks.

Etiology, Incidence, and Demographics

- Viral infections account for 90% of cases.
- *Bordetella pertussis*—second leading cause
- Less-common causes
  - Chlamydia pneumoniae
  - Mycoplasma pneumoniae
  - Moraxella catarrhalis
- Bacterial infection more common in smokers and those with preexisting chronic pulmonary disease
  - *Streptococcus pneumoniae*
  - *Haemophilus influenzae*
- Affects all ages and genders
- More common among smokers

Risk Factors

- Cigarette smoking
- Preexisting pulmonary disease

Prevention and Screening

- Smoking cessation

Assessment

- Severe cough
- Copious mucopurulent sputum production in most cases
- Low-grade temperature
- Occasional wheezing
- Substernal or costochondral pain
- Foul taste in mouth
- Cervical lymphadenopathy
- Upper airway rhonchi—clears with coughing
- No physical findings consistent with lower airway consolidation
  - No increase in tactile fremitus
  - No egophony
  - No dullness to percussion

Differential Diagnosis

- Pneumonia
- Chronic bronchitis
- Upper respiratory infection
- Tuberculosis
- Non-pulmonary cough
- Allergies
- Asthma

Diagnostic Studies

- Typically none—diagnosis based on clinical presentation
- Chest x-ray to assess for lower airway process
- Sputum culture if bacterial infection suspected
- Pulmonary function test if underlying obstructive disease suspected

Management

- Humidified air to loosen secretions
- Adequate hydration
- Smoking cessation
- NSAIDs for costochondral pain related to cough
- Expectorants and mucolytics have not demonstrated benefit—not recommended for routine use
- Short trial of antitussives generally indicated, particularly for
  - Those who cannot tolerate transient hypoxia of coughing
  - Patients who cannot work or sleep, or are otherwise impaired in activities of daily living
- Beta-adrenergic agonist bronchodilators may be useful in patients with wheezing.
- Antibiotics generally not indicated unless B. *pertussis* confirmed

When to Consult, Refer, or Hospitalize

- Admit
  - Patients with severe dyspnea, hypoxemia, respiratory failure, failed outpatient therapy
- Consult
  - Pulmonology for difficult-to-manage patients.

Follow-up

- Increase fluid intake to avoid dehydration.
- Humidifier may provide symptom relief.
- Stress the importance of completion of antibiotic regimen if prescribed.
- Report persistent symptoms or an increase in severity.

RESPIRATORY INFECTIONS

COMMUNITY-ACQUIRED PNEUMONIA

Description

- Community-acquired pneumonia is an acute pulmonary infection of the lower airway characterized by lung field consolidation. Pneumonia is considered community-acquired if the onset is outside the hospital setting or occurs within 48 hours hospital admission.

Etiology, Incidence, and Demographics

- Most deadly infectious disease—sixth leading overall cause of death
- 3 to 4 million cases each year in United States
- Bacterial causes are most common
  - *Streptococcus pneumoniae*
  - *Haemophilus influenzae*
  - *Mycoplasma pneumoniae*
  - *Chlamydia pneumoniae*
  - *Staphylococcus aureus*
  - *Neisseria meningitides*
  - *Moraxella catarrhalis*
  - *Klebsiella pneumoniae*
  - *Pneumocystis carinii*
  - *E. coli*
  - *Pseudomonas aeruginosa*
  - *Legionella species*
- Viral
- Fungal
- Chemical aspiration

Risk Factors

- Cigarette smoking
- Preexisting chronic pulmonary disease
- Age
- Nursing home residence
- Alcoholism
- Exposure to bats, birds, or soil with bird droppings; rabbits; farm animals; parturient cats
- Drug abuse
- Travel to the Southwest
- Poor dental hygiene

Prevention and Screening

- Should receive pneumococcal vaccination
  - All adults over age 65
  - All adults with chronic medical conditions
  - Asplenic individuals
  - Individuals receiving immunosuppressive therapy (chemotherapy)
  - May repeat dose in 5 years for those at greatest risk

Assessment

- Feels generally unwell
- Fever
- Fatigue
- Shaking chills
- Pleuritic chest pain
- Cough and purulent sputum not common features
- Rhonchi or rales in affected lung field(s)
- Evidence of lung consolidation
  - Increased tactile fremitus
  - Egophony present
  - Dullness to percussion

Differential Diagnosis

- Upper respiratory tract infections
- Reactive airway disease
- Decompensated heart failure
- Bronchiolitis
- Lung carcinoma
- Pulmonary vasculitis
- Atelectasis

Diagnostic Studies

- CBC: elevated WBCs (may be low in immunocompromised or elderly)
- Chest x-ray: pulmonary infiltrates (unilateral or bilateral)
- GS and culture not routinely indicated: useful if atypical or reportable organism suspected, or if patient is immunocompromised or has not responded to conventional treatment
- Routine electrolytes and LFTs of no value in the outpatient setting

Management

- CURB-65 or similar scale should be used to assess need for hospital admission
  - Confusion
  - Uremia
  - Respiratory rate
  - Blood pressure low
  - Age ≥ 65
- Previously healthy outpatients with no comorbidities
  - Macrolide (best evidence)
  - Doxycycline
- Presence of comorbidities or antibiotic use within the last three months
  - Respiratory fluoroquinolone
  - Beta-lactam with macrolide
- Hospitalization for the treatment of community-acquired pneumonia—use same antibiotics as for outpatients with comorbidities

When to Consult, Refer, or Hospitalize

- Admit
  - Failed outpatient therapy
  - Based on the following:
    - Clinical appearance, respiratory distress, $PAO_2 < 60$ mm Hg or $PACO_2 > 50$ mm Hg on room air, high risk for dehydration, patient reliability, more than 1 lung lobe involved, comorbid conditions
    - Fever > 101° F, immunocompromised status, age > 65, hypotension (BP 90/60 mm Hg) or tachycardia (HR > 140 bpm), altered LOC, abnormal renal function, anemia, additional chest x-ray findings (cavitary lung lesion or pleural effusion)
  - Must consider patterns of antimicrobial resistance and local bacteria spectra
  - Treatment for *S. pneumoniae* or other typical bacterial organisms is 7 to 10 days or until patient afebrile for at least 72 hours
- Consult
  - Pulmonology for cases with severe underlying lung disease or multiple comorbidities

Follow-up

- Increase fluid intake to avoid dehydration.
- Stress the importance of completion of antibiotic regimen.
- Report persistent symptoms or an increase in severity.

HOSPITAL-ACQUIRED PNEUMONIA (HAP) AND VENTILATOR-ASSOCIATED PNEUMONIA (VAP)

Description

- Hospital-acquired pneumonia (HAP) is a lower respiratory tract infection that occurs at least 48 to 72 hours after hospital admission.
- Ventilator-associated pneumonia (VAP) is a lower respiratory tract infection that begins in mechanically ventilated patients 48 hours or more after intubation.

Etiology, Incidence, and Demographics

- Most common organisms responsible for HAP/VAP
  - *Staphylococcus aureus*
  - *Klebsiella pneumoniae*
  - *Pseudomonas aeruginosa*
  - *Escherichia coli*
  - *Enterobacter*
  - *Haemophilus influenza*
  - *Serratia marcescens*

Risk Factors

- Poor oral integrity
- Altered immune system
- Comorbid states
- Immobility
- Age
- Trauma
- Decreased LOC
- Previous antibiotic therapy or inappropriate therapy
- Prolonged intubation
- NG/OG present

Prevention and Screening

- Meticulous hand-washing by hospital personnel and visitors
- See above (CAP Prevention and Screening) for recommendations on pneumococcal vaccination.
- See below for VAP bundle.

Assessment

- Findings for HAP/VAP are the same, except one or more of the following may be present in: purulent sputum, leukocytosis, or a new or worsening pulmonary infiltrate on CXR.

Diagnostic Studies

- Sputum gram stain and culture
- Blood cultures
- ABG
- Chemistry 12
- CBC with differential
- HIV serology if indicated
- Chest x-ray
- Lack of improvement or worsening infiltrates despite treatment should raise concern about additional pulmonary processes. It may take 6 weeks or longer for infiltrates to resolve.

Management

- Treatment is empirical
  - Severe early onset (within 5 days of hospitalization)
    - Beta-lactam and beta-lactamase inhibitor
  - Ticarcillin/clavulanate (Timentin) 3.1 g IV q. 4 hrs
  - *or*
    - Second- or third-generation cephalosporin (nonantipseudomonal)
  - Ceftriaxone 1 to 2 g IV q.d.
  - *or*
    - Fluoroquinolone
  - Gatifloxacin 400 mg IV q.d.
- Severe late onset (≥ 5 days of hospitalization) or VAP
- Treatment directed toward most virulent organisms (acinetobacter, enterobacter, *P. aeruginosa*)
  - Aminoglycoside (tobramycin 5 mg/kg IV q.d.) or fluoroquinolone (ciprofloxacin 400 mg IV q.d.) *plus*
  - Antipseudomonal PCN (piperacillin 3 to 4 g IM/IV q. 4 to 6 hrs), antipseudomonal cephalosporin (ceftazidime sodium 1 to 2 gm IV q. 8 to 12 hrs)
  - Add vancomycin 1 gm IV q. 12 hrs if MRSA is suspected.
- For patients at risk for anaerobic pneumonia, add clindamycin (600 mg IV q. 8 hrs) or beta-lactam/beta-lactamase inhibitor
- Prevention of HAP or VAP is key
  - Ensure proper hand-washing
  - VAP bundle
    - HOB elevation
    - PUD prophylaxis
    - DVT prophylaxis
    - Assess for readiness to extubate.
    - Oral care

When to Consult, Refer, or Hospitalize

- All patients are already hospitalized.
- Consult pulmonology for difficult-to-manage or complex cases, severe underlying lung disease, or multiple comorbidities.

Follow-up

- Educate the patient and family on the disease process.
- Educate the patient and family on the ICU environment and monitoring and assistive devices.

TUBERCULOSIS (TB)

Description

- Tuberculosis (TB) is a systemic disease caused by M. *tuberculosis*; pulmonary disease is the most common clinical presentation. Other sites of involvement include lymphatics, genitourinary, bone, meninges, peritoneum, and heart. Most cases of active TB in the United States are the result of reactivation rather than primary infection. **Your local health department should be notified of all cases of tuberculosis.**

Etiology, Incidence, and Demographics

- Inhalation of aerosolized droplets containing M. *tuberculosis*
- 2 billion people infected worldwide
- 10 to 15 million people in the United States have latent TB—approximately 10% will develop an active infection.

Risk Factors

- HIV infection
- Institutional living
- Chronic disease
- Malignancy
- Malnutrition
- Close contact with infected persons

Prevention and Screening

- Bacillus Calmette-Guerin (BCG) vaccination—not recommended in the United States because of low incidence of TB and variable effectiveness
- Report all cases (suspected and confirmed) to public health authorities.

Assessment

- Frequently asymptomatic in early disease
- Fatigue, anorexia
- Weight loss, low-grade fever, night sweats
- Dry cough progressing to productive and sometimes blood-tinged
- Pleuritic chest pain
- Examination findings consistent with lung consolidation
  - Adventitious lung sounds in affected fields
  - Increased tactile fremitus
  - Dullness to percussion
  - Egophony

Differential Diagnosis

- COPD
- Pneumonia
- Carcinoma
- Pleurisy
- Histoplasmosis
- Silicosis

Diagnostic Studies

- Purified protein derivative (PPD) to assess exposure
  - 5-mm induration is a positive result in HIV-infected persons, persons in close contact with infected persons, healthcare workers, and those with chest x-rays suspicious for TB.
  - 10-mm induration is a positive result in those living in high-risk groups or high-prevalence environments.
  - 15-mm induration is a positive result in all persons.
- Sputum for acid-fast bacilli (AFB)
  - Provides a presumptive diagnosis
  - Is an indication to begin treatment
- Chest x-ray is not diagnostic but may demonstrate typical findings
  - Small, homogenous infiltrates
  - Cavitation
  - Hilar and paratracheal lymph node enlargement
- Sputum culture for M. *tuberculosis*
  - Provides the only definitive diagnosis

Management

- Hospitalization is not required but should be considered if a client is noncompliant or is likely to expose susceptible individuals.
- Hospitalized clients with pulmonary disease should be in respiratory isolation in negative-pressure rooms.

Medication Regimen
- Dictated by the Centers for Disease Control and Prevention (CDC) and includes a variety of combinations of:
  - Isoniazid (INH)
  - Rifampin (Rifadin)
  - Pyrazinamide
  - Ethambutol (Myambutol)
- A variety of directly observed therapy (DOT) options are available at twice- and three-times weekly dosing.
- Treatment will vary from 6 to 9 months, depending upon a variety of circumstances.

Monitoring Therapy
- Weekly sputum smears and cultures for first 6 weeks after initiation of therapy
- Monthly sputum cultures until negative cultures are documented
- Continued symptoms or positive cultures after 3 months should raise suspicion of drug resistance

Baseline Evaluation
- Liver function studies
- CBC
- Serum creatinine
- Visual acuity and red-green color perception for patients taking ethambutol

Monitoring During Course of Treatment
- Routine monthly labs not necessary
- Question patients about symptoms of drug toxicity.
- LFTs indicated in those with symptoms of drug-induced hepatitis—LFTs > three times normal warrant consideration of changing therapy

Chemoprophylaxis
- Those with a positive PPD as defined above and under the age of 35 should receive 6 to 9 months of chemoprophylaxis with INH and B6.

When to Consult, Refer, or Hospitalize

- Admit or institute DOT for patients who are not capable of self-care and are potential danger for exposure to others.
- If hospitalized, will require isolation in negative pressure room until three consecutive morning sputum specimens are negative for MTB organism
- Consult for initiation of treatment plan

Follow-up

- Educate the patient and family on the underlying disease process.
- Discuss the importance of medication compliance.
- Discuss the importance of avoiding exposing others.

PULMONARY EMBOLISM

Description

- Pulmonary embolism is a thromboembolism other embolic material (e.g., air, amniotic fluid, bone marrow, foreign body) that becomes lodged in the pulmonary arterial circulation, thereby interrupting blood flow.

Etiology, Incidence, and Demographics

- > 600,000 case per year and 50,000 deaths
- Fatal PE occurs in 5% of high-risk patients
- See incidence in DVT section
- Most common cause is thromboemboli arising from the deep veins in pelvis and lower extremities

Risk Factors

- Virchow's triad—predisposing risk for thromboemboli
  - Venous stasis
  - Hypercoagulable state
  - Intimal injury
- Cancer
- Age
- Acquired hypercoagulable states
  - Antiphospholipid antibodies
  - Myeloproliferative disorders
- Inherited hypercoagulable states
  - Activated protein C resistance
  - Hyperhomocystinemia
  - Prothrombin gene mutation
  - Protein C deficiency, protein S deficiency
  - Antithrombin deficiency
- Estrogen
- Pregnancy
- History of VTE
- Prolonged immobility

- Surgery
- Trauma
- Obesity
- Major medical illnesses (myocardial infarction, heart failure)

Prevention and Screening

- VTE prophylaxis (see DVT section)

Assessment

- Dyspnea/tachypnea
- Pain
- Syncope
- Signs or symptoms of DVT
- Hemoptysis
- Anxiety
- Tachycardia
- Diaphoresis
- Initial hypertension
- Later hypotension and possible shock

Differential Diagnosis

- Acute coronary syndrome
- Pneumonia
- COPD exacerbation

Diagnostic Studies

- Arterial blood gas
  - Hypoxemia
  - Acute respiratory alkalosis
- ECG
  - Tachyarrhythmias (e.g., atrial fibrillation)
  - S1Q3T3
- Chest x-ray
  - May be normal
  - Hampton's hump—juxtapleural pulmonary soft tissue density
  - Westermark's sign—dilation of the pulmonary artery proximal to the embolism with oligemia (collapse of distal vessels)
- Ventilation/perfusion scan
  - If normal: Search for alternate diagnosis.

- If low or indeterminate probability: must correlate with clinical suspicion and investigate further
- If high probability: Treat with anticoagulation
- CT angiography (CTA), spiral CT, helical CT
  - If initial chest x-ray abnormal, CTA is test of choice
  - May not detect small emboli in branch or lobar arteries
- Pulmonary angiography
  - Gold standard

Management

- Anticoagulation
  - Low molecular weight heparin (e.g., enoxaparin) SC twice daily *or*
  - Unfractionated heparin IV bolus followed by drip
  - Warfarin
    - Continue heparin until INR therapeutic (2.0 to 3.0)
    - Length of treatment
      - 3 to 6 months
        - Limited risk factors
      - 6 to 12 months
        - Idiopathic PE
      - 12 months to lifetime
        - Malignancy
        - Some inherited thrombophilias
- Fibrinolytic therapy—typically reserved for massive PE
  - Be aware of contraindication (see contraindications to fibrinolytics in ACS section)
- Pulmonary embolectomy
- Inferior vena caval filter
  - Indicated in recurrent thromboembolism
  - Indicated if anticoagulation contraindicated
  - Indicated if high risk for future thromboemboli

When to Refer, Consult, or Hospitalize

- All patients with PE will require hospitalization for initiation of treatment and close hemodynamic monitoring.
- Consult for patients requiring procedures (e.g., embolectomy, inferior vena cava filter).

Follow-up

- Risk-factor modification as appropriate (e.g, discontinue oral contraceptives, weight loss, smoking cessation)
- Dietary modifications with use of warfarin
- Importance of close INR monitoring
- Report signs of bleeding.

ACUTE RESPIRATORY FAILURE

Description

- Acute respiratory failure is the inability of respiratory system to maintain normal state of gas exchange to meet cellular requirements
- Respiratory failure is present if:
  - PaO_2 is < 60 mm Hg on room air (SpO_2 90%) *or* hypoxemia present if on supplemental oxygen
  - $PaCO_2$ > 45 mm Hg, producing respiratory acidosis (Ph < 7.35), except when elevated $PaCO_2$ is compensation for metabolic alkalosis

Etiology, Incidence, and Demographics

- Disorders that affect the lung commonly present with *hypoxemia.*
- Disorders that affect parts of the respiratory system *other* than the lungs commonly present with *hypercapnia.*
  - Hypercapnia is the result of alveolar hypoventilation.
- Etiologies of hypercapnic respiratory failure
  - COPD-multiple mechanisms; structural and alveolar derangements
    - Increased work of breathing = increased CO_2 production
    - Fatigue of respiratory muscles—ventilation failure
    - Decreased central respiratory drive
  - Neuromuscular disease (e.g., Guillain Barré, myasthenia gravis)
  - Drug overdose (e.g., sedatives, opiates, hypnotics)
- Hypoxemic respiratory failure
  - More common than hypercapnic failure
  - Expect low PaO_2 *but normal/low PCO_2*
  - Indicates disease of
    - Lung parenchyma
    - Pulmonary circulation
- Hypoxemic respiratory failure
  - ARDS
  - Pneumonia
  - Pulmonary embolism
  - Asthma
  - Aspiration pneumonitis

Risk Factors

- See above etiologies

Prevention and Screening

- Smoking cessation
- Avoid drug use and overdose.

Assessment

- Hypercapnic respiratory failure
  - Elevated $PaCO_2$
  - Signs and symptoms
    - Somnolence
    - Lethargy
    - Restlessness
    - Headache
    - Slurred speech
- Hypoxic respiratory failure
  - Decreased PaO_2
  - Signs and symptoms
    - Anxiety
    - Restlessness
    - Tachycardia
    - Confusion or AMS
    - Hyper- or hypotension
    - Cardiac arrhythmias

Diagnostic Studies

- ABG (findings based on type of respiratory failure and underlying etiology)
- Chest x-ray (findings based on type of respiratory failure and underlying etiology)

Differential Diagnosis

- ARDS
- Cardiogenic pulmonary edema
- Pulmonary infection
- Pulmonary embolus
- COPD exacerbation

Management

- General initial approach to patient with respiratory failure
  - Administer oxygen.
  - Prepare for ventilatory support.
  - Review clinical history for suspected cause.
  - Chest x-ray
  - 12-lead ECG
  - Pulse oximeter
  - ABGs
  - Chemistry, CBC
- Determine the underlying etiology and treat as appropriate.

When to Consult, Refer, or Hospitalize

- All patients with acute respiratory failure require hospitalization.
- Consult
  - Pulmonology for complex, difficult-to-manage cases

Follow-up

- Educate patient and family regarding the underlying disease process and etiology of respiratory failure.
- Additional education will be based on the underlying etiology and presence of disease processes.

ACUTE RESPIRATORY DISTRESS SYNDROME

Description

- Acute respiratory distress syndrome (ARDS) is the most severe form of acute lung injury (ALI). ARDS is defined as an acute condition characterized by bilateral pulmonary infiltrates and severe hypoxemia in the absence of cardiogenic pulmonary edema. The severity of hypoxemia is determined by calculating the PaO_2/FiO_2 ratio. This is the partial pressure of oxygen in the arterial blood to the percentage of oxygen in the inspired air. In ARDS, the ratio is < 200. In ALI, the ratio is < 300.
Note. Refractory hypoxemia is a classic finding.

Etiology, Incidence, and Demographics

- Systemic causes
  - Trauma
  - Sepsis
  - Burns
  - Pancreatitis
  - Shock
  - DIC
  - TTP
  - Multiple blood transfusions
  - Head injury
  - Cardiopulmonary bypass
- Pulmonary causes
  - Gastric aspiration
  - PE
  - Pneumonia
  - Miliary TB
  - Pulmonary contusion
  - Near drowning
- Incidence is estimated at > 190,000 cases annually with > 74,000 deaths.
- Incidence in relation to demographics corresponds to the incidence of the underlying etiology.

Risk Factors

- Sepsis is the most common.
- Direct lung injury
- Systemic illnesses
- Injuries
- Pneumonia
- Near drowning
- Toxic inhalations

Prevention and Screening

- Strict fluid management in those at risk for ARDS
- Measures to prevent aspiration

Assessment

- Sudden onset severe dyspnea 12–48 hrs after insulting event
- Anxiety
- Restlessness
- Labored breathing
- Accessory muscle use
- Tachypnea
- Crackles
- Tachycardia
- AMS
- Hypotension
- Diffuse or patchy infiltrates on CXR, severe hypoxemia that does not respond to supplemental O_2, high ventilator pressures needed

Diagnostic Studies

- ABG
  - PaO_2 declines progressively
  - $PaCO_2$ decreases initially, then returns to normal or increases.
  - Initially respiratory alkalosis occurs, then respiratory acidosis.
- Hemodynamics
  - Cardiac output: initially increased
  - PAOP: normal or mildly decreased
  - PAP: increased
  - SVO_2: decreased
- PFTs
  - Tital volume: decreased
  - Compliance: decreased
  - Functional residual capacity: decreased
  - Dead space ventilation: increased
  - Peak inspiratory pressures: increased
  - End-tital PCO_2: decreased
  - O_2 saturation: decreased
  - Chest x-ray: bilateral infiltrates "white out"

Note. Essentials of diagnosis: bilateral pulmonary infiltrates on CXR, normal PAOP ($\leq$ 18 mm Hg), PaO_2/FIO_2 ratio < 200

Differential Diagnosis

- Cardiogenic pulmonary edema
- Pulmonary edema
- Pneumonia

Management

- Fluid resuscitation if hypotension present
- Intubation and mechanical ventilation with PEEP needed to treat hypoxemia
- Lowest level of PEEP and supplemental O_2 required to maintain $PAO_2 > 60$ mm Hg or $SaO_2 > 90\%$ should be used
- Maintain sedation for comfort.
- Nutritional support should be started early (within 24 to 48 hrs). Enteral route should be used if possible.

When to Consult, Refer, or Hospitalize

- All patients require hospitalization and ICU admission.
- Consult pulmonology to assist in management of difficult-to-treat patients

Follow-up

- Educate the patient and family about the disease process.
- Educate the patient and family about the use of mechanical ventilation.
- Provide comfort measures; educate patients on the use of call light and communication strategies.

PNEUMOTHORAX

Description

- Pneumothorax is the presence of gas in the pleural space.

Etiology, Incidence, and Demographics

- Spontaneous pneumothorax
  - Occurs with or without underlying disease
    - Primary pneumothorax: no underlying pulmonary disease present
    - Secondary pneumothorax: underlying pulmonary disease present (e.g., COPD, asthma, tuberculosis)
- Traumatic pneumothorax
- Tension pneumothorax: positive pressure in pleural space throughout respiratory cycle
  - Most commonly due to ventilator use and rescue efforts
  - Life-threatening
    - Positive pleural pressure compromises ventilation.
    - Positive pleural pressure shifts the mediastinum, which decreases venous return to heart.

Risk Factors

- Primary pneumothorax occurs most commonly in thin, young (age 10 to 30 years) males.
- Cigarette smoking
- Family history

Prevention and Screening

- Smoking cessation

Assessment

- Chest pain
- Spontaneous pneumothorax
  - Absent or reduced breath sounds on affected side
- Tension pneumothorax
  - Difficulty in ventilating or high-peak inspiratory pressure on ventilator
  - Absent breath sounds on affected side
  - Mediastinal shift to contralateral side

Diagnostic Studies

- ABG: most commonly reveals hypoxemia and acute respiratory alkalosis
- ECG: left-sided pneumothorax may cause T wave changes
- Chest x-ray: visceral pleural line on expiratory film is diagnostic, secondary pleural effusion may be present
  - Tension pneumothorax: large amount of air in hemithorax and possible contralateral shifting of mediastinum

Differential Diagnosis

- Pulmonary embolus
- Pneumonia

Management

- Supplemental oxygen
- Based on severity
  - Small (15% of a hemithorax), stable, spontaneous, primary pneumothorax may be observed. Small pneumothoraces often resolve spontaneously
  - Spontaneous pneumothorax
    · Needle aspiration if no underlying disease
    · Chest tube placement in most cases with underlying disease
  - Tension pneumothorax
    · Emergent needle aspiration
    · Chest tube placement after aspiration
  - Mechanical ventilation for severe cases

When to Consult, Refer, or Hospitalize

- Most patients will require hospitalization.
- Small spontaneous, primary pneumothoraces may be monitored on an outpatient basis in reliable patients.

Follow-up

- Educate patients on smoking cessation if appropriate (risk of reoccurrence is 50%).
- Avoid exposure to high altitudes.
- Educate regarding procedures (e.g., chest tube placement).

PLEURAL EFFUSION

Description

- Pleural effusion is the collection of fluid in the pleural space.

Etiology, Incidence, and Demographics

- Two types
  - Transudative pleural effusion: occurs in the absence of pleural disease
  - Exudative pleural effusion: most often secondary to pneumonia and malignancy

- Five causes of pleural effusions
  - Normal capillaries, increased production of fluid because increased hydrostatic or decreased oncotic pressure (transudative)
  - Abnormal capillary permeability (exudative)
  - Decreased clearance of lymphatic fluid (exudative)
  - Bleeding in pleural space (hemothorax)
  - Infected fluid in pleural space (empyema)

Risk Factors

- Transudative
  - Heart failure
  - Hypoalbumenemia
  - Cirrhosis
- Exudative
  - Pneumonia
  - Carcinoma
  - Bacterial, viral, or fungal pulmonary infections

Prevention and Screening

- Avoid the conditions that commonly cause pleural effusions (see Risk Factors).

Assessment

- Dyspnea
- Cough
- Pleuritic chest pain
- Small effusions less likely to produce symptoms
- Tachypnea
- Diminished or absent breath sounds
- Dullness to percussion
- Decreased tactile fremitus

Diagnostic Studies

- Chest x-ray: fluid in pleural space
- Laboratory testing: All pleural fluid must be sent for protein, glucose, LDH, total and differential WBC count, GS, and culture.
- Exudates have one of the following characteristics:
  - Ratio of pleural fluid protein to serum protein > 0.5
  - Ratio of pleural fluid LDH to serum LDH > 0.6
  - Pleural fluid LDH > 2/3 the upper limit of normal serum LDH (> 200 IU)
- Transudate characteristics
  - Pleural glucose = serum glucose
  - pH 7.40–7.55
  - Fewer than 1,000 WBC/mL with large number of mononuclear cells

Differential Diagnosis

- Pulmonary edema
- Pulmonary infection

Management

- Goal of treatment is directed at underlying cause
- Thoracentesis
- Transudative effusions
  - Therapeutic thoracentesis for severe dyspnea
  - Pleuradesis and tube thoracostomy

When to Refer, Consult, or Hospitalize

- Admit
  - Patients with moderate to large effusions may require hospitalization for treatment, including thoracentesis or chest tube placement.
  - Admit patients with significant symptoms such as dyspnea.
- Consult
  - Consult appropriate specialist based on underlying etiology of effusion (e.g., oncology if malignancy present).
  - Surgical for recurrent effusions if require pleuradesis

Follow-up

- Educate the patient and family on underlying disease process and etiology.
- Educate patients and prepare them for procedures or surgery as appropriate.

REFERENCES

Barkley, T. W., & Myers, C. (2008). *Practice guidelines for acute care nurse practitioners.* Philadelphia: W. B. Saunders.

Bongard, F., Sue, D., & Vintch, J. (2008). *Current diagnosis and treatment: Critical care* (3rd ed.). New York: Lange/McGraw Hill.

Buttaro, T., Trybulski, J., Bailey, P., & Sandberg-Cook, J. (2008). *Primary care* (3rd ed.). St. Louis, MO: Mosby.

Chesnutt, M.S. & Prendergast, T. J. (2007)Heart. In Tierney, L.M. Jr., McPhee, S.J., & Papadakis, M. A. (Eds.), *Current medical diagnosis and treatment* (p. 269), New York: Lange Medical Books/McGraw-Hill.

Fauci, A. S., Braunwalk, E., Kasper, D. L., Hauser, S. L., Longo, D. L., Jameson, J. L., et al. (2008). *Harrison's principles of internal medicine* (17th ed.). Philadelphia: McGraw Hill.

Fiebach, N. H., Barker, L. R., Burton, J. R., & Zieves, P. D. (2007). *Principles of ambulatory medicine* (7th ed.). Philadelphia: Lippincott, Williams, & Wilkins.

Marino, P. T. (2007). *The ICU book* (3rd ed.). Philadelphia: Lippincott Williams & Wilkins.

McPhee, S., & Papadakis, M. (2010). *Current medical diagnosis and treatment* (49th ed.). New York: Lange/McGraw Hill.

National Asthma Education and Prevention Program. (2007). *Expert panel report 3: Guidelines for the diagnosis and management of asthma.* Bethesda, MD: National Institutes of Health.

Parrillo, J., & Dellinger, R. (Eds.). (2008). *Critical care medicine: Principles of diagnosis and management in the adult* (3rd ed.). St. Louis, MO: Mosby.

Rabe, K. F., Hurd, S., Anzueto, A., Barnes, P. J., Buist, S. A., & Calverly, P., et al. (2007). Global strategy for the diagnosis, management, and prevention of chronic obstructive pulmonary disease: GOLD executive summary. *American Journal of Respiratory and Critical Care Medicine, 176,* 532–555.

6

Endocrine Disorders

Tiffany Boysen, RN, MSN, ACNP-BC, CCRN; Shirlee Drayton-Brooks, PhD, FNP-BC; and Melanie Smith, RN, MSN, ACNP-BC

GENERAL APPROACH

- An endocrine disorder is a defect in one aspect of the endocrine regulatory systems that can cause systemic consequences, morbidity, and death.
- Endocrine disorders generally manifest in one of four ways:
  - Excess hormone (e.g., Cushing's syndrome, excess cortisol secretion)
  - Deficit hormone (e.g., diabetes mellitus [DM] type 1, insulin secretion is low or absent)
  - Abnormal response of end organ to the hormone (pseudohypoparathroidism)
  - Gland enlargement (e.g., pituitary adenoma)
- Endocrine diseases may be associated with a deficiency or hypersecretion of hormones that affect target organs.
- There are basically three types of hormone: *steroids* such as cortisol (adrenal cortex), estrogen, progesterone (ovaries) and testosterone (testes); *amino acids*, tyrosine such as thyroxine (thyroid), catecholamines (adrenal medulla); and *proteins*, peptides such as insulin (pancreas).
  - Regulation of hormone secretion is through a negative feedback system.
  - Patients of all ages may need to carry or wear Medic Alerts or similar identification for many endocrine disorders.

RED FLAGS

- *Type 1 diabetics* may present with *acute ketoacidosis*: nausea, fatigue, abdominal pain, thirst, hunger, polyuria progressing to vomiting, confusion, lethargy, hypotension, fruity breath odor.
- *Type 2 diabetics* may present with hyperglycemic, hyperosmolar, nonketotic syndrome (HHNKS), characterized by confusion and lethargy, blood glucose > 600 mg/dL, minimal or no ketosis, serum osmolality > 320, and profound dehydration.
- *Hypoglycemia* may present as initial headache, hunger, difficulty with problem-solving, sweating, shakiness, tremor, anxiety, irritability, or behavior change; it progresses to coma and seizures without treatment.
- *Acute adrenal insufficiency* or Addisonian crisis may present as severe abdominal pain, nausea and vomiting, hypotension, hypoglycemia, and shock; it is precipitated by surgery, infection, exacerbation of comorbid illness, or sudden withdrawal of long-term glucocorticoid replacement.

DIABETES MELLITUS

Centers for Disease Control and Prevention (CDC) definition

Diabetes mellitus is a group of diseases marked by high blood glucose resulting from defects in insulin production, insulin action, or both (CDC, 2011).

Incidence

- 23.6 million people in the United States had diabetes mellitus in 2007; 1 million of these had type 1 and the rest had mostly type 2.

DIABETES MELLITUS TYPE 1

Description

- Diabetes mellitus type 1 is previously known as insulin-dependent diabetes mellitus (IDDM) or juvenile-onset diabetes.
- Develops as a result of an autoimmune response or environmental trigger that causes pancreatic islet beta cell destruction, resulting in an absence of or failure to produce insulin

Etiology

- Destruction of beta cells in pancreatic islets and absolute deficiency or failure to produce insulin related to autoimmune response or environmental trigger (e.g., virus)
- Human leukocyte antigens HLA, HLA-DR3, or HLA-DR4, associated with type 1
- May be triggered in susceptible individuals by viruses, toxic chemical agents, or cytotoxins
- Genetic susceptibility influenced by environmental factors
- Hyperglycemia results from inability of glucose to enter cell for use as energy.
- Ketoacidosis results from the use of free fatty acids for energy.

Incidence

- Type 1 accounts for 5% to 10% of all diabetes cases in the United States.
- Generally occurs in puberty between 8 and 14 years old
- Highest prevalence in Scandinavia, where 20% of diabetics are type 1; Japan and China < 1%
- Idiopathic etiology most common in individuals of Asian or African descent
- Can develop in adulthood but rarely occurs after age 30 and very rarely in older adults
  - 90% result of autoimmune response or environmental factor
  - 10% idiopathic

Risk Factors

- First-degree relative with type 1 diabetes mellitus
- Autoimmune
- Genetic
- Environmental

Preventions and Screening

- No prevention identified and no routine screening in childhood

Assessment

History
- Acute onset of
  - Polyuria, polydipsia, polyphagia
  - Weight loss with normal or increased appetite, anorexia
  - Blurred vision, fatigue
  - Abdominal pain, nausea and vomiting, dehydration, hypoglycemic or ketotic episodes
- Nocturnal enuresis
- Nightmares, night sweats, or headache may indicate nocturnal hypoglycemia in both children and adults.
- Family history of diabetes

Physical Examination
- Late disease: ophthalmic changes—microaneurysm with soft and hard exudates, deep retinal hemorrhages, neovascularization, cataracts, glaucoma; peripheral vascular insufficiency; diminished deep tendon reflex
- Possible cardiovascular changes occurring in late disease: postural hypotension, resting tachycardia, "silent" myocardial infarctions
- Possible peripheral vascular changes occurring in late disease: cool extremities because of decreased circulation, decreased pulses, edema, delayed capillary refill
- Possible neurological changes occurring in late disease: diminished pain sensation, proprioception, vibration, light touch, absent lower extremity reflexes, dysfunction in extraocular movements, weakness, ataxic gait, paresthesias, change in level of consciousness

Diagnostic Studies
- Random glucose level > 200 mg/dL plus symptoms of polyuria, polydipsia, and weight loss or subsequent day fasting plasma glucose (FPG) > 126 mg/dL
- FPG > 126 mg/dL on two occasions
- FPG from 100 to 126 mg/dL classified as impaired fasting blood glucose.
- Blood glucose between 140 and 199 mg/dL after a 2-hr oral glucose tolerance test considered impaired glucose tolerance
- Glucosuria
- Ketonuria (only in type 1)
- May consider C peptide or insulin level (decreased)
- Islet cell antibodies present in approximately 90% of patients
- Baseline diagnostic studies: BUN, serum creatinine, urinalysis, urine microalbumin, and fasting lipid profile; glycosylated hemoglobin (HbA1c) (5.5% to 7% good control)
- ECG and chest x-ray for coronary and pulmonary pathology in adults
- Elevated BUN and creatinine if dehydrated; hypertriglyceridemia: triglyceride levels > 150 mg/dL
- Thyroid-stimulating hormone (TSH) level

Differential Diagnosis

- Diabetes mellitus type 2
- Diabetes insipidus
- Pancreatitis or pancreatic disease
- Pheochromocytoma
- Cushing's syndrome
- Acromegaly
- Liver disease
- Salicylate poisoning
- Glycosuria without hyperglycemia in renal tubular disease or benign renal glycosuria
- Secondary effects of oral contraceptives, corticosteroids, thiazides, phenytoin, nicotinic acid
- Severe stress from trauma, burns, or infection
- Urinary tract infection (UTI)

Management

Nonpharmacologic Treatment
- Obtain history and baseline studies
  - Family history, age on onset
  - Obesity
  - Cardiovascular risk factors: smoking, hypertension, hyperlipidemia, oral contraceptive use
  - Fasting triglycerides, total cholesterol, HDL-cholesterol, electrocardiogram, BUN/creatinine
  - Peripheral pulses assessment
  - Neurologic, podiatric, and ophthalmologic exams
- Patient education
  - Basic pathophysiology, cause, general management
  - Long-term complications of type 1 DM
  - Administration of insulin and medications
- Short- and long-term treatment goals: blood glucose average 80 to 120 mg/dL preprandially and 100 to 140 mg/dL at bedtime; HgbA1c < 7%
- Lifestyle modifications: diet, exercise, smoking cessation (if appropriate), avoid alcohol
- Medical nutrition therapy prescribed by a registered dietician, following American Diabetes Association (ADA) guidelines; constant reinforcement from all providers
- General ADA dietary guidelines for adults
  - 45 to 65% of calories from carbohydrates
  - 25 to 35% from fat (7% of this from saturated fat)
  - 10 to 35% from protein
  - Limit cholesterol to 300 mg daily.
- Daily exercise regimen for adults
- Multidisciplinary approach to care of patient
  - Involve family, parents (if appropriate), significant others (if appropriate), primary care physician, nurse educator, endocrinologist, dietician
  - Teach family, parents, significant others the signs of hypoglycemia
  - Glucose monitoring education: AC and HS, check for urine ketones if blood glucose > 300 mg/dL, during illness, stress, pregnancy, or symptoms of ketosis such as nausea, vomiting, or abdominal pain
  - Keep self-monitoring glucose log (SMBG)
- Establish foot care plan
- Establish dental care plan
- Annual eye examination
- Teach patient, parent, or both how to modify therapy if patient is ill. "Sick day guidelines" require continuing usual dose of insulin, frequent SMBG, and adjustment of insulin if necessary; check urine for ketones if SMBG >300 mg/dL; increase intake of fluids.
- Referral to local support groups and American Diabetes Association
- Medic Alert or similar identification bracelet or necklace
- Inform school, work, and friends of condition
- Pneumococcal vaccine and annual influenza vaccines

Pharmacologic Treatment

- Individual presenting with ketones must be started on insulin. Goal of therapy is to maintain blood sugar as follows:
  - Fasting: 70 to 130 mg/dL
  - Preprandial: 70 to 130 mg/dL
  - Postprandial: < 180 mg/dL
- Insulin regimens are individualized
  - Total daily dose (TDD)—usually start at 0.2 to 0.8 units/kg/day
  - Basal: 40%–50% is given as intermediate or long-acting (NPH twice daily, insulin detemir once or twice daily, or glargine once daily).
  - Basal should be given despite NPO status.
  - Premeal insulin (remaining portion of TDD): one-third of this should be given before or after each meal.
  - Premeal insulin is held when patient is NPO.
  - Sliding scale should be a part of the insulin regimen and combined with premeal insulin injections.
- Insulin doses in general can be divided into 2 to 4 injections per day or continuous subcutaneous insulin infusion (insulin pump) once stabilized; typical regimen for adults is two injections per day.
- Adjust insulin doses according to glucose monitoring.
- Honeymoon period or remission phase after diagnosis may last from several months to 2 years.
- Insulin glargine (Lantus) is a long-acting preparation designed for once-a-day administration at bedtime. It cannot be mixed with other types of insulin.

When to Consult, Refer, or Hospitalize

- Hospitalize adults with diabetic ketoacidosis (DKA) and severe infections.
- Refer unstable adult or geriatric patients; consider co-management of all type 1 DM patients.
- Refer all families to diabetic educator, and registered dietitian.
- Ophthalmologist: initial screening and annual exam for diabetic retinopathy and visual problems; all patients > 30 years
- Dentist: routine check-ups and for dental complaints
- Podiatrist: routine foot care in older adults and for foot problems as indicated
- Consider psychological counseling if needed to address issues of altered body image and individual and family stressors related to disease and management.

Follow-up

- Continue ongoing follow-up and consultation with endocrinologist and diabetic educator.
- Routine diabetes visits: daily for initiation of insulin or change in regimen, at least quarterly for patients not meeting their goals, and semiannually for other patients
- HbA1c every 3 to 6 months

- Glycosylated hemoglobin (HbA1c): target goal is 6%; normal range 4% to 6%; each % correlates to 30 mg/dL FPG elevation; provides index of glycemic control for life of red blood cell, 8 to 12 weeks
- Serum fructosamine: glycosylated protein (primarily albumin); normal value is 1.5–2.4 mmol/L; provides index of glycemic control for preceding 2 to 3 weeks; low albumin levels will lower fructosamine levels; useful when hemolytic states affect HbA1c measures
- Annual physical exam with primary care provider
- Thyroid function tests initially, then every 2 to 3 years for adults

Expected Outcomes
- Chronic, lifelong disease with no cure

Complications
- Hypoglycemia signs and symptoms: shakiness, weakness, sweating, headache, tachycardia, nervousness, dizziness, hunger, irritability, convulsions, coma
- **Somogyi effect**: early morning rebound hyperglycemia because of nocturnal hypoglycemia; around 3:00 a.m., serum glucose falls and patient is hypoglycemic; counterregulatory hormones compensate by mobilizing glucose stores; patient rebounds and becomes hyperglycemic by early morning; *treated by reducing or eliminating p.m. or hs doses to eliminate nocturnal hypoglycemia*
- **Dawn phenomenon**: hyperglycemia because of hepatic gluconeogenesis in early morning. Peripheral tissue insulin receptors become desensitized to insulin nocturnally, believed to be result of insulin receptor desensitizing property of growth hormone. Around 3:00 a.m., blood sugar measures either normal or high normal and get progressively higher throughout the night, is elevated at 7 a.m. *Treatment is to increase p.m. long-acting insulin or add an hs dose.*
- Lipodystrophy (destruction of subcutaneous fat at injection sites): seen less with use of synthetic human insulin than beef or pork insulin
- Retinopathy
- Nephropathy and renal failure
- Cardiovascular disease with lipid abnormalities; premature atherosclerosis
- Cerebrovascular disease
- Diabetic ketoacidosis
- Insulin resistance with long-term, high-dose therapy
- Peripheral neuropathy
- Autonomic nervous system problems, incontinence, and erectile dysfunction
- Infections
- Foot and skin ulcerations
- Insulin allergy

DIABETES MELLITUS TYPE 2

Description

Diabetes mellitus type 2 is a metabolic disease that causes hyperglycemia, characterized by insulin resistance in target tissues, decrease in insulin receptors, impairment of insulin secretion, or a combination of these. It was formerly known as non-insulin-dependent diabetes mellitus (NIDDM), adult onset, type 2, nonketotic diabetes.

Etiology

- Genetically and clinically, a heterogeneous disorder with familial pattern
- Influenced by environmental factors, physical inactivity, and diet high in refined carbohydrates and fat with low fiber
- Two major types
  - Obese type 2 diabetes: most common
    - Initial peripheral insulin receptor insensitivity, possibly because of cellular distention secondary to increased fat accumulation
    - Beta cell compensates by increasing insulin release; hyperglycemia does not occur
    - Over time, beta cells may "burn out," insulin release falls, and hyperglycemia occurs as a result of the insulin receptor insensitivity.
  - Non-obese type 2 diabetes
    - Initial problem may be blunted response of beta cells to glucose
    - Glucose does not trigger adequate insulin release.
    - Insulin resistance is not clinically significant.
    - More common in Asian populations
- No human leukocyte antigen or islet cell antibodies
  - Associated with metabolic syndrome or syndrome X:
    - Involves abdominal obesity, hypertension, glucose intolerance, increased triglycerides, low HDL cholesterol, and small, dense LDL cholesterol
  - Diagnostic criteria
    - Fasting glucose > or equal to 110 mg/dL
    - Waist circumference > 40 inches in men and > 35 inches in women
    - Triglycerides > or equal to 150 mg/dL
    - HDL cholesterol < 40 mg/dL in men and < 50 mg/dL in women
    - BP > or equal to 130/85 mm Hg
    - Effects approximately 22% of Americans and prevalent in older people, women, Hispanics, and Blacks
    - Increase of cardiovascular events and death

Incidence

- Associated with obesity, family history of diabetes mellitus, age, history of gestational diabetes, impaired glucose metabolism, physical inactivity, and race and ethnicity
- At-risk racial and ethnic groups: Blacks, Hispanic and Latino Americans, Native Americans, some Asian Americans, and some Native Hawaiians or other Pacific Islanders
- Usually occurs in obese adults > 30 years
- Female > male
- Accounts for 90% to 95% of all cases of diabetes mellitus

Risk Factors

- Obesity/inactivity, > 20% ideal body weight, or body mass index (BMI) > 27 kg/m$_2$
- Family history of diabetes type 2
- Gestational diabetes—at risk for developing type 2 diabetes within 5 to 10 years postparturition
- Delivery of macrosomic infant, > 9 lbs
- Previously impaired glucose tolerance
- > 45 years old
- Member of one of the at-risk racial or ethnic groups
- Metabolic syndrome or syndrome X
- HDL cholesterol < or equal to 35 mg/dL, triglycerides > 250 mg/dL, or both
- Hypertension
- Polycystic ovary disease
- History of vascular disease

Prevention and Screening

- Should be done at 3-year intervals starting at age 45, particularly for patients with BMI > 25 or earlier for at-risk patients; more often if FPG near 126 mg/dL
- Fasting plasma glucose preferred over oral glucose tolerance test
- Secondary prevention of complications is essential.

Assessment

History
- More insidious onset than type 1 diabetes
- Obesity, blurred vision, chronic skin infections, polyuria, polydipsia, polyphagia, weight loss, fatigue, slow-healing wounds, recurrent infections (especially *Candida* and UTIs), spontaneous abortion
- History related to type 2 diabetes: more prominent macrovascular changes than microvascular, such as vascular insufficiency, cardiovascular/cerebrovascular disease, and atherosclerosis
- History of HHNKs: precipitating factors, including treatment with calcium channel blockers, propranolol, corticosteroids, thiazides, phenytoin

Physical Examination

- Usually discovered on routine exam with elevated glucose level
- *Candida* vaginitis may be presenting factor in some women
- Central obesity
- Hypertension
- Advanced stages
  - Orthostatic blood pressure changes
  - Weight loss
  - Skin infections present
  - Visual and funduscopic changes: microaneuryms with soft (cotton wool) and hard exudates, deep retinal hemorrhages, neovascularization, cataracts, glaucoma
  - Oral *Candida* infections
  - Peripheral vascular: decreased circulation, cool extremities, decreased pulses, edema, capillary refill > 3 seconds
  - Neurologic: decreased sensation of pain, proprioception, vibration, light touch, absent lower extremity reflexes, dysfunction in extraocular movements, weakness, ataxic gait

Diagnostic Studies

- Random glucose level > 200 mg/dL plus symptoms of polyuria, polydipsia, and weight loss or subsequent day fasting plasma glucose (FPG) > 126 mg/dL
- FPG > 126 mg/dL on 2 occasions
- FPG from 100 to 126 mg/dL classified as impaired fasting blood glucose
- Blood glucose between 140 and 199 mg/dL after a 2-hr oral glucose tolerance test considered impaired glucose tolerance
- Glucosuria
- An individual with an impaired fasting glucose, impaired glucose tolerance test, or both is thought to be "prediabetic," meaning their blood glucose levels are higher than normal, but not high enough to be diabetic; at increased risk for developing type 2 diabetes, stroke, and heart disease
- Baseline studies: urinalysis for protein, glucose, and ketones (ketones present only in type 1); microalbuminuria screening at initial diagnosis
- Other baseline studies: BUN, urine and serum creatinine, fasting serum cholesterol and lipid profile, TSH, ECG; chest x-ray if clinically indicated

Differential Diagnosis

- Diabetes mellitus type 1
- Diabetes insipidus
- Pancreatitis or pancreatic disease
- Pheochromocytoma
- Cushing syndrome
- Liver disease
- Glycosuria without hyperglycemia in renal tubular disease or benign renal glycosuria
- Secondary effects of oral contraceptives, corticosteroids, thiazides, phenytoin, or nicotinic acid
- Severe stress from trauma, burns, or infection

Management

Common Treatment Plan With Goal of FPG 80 to 100 mg/dL and HbA1c < 7.0%
- Diet and exercise
- Oral monotherapy
- Add second drug class
- Add third drug class or insulin

Goals of Therapy
- Preprandial blood glucose 90 to 130 mg/dL
- Postprandial blood glucose < 180 mg/dL
- HgbA1C < 7.0 %
- Lipids
  - LDL < 100 mg/dL
  - HDL > 40 mg/dL
  - Triglycerides < 150 mg/dL
- Blood pressure < 130/80 mm Hg
- Reduce or eliminate micro- and macrovascular effects of DM.
- Eliminate symptoms of hyperglycemia.
- Maintain quality of life.

Nonpharmacologic Treatment
- Patient education
  - Basic pathophysiology, cause, general management
  - Long-term complications of type 2 DM
  - Administration of insulin and medications
- Lifestyle modifications: diet, exercise, smoking cessation (if appropriate), alcohol avoidance
- Patients with fasting plasma glucose levels < 250 mg/dL should be treated initially with medical nutrition therapy and lifestyle modifications.
- Medical nutrition therapy prescribed by a registered dietician, following American Diabetes Association (ADA) guidelines; constant reinforcement from all providers
- Weight reduction of 5 to 10 lbs increases insulin sensitivity.
- General ADA dietary guidelines for adults
  - 45% to 65% of calories from carbohydrates
  - 25% to 35% from fat (7% of this from saturated fat)
  - 10% to 35% from protein
  - Limit cholesterol to 300 mg daily.
- Multidisciplinary approach to care of patient
  - Involve family, significant others, other identified support systems, PCP, nurse educator, endocrinologist, dietician
  - Teach family, significant others, those in support systems, the signs of hypoglycemia
  - Teach glucose monitoring; should be done daily and more frequently when altering or initiating therapy
- Perform stress test if > 35 years old with DM
- Referral to local support groups and ADA
- Medic Alert or similar identification bracelet or necklace
- Foot care plan
- Annual influenza and pneumococcal vaccinations

Pharmacologic Treatment

- Should be initiated once medical nutrition therapy and lifestyle modifications are no longer effective
- Sulfonylureas
  - Glipizide, glimepiride
  - Pancreatic islet beta cell insulin-release stimulator
  - Good in controlling postprandial hyperglycemia
  - Can cause hypoglycemia and weight gain of 2 to 5 kg
- Meglitinides
  - Prandin
  - Pancreatic islet beta cell insulin-release stimulator
  - Short-acting
  - Good postprandial blood glucose control with less risk of hypoglycemia than the sulfonylureas
- Biguanides
  - Metformin
  - Decrease hepatic glucose production; increase action on muscle glucose uptake
  - Contraindicated in renal dysfunction, chronic heart failure requiring treatment, use cautiously in many conditions that may predispose to lactic acidosis
- Thiazolidinediones
  - Avandia, Actos
  - Increase insulin action on muscle and fat glucose uptake
  - Take precautions with those with hepatic dysfunction, cardiac disease, or anovulatory conditions
- Alpha-glucosidase inhibitors
  - Precose, glyset
  - Short-acting
  - Take before meals; contraindicated in those with inflammatory bowel disease and other intestinal conditions—use glucose rather than sucrose for hypoglycemia
- Incretins
  - Byetta, Januvia
  - Given by injection
  - Stimulate insulin secretion, lowers post prandial blood glucose and has less side effects of hypoglycemia and weight gain
- Dipeptidyl peptidase-4 inhibitors
  - Januvia
  - Inhibits dipeptidyl peptidase, the enzyme that breaks down glucogan—like peptide-1; GLP-1 is a "gut hormone," which stimulates insulin secretion in relation to glucose
  - Adverse effects: angioedema, Stevens-Johnson syndrome, upper respiratory infection
- If blood glucose is not controlled two oral agents, then insulin should be initiated.
  - Start with 0.6 to > 1.0 units/kg/day.
  - Can be added to oral agent and given as once-daily dose at bedtime or before breakfast
  - If oral agent plus basal insulin not effective, then add premeal insulin before breakfast and dinner (short or rapid acting)
  - Goal: ensure patient is receiving appropriate amount of insulin each day, rather than the pattern in which it is given
  - May require up to > 2 units/kg/day
- If FPG > 400 mg/dL or patient has signs of ketoacidosis, insulin therapy required

- Patients with metabolic syndrome (syndrome X or insulin-resistance syndrome) require treatment for hyperglycemia, hypertension, dyslipidemia, and weight loss.
- Other agents
  - ACEI or ARBs—for patients with early nephropathy even without hypertension, or as treatment of hypertension in diabetics
  - Aspirin daily (75, 81, 162, or 325 mg)—cardiovascular protection in patients who are 40 years old and older or have other risk factors
  - Medications to treat dyslipidemia

Special Considerations

- Older adults
  - Frail or mentally disabled older adults are likely to have hypoglycemic events as a result of forgetting to take medication as prescribed; incidence of falls may increase.

When to Consult, Refer, or Hospitalize

- Endocrinologist referral for uncontrolled hyperglycemia
- Hospitalize for severe infections, HHNKS characterized by blood glucose > 600 mg/dL, minimal ketosis, serum osmolality > 320, and profound dehydration
- Diabetic educator for further teaching for all patients
- Registered dietitian for further nutritional teaching
- Ophthalmologist: initial screening and annual exam for diabetic retinopathy and visual problems; all patients > 30 years
- Podiatrist for routine foot care in older adults and foot problems as indicated

Follow-up

- When first diagnosed or when adjusting medications, see weekly, then biweekly, monthly; well-controlled diabetic patients, see every 6 months
- Annual urine protein, FPG, lipid profile, creatinine, ECG, full physical exam with funduscopic and neurologic exams, complete foot inspection
- If treated with medication, obtain HbA1c every 3 to 6 months; goal < 7%
- Thyroid function tests as indicated

Expected Outcomes
- Chronic, lifelong disease with no cure

Complications
- Hypoglycemia
- Lipodystrophy (destruction of subcutaneous fat at injection sites)
- Retinopathy
- Nephropathy and renal failure
- Cardiovascular disease with lipid abnormalities; premature atherosclerosis
- Cerebrovascular disease

- Hyperglycemic hyperosmolar nonketotic coma (HHNK)
- Diabetic ketoacidosis (DKA)
- Insulin resistance with long-term, high-dose therapy
- Peripheral neuropathy

- **Somogyi effect**
  - Early morning rebound hyperglycemia because of nocturnal hypoglycemia
  - Around 3:00 a.m., serum glucose falls and patient is hypoglycemic.
  - Counterregulatory hormones compensate by mobilizing glucose stores.
  - Patient rebounds and becomes hyperglycemic by early morning.
  - Treated by reducing or eliminating p.m. or hs doses

- **Dawn phenomenon**
  - Hyperglycemia because of hepatic gluconeogenesis in early morning
  - Peripheral tissue insulin receptors become desensitized to insulin nocturnally; believed to be result of insulin receptor desensitizing property of growth hormone
  - Around 3:00 a.m., blood sugar measures either normal or high normal, progressively higher throughout the night and elevated at 7:00 a.m.
  - Treatment is to increase p.m. long-acting insulin or add hs dose

DIABETIC KETOACIDOSIS

Description

- Diabetic ketoacidosis (DKA) is an insulin deficiency associated with infection, trauma, myocardial infarction, or surgery.
- Insulin deficiency results in hyperglycemia, which causes intracellular dehydration.
- Insulin deficiency, which triggers the body to burn fatty acids, results in the production of ketones.

Etiology

- Usually occurs as a result of infection, trauma, surgery, or myocardial infarction
- May be presenting factor for type 1

Incidence

- Occurs more frequently in type 1
- Occurs in 46 of 10,000 diabetic patients
- Mortality between 1% and 10%

Risk Factors

- Sepsis
- Trauma
- Infection
- Myocardial infarction
- Interruption in insulin therapy

Prevention and Screening

- Instruct patients on importance of compliance and insulin adjustment for "sick days" and times of increased metabolic demands

Assessment

History
- Similar to presentation of type 1 diabetes
- Presence of a risk factor
- Polyuria, polydipsia, polyuria
- Weight loss, nausea and vomiting, abdominal pain

Physical Examination
- Altered level of consciousness
- Kussmaul respirations
- Fruity breath odor
- Decreased capillary refill
- Tachycardia

Diagnosis
- Acidosis (pH < 7.30)
- Serum bicarbonate < 15 mEq/L
- Ketonemia
- Hyperglycemia > 250 mg/dL (usually 350 to 900 mg/dL)
- Hyperkalemia
- Elevated BUN/creatinine
- PCO_2 low (hyperventilation)
- Increased serum osmolality

Differential Diagnosis
- Hyponatremia
- Severe dehydration
- Uremia
- Hyperammonemia
- Drug overdose
- Sepsis

Management

Nonpharmacologic Treatment
- Patient should be in ICU for moderate or severe ketoacidosis
- Maintain airway and provide supplemental oxygen as needed.
- Supportive care
- Nasogastric tube in comatose patient due to risk of aspiration from gastric atony
- Indwelling catheter for accurate intake and output
- Central venous catheter to assess the degree of hypovolemia in patients with renal or cardiovascular disease or those with severe cardiovascular collapse
- Record plasma glucose hourly during initial treatment period
- Identify and treat underlying cause

Pharmacologic Treatment
- Fluid replacement
  - Start with 1 liter NS bolus followed by 1 liter, 500 cc/hour to maintain urine output and stable hemodynamics
  - After above, fusion rate may be decreased to between 150 and 500 cc/hour depending on patient needs
  - Use ½ NS for normal or elevated sodium levels and 0.9% NS for low sodium levels
  - Once blood glucose is < 250 mg/dL, change to D5 ½ NS to prevent hypoglycemia
- Hyperglycemia
  - Start with 0.15 unit/kg IV bolus of regular insulin
  - Start continuous infusion of regular insulin at 0.1 unit/kg/hr in 0.9% saline
  - Goal is to decrease blood glucose levels at a rate of 50–75 mg/dL/hr
  - Once blood glucose is < 250 mg/dL, decrease rate of infusion to 0.05 unit/kg/hr to prevent hypoglycemia
- Sodium bicarbonate
  - If pH < 7.1, initiate infusion of 1 liter ½ NS with 50–100 mEq of sodium bicarbonate; can be given over 1 hr
  - Monitor for hypokalemia; consider 10 mEq KCL with each liter

Potassium
- Total body potassium loss maybe as high as 200 mEq
- If the patient is not uremic and has adequate urinary output, potassium chloride in doses of 10–30 mEq/hr should be infused during the second and third hours after the initiation of therapy.
  - Start sooner if the initial serum potassium is inappropriately normal or low; should be delayed if the serum potassium does not respond to initial therapy and the potassium level remains above 5 mEq/L (usually in the presence of chronic kidney disease)
  - Monitor electrocardiogram; peaked T waves are a sign of hyperkalemia, flattened T waves with U waves indicate hypokalemia.

Phosphate
- Replacement seldom required in treatment of DKA and reserved for severe cases Hypophosphatemia < 1 mg/dL

When to Consult, Refer, or Hospitalize

- DKA patients should be hospitalized and have endocrinology involved in care.

Follow-up

Expected Outcomes
- Mortality rate 1% to 10%
- Shock and coma on admission increase mortality.
- Rapid initiation of therapy improves outcome.

Complications
- Lactic acidosis
- Arterial thrombus
- Cerebral edema (more in children than adults)
- Rebound ketoacidosis

HYPEROSMOLAR HYPERGLYCEMIC NONKETOSIS

Description
- In hyperosmolar hyperglycemic nonketosis (HHNK), dehydration and hyperosmolality develop as a result of hyperglycemia-induced osmotic diuresis.
- The patient is unable to keep up with his or her fluid needs because of the osmotic diuresis.

Etiology

- Usually occurs as result of acute infection, glucocorticoid administration, diuretics, noncompliance, stroke, myocardial infarction, or surgery

Incidence

- Occurs more in type 2
- Affects older adults and middle-aged patients
- Mortality rate of up to 40%
- Underlying congestive heart failure or chronic kidney disease usually present

Risk Factors

- Acute infection
- Glucocorticoids
- Diuretics
- Medical noncompliance
- Stroke
- Recent surgery
- Myocardial infarction

Prevention and Screening

- Instruct patients on importance of compliance and insulin adjustment for "sick days" and times of increased metabolic demands

Assessment

History
- Presence of one of the risk factors
- Onset is over days or weeks
- Recent inability to control blood glucose
- Increasing weakness/fatigue
- Polyuria, polydipsia
- Reduced oral fluid intake
- Nausea

Physical Examination
- Decreased level of consciousness
- Signs of dehydration

Diagnostic Data
- Hyperglycemia > 600 mg/dL (sometimes > 1,000 mg/dL)
- Hyperosmolality > 320 mOsm/L
- No ketones present
- Elevated BUN/creatinine
- pH > 7.3

Differential Diagnosis

- Hyponatremia
- Severe dehydration
- Uremia
- Hyperammonemia
- Drug overdose
- Sepsis

Management

Nonpharmacologic Treatment
- Patient should be in ICU setting
- Maintain airway
- Identify and treat underlying cause
- Supportive care

Pharmacologic Treatment
- Fluid replacement
  - May require up to 4–6 L in the first 8–10 hrs
  - Start with 0.9% normal saline or ½ NS
  - When blood glucose reaches 250 mg/dL, dextrose 5% should be added to IV solution
  - Goal is to keep blood glucose between 250 and 300 mg/dL
  - Adequate fluid replacement is accomplished when urine output is at least 50 cc/hr
  - Hyperglycemia
  - 0.15 units/kg IV bolus
  - Then 0.1 unit/kg/hour infusion
  - Goal is to lower blood glucose by 50–70 mg/dl/hr

Follow-up

Expected Outcomes
- Mortality rate up to 40%
- Outcomes improve with rapid initiation of treatment.

Complications
- Adult respiratory distress syndrome
- Rhabdomyolysis
- Cerebral edema
- Pulmonary embolism
- Disseminated intravascular coagulation

HYPOGLYCEMIA

Description

- Hypoglycemia is defined as plasma glucose concentration < 50 mg/dL (value may vary by lab); may be asymptomatic; plasma glucose level of < 30 mg/dL is usually symptomatic.
- Can be classified as reactive (within 5 hours of eating) or fasting (occurs > 5 hours after a meal)
  - Reactive hypoglycemia is rare; more likely is pseudo-hypoglycemia (symptoms without drop in blood glucose; cause unclear)

Etiology

- Most commonly caused by excess exogenous insulin in diabetics, but may result from use of some oral antihyperglycemic agents; precipitated by change in quantity and timing of activity and food
- At the onset of hypoglycemia, the parasympathetic nervous system is activated, causing hunger, which is followed by activation of the sympathetic nervous system (nervousness, sweating, tachycardia); known as "Whipple's Triad," which consists of low plasma glucose, parasympathetic and sympathetic symptoms, and relief with ingestion of carbohydrates
- Other causes: benign functional disturbance of insulin secretion, pancreatic beta cell tumor (insulinoma); autoimmune process (very rare); ethanol ingestion; glucocorticoid and growth hormone deficiencies; malnutrition; gastrointestinal surgery; chronic disease states (hepatic, renal, chronic heart failure [CHF])

Incidence

- Most prevalent in diabetic patients on insulin and sulfonylureas

Risk Factors

- Type 1 DM, type 2 DM on insulin or sulfonylureas
- Enzyme defects
- Liver disease, insulinoma
- Medication use such as disopyramide (Norpace), pentamidine, quinine
- Pregnancy (third trimester)
- Pituitary or adrenal insufficiency
- Alcohol abuse

Assessment

History
- Symptom history, especially if occurs postprandially or when fasting; may occur following excessive exercise
- Initial symptoms of headache, hunger, difficulty problem-solving; may have sweating, shakiness, tremor, anxiety, irritability, behavior change
- Progresses to coma and seizures without treatment
- Insulinoma: morning headaches, morning confusion, nocturnal or early-morning seizures

Physical Examination
- Altered mental status; tachycardia; hypotension; pale, cool, and clammy skin; coma

Diagnostic Studies
- Serum glucose level < 50 mg/dL indicates hypoglycemia (varies by laboratory)
- Consider drug testing for ethyl alcohol or sulfonylurea, liver function, BUN, creatinine, cortisol tests to identify associated factors in a diabetic patient
- In nondiabetic patient, also get C peptide levels, insulin, insulin antibodies, oral glucose tolerance test
- If cause not identified, additional testing after 72-hour fast may be done by specialist

Differential Diagnosis

- Pseudo-hypoglycemia
- Anxiety and panic
- Factitious hypoglycemia
- Other causes of coma
- See conditions listed under Etiology

Management

Nonpharmacologic Treatment
- Avoid fasting, alcohol use; snack before exercise
- Caffeine restriction (mimics symptoms)
- Avoid simple carbohydrates or beverages with high sugar content
- Diet: high protein with complex carbohydrates, frequent small meals approximately 6x/day
- Avoid causative agents
- Insulinomas and nesidioblastosis: surgery

Pharmacologic Treatment
- If able to take oral substances, consume two glucose tablets or five Life Savers candies (equivalent to 10 to 15 g glucose) at onset of symptoms, followed by complex carbohydrates after acute reaction is controlled

- If patient is unconscious or unable to swallow, home or office management could include 1 mg glucagon IM or SC (adult and adolescent: roll on side in case of vomiting; patient should be transported to an acute care facility for further monitoring and treatment

Special Considerations

- Some drugs, such as beta-adrenergic antagonists, mask the symptoms of hypoglycemia.
- Men can fast for 72 hours and maintain plasma glucose level above 50 mg/dL, whereas women exhibit progressive decrease in plasma glucose during prolonged fasting.
- Geriatric patients may have blunted autonomic response and present with confusion and impaired central nervous system (CNS) function.

When to Consult, Refer, or Hospitalize

- Refer for suspected insulinoma and nesidioblastosis to adult or pediatric surgeon as appropriate.
- Consult with physician or refer to endocrinologist for any unknown or uncontrollable cause.
- Activate the emergency medical system for all unconscious patients.

Follow-up
- Educate patient and family about prevention, symptoms, and treatment of hypoglycemia
- Monitor insulin and sulfonylurea dosage carefully based on patient's diet and activity

Expected Outcomes
- Variable and dependent on etiology, but favorable prognosis with appropriate treatment

Complications
- Brain damage and tissue death from prolonged low glucose level

THYROID DISORDERS

HYPERTHYROIDISM (THYROTOXICOSIS)

Description

- Hyperthyroidism (thyrotoxicosis) is a clinical condition that is associated with elevated levels of T_4 or T_3.
- Manifestations include excessive metabolic activities.

Etiology

- Graves' disease (most common cause)
- Thyroiditis
- Hyperfunctioning single nodular and multinodular goiter (toxic nodular goiter, Plummer's disease)
- Pituitary tumor
- Drug-induced—with iodide and iodide-containing drugs (amiodarone) and contrast media
- Exogenous ingestion of thyroid hormone (factitia)
- Struma ovarii
- Thyroid cancer
- HCG-secreting tumors
- Testicular embryonal carcinoma
- Pregnancy

Incidence

- Graves' disease accounts for 85% of cases of hyperthyroidism; autoantibodies against diffuse fractions of the gland catalyze accelerated hormone production and release
- Affects women > men, 8:1
- Typical age at onset in adulthood is mid-20s through 30s, but can occur in the elderly

Risk Factors

- Family history of thyroid disorders and autoimmune disorders
- Thyroid replacement hormone ingestion
- Other history of autoimmune disorder

Prevention and Screening
- Monitor TSH and T4 for patients taking thyroid replacement hormones.

Assessment

History
- Heat intolerance, weight loss, weakness, palpitations, oligomenorrhea, fatigue, hypersensitivity to heat
- Mental: insomnia, nightmares, irritability, anxiety, psychosis; in elderly, severe depression
- GI: increased appetite, loose stools, increased frequency of bowel movements, pernicious vomiting
- Medication history, past medical history, family history of autoimmune disease

Physical Examination
- Adrenergic: nervousness, sweating, tachycardia, tremor, lid lag, excitability
- Skin: onycholysis, myxedema, hyperpigmentation, flushes, diaphoresis, thin or fine hair, spider angiomas
- Eyes (only in Graves' disease): periorbital edema, exophthalmos, chemosis, ophthalmoplegia, papilledema, blurred vision, photophobia, diplopia
- Neck: goiter smooth or nodular, thyroid bruit or thrill
- Cardiac: sinus tachycardia, atrial fibrillation, worsening of coronary artery disease or heart failure, systolic flow murmurs, widened pulse pressure
- Respiratory: dyspnea on exertion, tachypnea
- Muscle: proximal myopathy, periodic paralysis, progressive wasting of muscles
- Lymph nodes: lymphadenopathy, splenomegaly
- Bone: osteoporosis, hypercalcemia
- Reproductive: abortion, infertility, abnormal menses, testicular atrophy, gynecomastia
- Neurological: brisk tendon reflexes, fine tremor, proximal weakness

Diagnostic Studies
- Decreased TSH–best initial test
- Elevated T4
- Elevated T3
- Elevated erythrocyte sedimentation rate
- ANA levels elevated without evidence of autoimmune disease
- Hypercalcemia
- Decrease Hgb/Hct
- MRI of orbits if indicated to assess Graves' ophthalmopathy

Differential Diagnosis

- Psychological disorders
- Pheochromocytoma
- Infection
- Thyrotoxic phase of Hashimoto's thyroiditis
- Hormone ingestion
- Plummer's disease
- Acromegaly
- Malignancy
- Chronic heart failure
- New onset or worsening angina
- Orbital tumors
- Myasthenia gravis

Management

Nonpharmacologic Treatment
- Treatment may not be necessary in mild cases.
- Surgery is last option because of complications of hypoparathyroidism and vocal cord paralysis
- Educate parents about thyroid disease if appropriate.

Pharmacologic Treatment
- Radioactive iodine ablation (RAI) is most-preferred treatment choice for Graves' disease, symptomatic multinodular goiter, and single hyperfunctioning adenoma; treatment of choice in elderly; takes 3 to 4 months for patient to become euthyroid
- Symptomatic relief
  - Propanolol can be used for symptom relief until the hyperthyroidism is resolved. Begin with propanolol ER 60 mg orally twice a day, increase every 2–3 days to a daily max of 320 mg; atenolol may also be used at 25 to 100 mg orally daily.
  - If beta-blockers are contraindicated, may use verapamil at an initial dose of 40 to 80 mg orally three times a day
- Antithyroid drugs (ATDs)
  - Propylthiouracil (PTU): start with 100 to 150 mg orally every 8 hours; 6 to 12 weeks to reach euthyroid state
  - Methimazole: start with 5 to 20 mg orally t.i.d.; 4 to 6 weeks to reach euthyroid state
  - Once T4 and T3 reach normal levels, decrease each drug to maintance doses and continue for one or more years depending on clinical picture.
  - Maintance doses: PTU 50 mg orally t.i.d.; methmizole 5 to 15 mg orally daily
  - Agranulocytosis: rare side effect of drugs; monitor WBC
- Other medications as needed
  - Diltiazem (Cardizem) for patients unable to take beta-blockers
  - Multivitamin, calcium replacement, and vitamin D to rebuild bone density
  - Ophthalmopathy: eye lubricants for mild cases

Special Considerations

- Older adults may develop arrhythmia (usually atrial fibrillation), CHF, and angina.
- Nonthyroidal illnesses, such as active hepatitis, cirrhosis, nephrotic syndrome, infections, malnutrition, and severe acute illness, can affect thyroid functioning serum tests.

When to Consult, Refer, or Hospitalize

- Refer to endocrinologist for management of all patients; may co-manage after initial therapy
- Hospitalize for thyroid storm
- Pituitary tumor: immediate referral to neurosurgeon
- Surgical referral for thyroidectomy
- Ophthalmologist for evaluation of eye pathology

Follow-up

- Monitor free T4 and TSH every 4 to 8 weeks until patient becomes euthyroid or hypothyroid, then thyroid replacement therapy
- Maintenance visits every 3 months, then 6 months, then annually
- After radioactive iodine therapy, order TSH every 6 weeks, 12 weeks, 6 months, then annually
- Baseline CBC, LFT every 3 to 6 months, ECG

Expected Outcomes

- Usually requires long-term maintenance for replacement therapy or follow-up for recurrence after remission

Complications

- Hypothyroidism following surgery or radiation
- Severe depression posttreatment
- Visual disturbance from ophthalmopathy
- Hypoparathyroidism and vocal cord paralysis postsurgery

Thyroid Storm

- Hospitalize; endocrinology involved
- High mortality rate
- Signs: hyperpyrexia, tachyarrhythmia, encephalopathy, diaphoresis, palpitations, agitation, delirium, psychosis, stupor or coma, hyperdefecation, hyperglycemia
- Causes: infection, trauma, noncompliance with antithyroid drugs, thyroid surgery, uncontrolled diabetes, pregnancy, major stress
- Treatment
  - PTU (treatment of choice): give 150 to 200 mg orally every 6 hours *or*
  - Methimazole 15 to 25 mg orally every 6 hours—must have one of the following 1 hour later:
    - Lugol's solution 10 drops orally t.i.d. *or*
    - Sodium iodine 1 gm slowly IV with beta-blocker and hydrocortisone (see below)
    - Ipodate sodium 500 mg orally daily; is helpful with both PTU and methimazole
  - Beta-blockade: propanolol drug of choice—0.5 mg to 2.0 mg IV every 4 hours, or 20 to 120 mg orally every 6 hours (use caution in heart failure patients)
  - Hydrocortisone 50 mg IV every 6 hours; rapidly taper as patient improves
- Other
  - Avoid aspirin—displaces T4 from TBG, thus raising FT4 levels.
  - Decrease environmental stimulation.

HYPOTHYROIDISM

Description

- Hypothyroidism involves decreased secretion of the thyroid hormone because of dysfunction in the thyroid gland or pituitary gland.

Etiology

Primary: Inability of Thyroid Gland to Produce TSH

Autoimmune thyroiditis (Hashimoto's) is the most common

- Transient hypothyroidism in acute or subacute thyroiditis (viral etiology): transient postpartum thyroiditis
- Ablation of gland because of surgery, radiation, thioamide drugs, radioactive iodine
- Congenital: ectopic thyroid gland, aplasia of the thyroid gland, ineffective synthesis or use of thyroid hormones, transient hypothyroidism related to maternal antithyroid medications or fetal or neonatal exposure to high levels of thyroid hormone, congenital hypopituitarism
- Iodine deficiency

Secondary: Lesions in Pituitary Gland (Less Common)

- Pituitary adenoma
- Certain drugs such as lithium and para-aminosalicylic acid; previously treated hyperthyroidism, especially postpartum; coexisting autoimmune disorders (lupus, pernicious anemia, rheumatoid arthritis)

Tertiary: thyrotropin-releasing hormone (TRH) deficiency from hypothalamus

Incidence

- Predominant age > 40; more frequent in women
- Hashimoto's thyroiditis can occur < age 3 years but usually > age 6 years, with increasing incidence in adolescence
- Congenital hypothyroidism occurs in 1 in 3,700 live births in North America; more frequent, in those of Far Eastern and Hispanic descent

Risk Factors

- Previous hyperthyroidism treatment
- Autoimmune diseases; presence of thyroid antibodies
- Family history of thyroid or autoimmune disorders
- Pituitary disease; hypothalamic disease
- Postpartum women, maternal TSH-binding antibodies
- Lithium treatment
- Diabetes mellitus type 1 (10% will develop hypothyroidism)
- Infertility problems, repeated spontaneous abortions

Prevention and Screening

- No official screening guidelines; however, periodic TSH screening for patients treated for hyperthyroidism or those who are symptomatic; some clinicians screen adult women > 45 or 50
- Screen those with autoimmune diseases.

Assessment

History
- Anorexia, dry skin, coarse/dry hair, alopecia, receding hairline, constipation, cold intolerance, lethargy, weight gain, irregular or heavy menses, memory loss, depression, muscle aches, paresthesias, medication history (especially lithium), arthralgias or myalgias, muscle cramps

Physical Examination
- Weight gain, subnormal temperatures, decreased level of consciousness
- Face: dull, blank expression; periorbital edema; decreased auditory acuity
- Skin: dry skin, coarse/dry hair, brittle nails, hair loss, temporal thinning of eye brows
- Mouth: swollen tongue, slow speech, hoarseness
- Thyroid—enlarged gland or atrophy, tender, nodules
- Cardiac: bradycardia, decreased heart tones, mild hypotension or diastolic hypotension, cardiomegaly
- Respiratory: dyspnea, pleural effusion
- Breasts: galactorrhea
- Extremities: swollen hands or feet, leg edema
- Neurological: dementia, paranoid ideation, slow or delayed reflexes, cerebellar ataxia, carpal tunnel syndrome
- Hematologic: anemia, hyperlipidemia, hypercholesterolemia

Diagnostic Data
- Elevated TSH in primary hypothyroidism
- Decreased TSH in cases that are the result of pituitary insufficency
- Decreased free T4
- Antithyroperoxidase antibodies or anti-Tg antibodies present with autoimmune thyroiditis
- Other lab abnormalities
  - Increased LDL cholesterol
  - Increased triglycerides
  - Hyponatremia
  - Hypoglycemia
  - Anemia
  - ANA present without evidence of lupus

Differential Diagnosis

- Depression
- Obesity
- Dementia
- Ischemic heart disease
- Chronic heart failure
- Kidney failure
- Cirrhosis
- Nephrotic syndrome

- Chronic renal disease
- Transient hypothyroidism
- Hypopituitarism
- Sick euthyroid
- Iodine ingestion
- Thyroid hormone resistance

Management

Nonpharmacologic Treatment
- Education, high-fiber diet for constipation; diet and exercise for weight loss if obese
- Avoid drug interactions: cholestyramine; ferrous sulfate; aluminum hydroxide antacids; sucralfate; foods such as cabbage, turnips, kale, and soybeans that increase the loss of thyroid hormone as they may interfere with levothyroxine absorption—should be spaced 4 hours from these medications
- Take medication in the morning on an empty stomach to increase absorption.

Pharmacologic Treatment
- Oral replacement: levothyroxine
- Starting dose:
  - If < 60 years old without CAD, then 50 to 100 mcg orally daily
  - If > 60 years old or with CAD, then 25 to 50 mcg orally daily
  - Dose increased 25 mcg every 1 to 3 weeks until euthyroid

Special Considerations

- Adults and geriatric patients: concomitant use of CNS depressants, digoxin, or insulin may decrease efficacy of thyroid replacement dosage; older adults at risk for angina as thyroid levels increase

When to Consult, Refer, or Hospitalize

- Refer to an endocrinologist for developing myxedema coma, hypothermia, decreased mentation, respiratory acidosis, hypotension, hyponatremia, hypoglycemia, hypoventilation, significant cardiac disease, secondary hypothyroidism, or radically abnormal thyroid function tests.
- Consult or refer for co-management of congenital hypothyroidism.
- Refer pregnant and pediatric patients to an endocrinologist for ongoing management.
- Hospitalization is not usually required.

Follow-up

- Adults: measure TSH 4 to 6 weeks after initial dosage, then every 2 months until within normal limits, then every 6 to 12 months (TSH levels may remain elevated for several months despite effective treatment); if drug dosage changed, recheck TSH levels in 2 to 3 months
- Annual lipid levels

Expected Outcomes

- Improvement within 1 month of starting medication; symptoms resolve within 3 to 6 months
- Treatment usually lifelong; maintain medication at lowest dosage to maintain euthyroid state
- Excellent prognosis with appropriate treatment

Complications

- Chronic heart failure
- Depression, psychoses
- Miscarriages during pregnancy
- Bone demineralization because of overtreatment

Myxedema Coma

- Hospitalized; endocrinology involved
- Results from uncompensated hypothyroidism
- Causes: illness, infection, trauma, exposure to cold, CNS depressants, noncompliance with thyroxine medication
- Clinical manifestations: coma with extreme hypothermia, hyponatremia, seizures and respiratory depression, hypotension, bradyarrhythmia; serious precipitating illness
- Presents most often in elderly and women in winter months
- Treatment
  - IV thyroid replacement
    - Levothyroxine, one dose of 400 mcg IV, then 50–100 mcg daily; lower dose for patients with coronary insufficiency
    - If adrenal insufficiency is present: hydrocortisone 100 mg IV bolus, then 25 to 30 mg every 8 hours
  - Rewarm slowly—rapid re-warming places patient at risk for hypotension and arrhythmias.
  - Oxygen supplementation and mechanical ventilation if necessary
  - Severe hyponatremia: fluid restriction and hypertonic saline

ADRENAL DISORDERS

CUSHING'S SYNDROME

Description

- Cushing's syndrome involves clinical abnormalities resulting from excessive amounts of glucocorticoids.

Etiology

- Prolonged use of glucorticoids
- Excess pituitary secretion of ACTH
- 80% of cases caused by ACTH-secreting pituitary microadenomas; others include small cell carcinoma of the lung, carcinoids, and adrenal adenomas

Incidence

- Pituitary adenoma three times more likely in women than in men
- Age of onset 20 to 40 years
- Rare in childhood and infancy

Risk Factors

- Prolonged glucocorticoid use
- Nonpituitary neoplasms
- Pituitary adenomas
- Adrenal adenoma/carcinoma

Assessment

History
- Weakness, headache, backache, oligomenorrhea or amenorrhea, erectile dysfunction in males, osteoporosis, avascular bone necrosis, acne, superficial skin infections, thirst, polyuria, renal calculi, glaucoma, easily bruised, impaired wound healing, mental changes ranging from inability to concentrate to psychosis, increased susceptibility to infection
- Prolonged use of corticosteroids

Physical Examination
- Hypertension
- Central or truncal obesity
- Moon face
- Buffalo hump
- Supraclavicular fat pads
- Thin extremities
- Acne
- Thin skin
- Ecchymosis
- Purple striae around breasts, abdomen, and thighs
- Hirsutism
- Hyperpigmentation
- Increased intraocular pressure
- Muscle atrophy and weakness

Diagnostic Studies
- Elevated free urine cortisol (24-hr urine for free cortisol)
- Elevated serum cortisol
- Hyperglycemia, hypokalemia without hypernatremia
- Glycosuria
- CT scans of chest and abdomen for adrenal tumors, MRI for pituitary tumors
- Screening—refer to an endocrinologist
  - Dexamethasone suppression test
  - Drugs such as Phenytoin, phenobarbital, and primidone can cause false positive results

Differential Diagnosis

- Alcoholism
- Obesity
- Depression
- Familial cortisol resistance
- Hirsutism
- Anorexia nervosa

Management

Nonpharmacologic Treatment
- Consult or refer to endocrinology
- High-protein diet
- Transphenoidal selective resection of the pituitary adenoma
- Stereotactic pituitary radiosurgery
- Resection of adrenal neoplasms and ectopic ACTH-secreting tumors
- Bilateral adrenalectomy

Pharmacologic Treatment
- Replacement glucocorticoid therapy for up to 1 year post-adrenal surgery and lifelong if bilateral adrenalectomy
- Monitor and treat electrolyte inbalances as needed

Special Considerations

- Pregnancy can exacerbate symptoms.

When to Consult, Refer, or Hospitalize

- Refer all cases to endocrinologist and coordinate their primary care.
- Refer to surgeon and oncologist for adrenal or pituitary tumor.

Follow-up

- For recurrent symptoms, measure urinary-free cortisol.

Expected Outcomes
- Posttreatment for pituitary adenoma: normal ACTH suppressed and requires 6 to 36 months to recover to normal function; hydrocortisone replacement therapy necessary
- Normal HPA function returns within 3 to 24 months after surgery if one adrenal gland is left.
- 10% to 20% failure rate with transsphenoidal surgery; those with complete remission will have 15% to 20% recurrence rate over next 10 years

Complications
- Hypertension, CAD
- Osteoporosis, compression fractures of spine, aseptic necrosis femur head
- Diabetes mellitus
- Overwhelming infection
- Nephrolithiasis
- Psychosis
- If untreated, morbidity and death

ADDISON'S DISEASE/ADRENAL INSUFFICIENCY

Description

- Addison's disease is adrenal insufficiency.
- An insidious, chronic disease of adrenal destruction, also known as primary adrenal failure.
- Primary adrenal insufficiency is a loss of all adrenal hormones, including mineralocorticoids, glucocorticoids, and adrenal androgens.
- Secondary adrenal insufficiency is a lack of glucocorticoids because of primary dysfunction; tertiary adrenal insufficiency is a lack of glucocorticoids caused by hypothalamic failure.

Etiology

- 80% of cases in the United States caused by autoimmune destruction of the adrenals
- Other, rarer causes include tuberculosis, genetic disorders, adrenal hemorrhage, lymphoma, metastatic carcinoma, cytomegalovirus (in AIDS patients), amyloid disease, scleroderma, syphilitic gummas, coccidioidomycosis, histoplasmosis, and hemachormatosis.
- Secondary and tertiary adrenal insufficiency result from suppression of HPA axis through glucocorticoid replacement, adrenalectomy, pituitary tumor, trauma, surgery, infarction, or hypothalamic disease.

Incidence

- Prevalence approximately 4:100,000
- Affects females > males
- Affects all age groups; usually occurs between ages 30 and 50

Risk Factors

- Autoimmune disease
- Family history of adrenal insufficiency
- Prolonged steroid use followed by infection, surgery, or trauma
- Medications such as ketoconazole, dilantin, rifampin, and opiates

Assessment

History
- Weakness, fatigue, weight loss, myalgias, arthalgias, fever, anorexia, nausea, vomiting, emotional changes, abdominal pain, cold intolerance, dizziness

Physical Examination
- Orthostatic hypotension: 90% have systolic < 110 mm Hg, > 130 mm Hg is rare
- Hyperpigmentation: most noticeable over the knuckles, elbows, knees, posterior neck, and in palmar creases; new scars, pressure areas such as belt or brassiere lines, and buttocks also darkened
- Areas of vitiligo in about 10% of cases
- Bluish-black discoloration of areolae and mucus membranes of lips, mouth, rectum, vagina
- Scant axillary and pubic hair (more common in women)
- Lymphoid tissue hyperplasia
- Small heart
- **RED FLAG**
  - Acute adrenal insufficiency or Addisonian crisis may present with profound fatigue, dehydration, severe abdominal pain, nausea and vomiting, hypotension, hypoglycemia, and shock with vascular collapse and renal shutdown. This event is precipitated by surgery, infection, exacerbation of comorbid illness, or sudden withdrawal of long-term glucocorticoid replacement.

Diagnostic Studies
- Low plasma cortisol levels < 3 mcg/dL at 8:00 a.m.
- Cosyntropin stim test: Normal peak plasma cortisol levels are > 20 mcg/dL
- Hyponatremia
- Hyperkalemia
- Low fasting glucose
- Neutropenia
- Lymphocytosis
- Abdominal CT scan: small adrenals

Differential Diagnosis

- Hyperpigmentation is seen in other disease processes, such as bronchogenic carcinoma, ingestion of heavy metals, chronic skin conditions, hemochromatosis, and Peutz-Jeghers syndrome.
- Neuropsychiatric weakness—worse in the morning than with activity; in Addison's, weakness subsides with rest
- Myopathies
- Salt-wasting nephritis
- Depression
- Mild thyrotoxicosis in older patients
- GI malignancy
- Chronic infection
- ACTH-secreting tumors

Management

Nonpharmacologic Treatment
- Management initiated by endocrinologist
- Patient should have wallet card and/or Medic Alert bracelet
- Patient education on indications for dose adjustments and signs/symptoms of adrenal crisis

Pharmacologic Treatment
- Treat all infections immediately and raise cortisol dose
- Chronic therapy, initiated by endocrinologist
  - Hydrocortisone 15–25 mg p.o. in two divided doses daily; 2/3 in a.m. and 1/3 in afternoon *or*
  - Prednisone 3 mg p.o. every a.m., 2 mg p.o. every p.m.
    - Increase dose in case of stress, trauma, surgery, or stressful diagnostic procedures
    - Adequate therapy when WBC is normal.
  - Fludrocortisone acetate 0.05–0.3 mg p.o. every day or every other day for cases of primary adrenal insufficiency if insufficient sodium retention with cortisol alone.
    - Lower dose in the presence of edema, hypokalemia, or hypertension
    - Increase dose in the presence of hyponatremia, hyperkalemia, or postural hypotension
    - Salt additives for excess heat or humidity

When to Consult, Refer, or Hospitalize

- Refer all suspected cases to endocrinologist for management.
- Hospitalization with acute crisis, dehydration, severe stress

Follow-up

- Periodic evaluations of blood pressure, weight, electrolytes and other labs, muscle strength, appetite, cardiac status
- Medic Alert or similar identification bracelet or necklace

Expected Outcomes
- Excellent prognosis with lifelong steroid replacement therapy

Complications
- Complications of steroid therapy: osteoporosis, psychosis, hyperglycemia, Cushing's syndrome
- Acute adrenal crisis
  - Present with profound fatigue, dehydration, severe abdominal pain, nausea and vomiting, hypotension, hypoglycemia, confusion, fever
  - Precipitating events include surgery, infections, trauma, sudden withdrawal of long-term glucocorticoid replacement, bilateral adrenalectomy, removal of functioning adrenal tumor
  - Patient must be hospitalized
  - Managed by endocrinologist
  - Obtain blood, urine, and sputum cultures because infection is a causative factor
  - Obtain cortisol level

- Start hydrocortisone 100 mg every 8 hr
- Rapid IV infusion (500 cc/hr) of D5NS; taper has hypotension resolves
- Taper dose of hydrocortisone as condition improves and eventually start oral therapy when patient is able to tolerate p.o.
- Consider broad spectrum antibiotics while waiting on culture results

DIABETES INSIPIDUS

Description

- Diabetes insipidus (DI) is a condition in which regulation of the body's water balance is impaired, secondary to either decreased pituitary secretion of antidiuretic hormone (ADH) or the inability of the kidneys to respond normally to ADH.
- Central DI: ADH deficit
- Nephrogenic DI: ADH resistance
- Psychogenic DI
- Can be a transient or permanent condition

Etiology

- Central DI: CNS disorders that damage the hypothalamus or pituitary gland can impair ADH production or secretion, thus precipitating central DI.
  - Brain tumors, neurosurgical procedures, head trauma, and CNS infections are leading causes; however, literature indicates that approximately 30% of cases are idiopathic, tuberculosis, syphilis, anoxic encephalopathy, vasopressin-induced (seen in the last trimester of pregnancy)
- Nephrogenic DI: secondary to a defect in the renal tubules that causes renal resistance to ADH; interferes with water absorption and is unresponsive to vasopressin
  - Associated with drugs such as lithium, opiate antagonists, phenytoin, and ethanol.
  - Can also develop as a result of chronic kidney disease, hypercalcemia, or hypokalemia.
  - Can be hereditary, but this is rare
- Other causes: cancer (primary intracranial tumors, lung cancer, leukemia, and lymphoma), anorexia nervosa, hypoxic encephalopathy, and vascular lesions

Incidence

- Found in 1 case per 25,000 in the general population
- Postoperative transphenoidal adenoma resection is as high as 60% to 80% if a large tumor was removed.
- Equal occurrence in males and females
- Familial DI is rare and the majority of these cases of nephrogenic DI are related to an X-linked defect of an ADH receptor gene.

Risk Factors

- Postoperative transphenoidal adenoma resection
- Cancer (primary intracranial tumors, lung cancer, leukemia, and lymphoma)
- Anorexia nervosa
- Hypoxic encephalopathy
- Vascular lesions

Assessment

History
- Extreme thirst—craving for ice water
- Irritability
- Polyuria
- Nocturia
- Symptoms of dehydration

Physical Examination
- Physical exam may be completely normal
- Distended bladder
- Dry mucus membranes
- Poor skin turgor
- Elevated temperature, fever
- Orthostatic hypotension
- Postural tachycardia
- Increased urine output

Diagnostic Data
- Serum osmolality > 287 mOsm/kg
- Urine osmolality < 200 mOsmo/kg
- Urine-specific gravity < 1.00
- Hypernatremia
- Water deprivation test: This is a semi-quantitative test in which dehydration is established in a controlled setting, challenging the body to produce ADH. Serial testing of urine osmolality and ADH levels and measurement of urine output and body weight quantifies ADH activity and helps to determine whether DI is a result of excess fluid intake, an ADH deficit, or a defect in the kidneys' response to ADH.

Differential Diagnosis

- Diabetes mellitus
- Psychogenic polydipsia
- Diuretic use
- Cushing's syndrome

- Corticosteroid treatment
- Lithium use
- Hypercalcemia
- Hypokalemia
- Parkinson's disease

Management

Nonpharmacologic Treatment
- Patient education at discharge should include teaching intranasal administration of DDAVP and maintaining awareness of fluid and salt intake

Pharmacologic Treatment
- Goal of clinical management of DI is to prevent circulatory failure and prevent hyperosmolar encephalopathy.
- Volume replacement is carried out over 24–48 hours to allow for slow correction of hypernatremia and titration to electrolyte levels and ongoing urine losses
- DDAVP is the ADH replacement of choice in treating central and gestational DI:
  - Give 5–20 mcg intranasally, daily or b.i.d., or
  - 0.05–0.8 mg orally daily
- Thaizide diuretics or indomethacin may be used to treat nephrogenic DI because desmopressin will be ineffective and amiloride has been shown to be helpful in treating lithium-induced nephrogenic DI. No matter which agent is used for medical management, the therapeutic effect should be measurable, as evidenced by an increase in urine-specific gravity and a decrease in urine output within 1 hour of the dose. Close monitoring of hemodynamics, intake and output, neurological status, and serial lab work should be ongoing until euvolemia has been restored.

When to Consult, Refer, or Hospitalize

- May be hospitalized due to precipitating factor of diabetes insipidus (e.g., head trauma, neurosurgical procedures)
- Management of hypernatremia

Expected Outcomes
- Central DI secondary to pituitary surgery: usually remits in days to weeks
- Chronic DI: responds well to treatment with desmopression; no effect on life expectancy

Complications
- Severe dehydration
- Hypernatremia
- Induced water intoxication in patients who are on desmopression acetate therapy

SYNDROME OF INAPPROPRIATE ANTIDIURETIC HORMONE

Description

- Release of antidiuretic hormone (ADH) without appropriate stimuli such as hypovolemia and hyperosmolality
- Results in evolemic, hypotonic hyponatremia

Etiology

- Central nervous system disorders: meningitis, encephalitis, cerebrovascular accident, head trauma, Guillain-Barré syndrome
- Pulmonary diseases: bacterial pneumonia, aspergillosis, bronchiectasis, acute respiratory failure, positive pressure ventilation, tuberculosis
- Malignancies: most commonly small-cell lung cancer; also, pancreatic, prostatic, or renal carcinoma, and malignant lymphoma
- Some drugs can either potentiate ADH action or increase ADH production. A few examples of these are NSAIDs, antidepressants, antineoplastics, carbamazepine, and amiodarone.
- Other contributing factors: AIDS, pain, and physiologic stress

Incidence

- Affects 1% to 2% of cancer patients
- Hyponatremia due to SIADH commonly seen in hospitalized patients

Risk Factors

- Central nervous system disorders
- Pulmonary diseases
- Malignancies
- Drugs
- AIDS
- Pain
- Physiologic stress

Assessment

History
- Presence of one or more of the risk factors
- Many patients are asymptomatic.
- Headache, fatigue
- Nausea, vomiting, abdominal cramping, anorexia

Physical Assessment
- Weight gain and edema
- Decreased urinary output
- Decreased deep tendon reflexes
- Can progress to altered mental status, coma, seizures, and death
- Symptoms correlate with serum sodium less than 125 mg/dL.

Diagnostic Data
- Hyponatremia—patient is euvolemic
- Urine osmolality > mOsm/kg
- Urine sodium > 20 mEq/L
- Serum osmolality < 280 mOsm/kg
- BUN < 10 mg/dL
- Patient does not have heart, kidney, or liver disease.

Differential Diagnosis
- Hypothyroidism
- Adrenal insufficiency
- Diuretic use
- Renal disease
- Volume depletion

Management

Nonpharmacologic Treatment
- Identify and treat underlying cause
- Water restriction if hyponatremic and asymptomatic (800 to 1000 mL per day)
- Requires hospitalization for correction of sympotomatic hyponatremia.
- Consult nephrology.
- Monitor sodium levels hourly during replacement therapy.
- Seizure precautions

Pharmacologic Treatment
- Asymptomatic hyponatremia
  - Fluid restriction < 1,000 mL/day if sodium > 120 mEq/L
  - Fluid restriction to < 500 mL/day if sodium 110–120 mEq/L
- Acute symptomatic hyponatremia
  - Fluid restriction to 500 mL/day
  - Calculate sodium deficit
  - Use hypertonic (3%) saline to correct sodium level (usual infusion rate is 0.5 mL/kg/hr)
  - Replacement should not exceed 1–2 mEq/L/hr and reduce the rate to 0.5 mEq/L/hr once neurologic symptoms improve
  - Give furosemide (0.5–1 mg/kg) with saline infusion to inhibit free water reabsorption
  - Goal is a sodium level of 125–130 mEq/L
- Chronic SIADH
  - Fluid restriction
  - In cases in which the underlying cause is not able to be treated and the patient is unable to adhere to strict fluid restrictions, demeclocycline (300–600 mg p.o. b.i.d.) may be used. Takes 1–2 weeks for best effect. Caution: May cause renal failure.

When to Consult, Refer, or Hospitalize

- Hospitalize for symptomatic hyponatremia
- Consider nephrology, endocrine consult, or both, in severe cases.
- If treatment of underlying cause warrants hospitalization

Follow-up

Expected Outcomes
- Prognosis is in relation to underlying cause

Complications
- Cerebral edema from rapid replacement of sodium

PHEOCHROMOCYTOMA

Description

- Pheochromocytoma is a rare catecholamine-secreting tumor of chromaffin cells.
- 85% to 90% arise from medulla (pheochromocytomas)
- 10% to 15% are found on sympathetic ganglia (extra-adrenal pheochromocytoma)

Etiology

- Rare condition
- Adrenal medullary tumor is a common cause
- Can also be related to multiple endocrine neoplasia (familial cause)

Incidence

- Found in < 0.3 % of hypertensive patients
- 2 to 3 new cases per million annually
- 250 to 1,300 cases per million diagnosed during autopsy
- Occurs at any age, but peak ages 30 to 60
- Occurs equally in males and females
- 10% are bilateral or multiple tumors
- < 10% of adrenal tumors are malignant.
- About 10% of cases are the result of familial causes, and are a component of four autosomal dominant syndromic diseases:
  - Multiple endocrine neoplastic type 2
  - Von-Hippel-Lindau disease
  - Hereditary paraganglioma syndrome
  - Neurofibromatosis type 1

Prevention and Screening

- Suspect pheochromocytoma if patient has severe, sudden, unexplained hypertension

Assessment

History
- Headache
- Polydipsia
- Polyuria
- Panic attack symptoms
- Palpitation
- Generalized weakness
- Dyspnea
- Weight loss
- Increased appetite

Physical Examination
- Sustained or paroxysmal hypertension
- Generalized sweating
- Tachycardia
- Postural hypotension
- Tremor
- Hypertensive retinopathy

Diagnostic Studies
- Plasma fractionated free metanephrines—single most sensitive test
- 24-hr urine measurement of catecholamines and total metanephrines
  - > 2.2 mcg of total metanephrine per mg of creatinine
  - > 135 mcg total catecholamines per gram of creatinine
  - Certain drugs can alter these results, such as alcohol, sympathomimetics, vasodilators, levodopa, methyldopa, methylxanthines, isoproterenol, lithium, TCAs, chlorpromazine, sotalol, amphetamines, buspirone, and benzodiazepines.
  - Disease processes that can influence results include Guillain-Barré syndrome, hypoglycemia, quadriplegia, intracranial lesions, and acute psychosis.
- MRI for localization of the pheochromocytoma
- Nuclear medicine MIBG scan can localize tumors.
- Diagnosis of pheochromocytoma is rarely confirmed.

Differential Diagnosis

- Labile essential hypertension
- Anxiety
- Paroxysmal cardiac arrhythmias
- Thyrotoxicosis
- Amphetamine or cocaine use

Management

Nonpharmacologic Treatment
- Acute treatment should take place in a critical care setting.
- Target blood pressure is less than 140/90 mm Hg.

Pharmacologic Treatment

- Immediately institute alpha blockade with an agent such as phentolamine. Nitroprusside also can be used for uncontrolled hypertension. Initial use of beta-blockers for blood pressure control can exacerbate hypertension or cause rebound tachycardias or pulmonary edema. They can be added as a second agent once alpha blockade has been established, particularly in the setting of cardiac arrhythmias. Low dose, short-acting beta-blockers should be chosen. Brisk fluid resuscitation may also be need once vasoconstriction is relieved. When ready to transition to oral therapy, alpha blockade should continue with agents such as prazosin, terazosin, or doxazosin. Patients who are surgical candidates should be scheduled only after catecholamine excess has been successfully blocked preoperatively.
- Surgical removal of pheochromocytoma is the treatment of choice. It should be a multidisciplinary approach to the procedure and should include endocrinology, anesthesiology, and surgery teams.

Follow-up

- Discharge teaching should include blood pressure monitoring.
- 2-week and then annual post-operative urine assessment for catecholamines and metanephrines.

Expected Outcomes

- Symptoms and hypertension usually resolve or improve with treatment, removal of pheochromocytoma, or both.
- Requires lifelong surveillance.
- Patients with benign tumors have a good survival rate.
- There is a less than 50% 5-year survival rate if tumors are malignant.

Complications

- Severe hypertension
- Catecholamine-induced cardiomyopathy
- Sudden death caused by arrhythmias
- Hypertension-induced blindness and CVA

REFERENCES

Barkley, Jr., T. W. (2009). *Acute care nurse practitioner certification review manual.* West Hollywood, CA: Barkley & Associates.

Barkley, Jr., T., & Myers, C. (2008). *Practice guidelines for acute care nurse practitioners* (2nd ed.). Philadelphia: Elsevier Saunders.

Beers, M. H., Porter, R. S., Jones, T. V., Kaplan, J. L., & Berkwits, M. (2006). *The Merck manual of diagnosis and therapy* (18th ed.). Whitehouse Station, NJ: Merck Research Laboratories.

Centers for Disease Control and Prevention. (2011). *2011 national diabetes fact sheet.* Retrieved from http://www.cdc.gov/diabetes/pubs/factsheet11.htm

Dambro, M. R. (2007). *Griffith's five-minute clinical consult.* Philadelphia: Lippincott Williams & Wilkins.

Edmunds, M. W., & Mayhew, M. S. (2004). *Pharmacology for primary care providers* (2nd ed.). St. Louis, MO: Mosby.

Foster, C., Mistry, N. F., Peddi, P. F., & Sharma, S. (2010). *The Washington manual of medical therapeutics* (33rd ed.). Philadelphia: Wolters Kluwer/Lippincott Williams & Wilkins.

Goroll, A. H., & Mulley, A. G. (2006). *Primary care medicine* (4th ed.). Philadelphia: Wolters Kluwer/Lippincott Williams & Wilkins.

Kleigman, R. M., Marcdante, K. J., Jensen, H. B., & Behrman, R. E. (2006). *Nelson essentials of pediatrics* (5th ed.) Philadelphia: Elsevier Saunders.

McPhee, S. J., Papadakis, M. A., & Tierney, L. M. (2008). *Current medical diagnosis & treatment* (44th ed.). Norwalk, CT: Appleton & Lange.

McPhee, S. J., Papadakis, M. A., & Tierney, L. M. (2011). *Current medical diagnosis & treatment* (50th ed.). New York: Lange Medical Book/McGraw Hill.

National Center for Chronic Disease Prevention and Health Promotion. (n.d.). *Body mass index-for-age: BMI is used differently with children than it is with adults.* Retrieved from www.cdc.gov/obesity/downloads/BMIforPactitioners.pdf

National Guideline Clearinghouse. (2004). Standards of medical care for patients with diabetes mellitus. *Diabetes Care, 27,* S15–S35. Retrieved from http://www.guidelines.gov/summary/summary.aspx?ss=15&doc_id=10400&nbr=005446&string=diabetes

Riddle, M. C., Rosenstock, J., & Gerich, J. (2003). Treat to the target trial: Randomized addition of glargine or human NPH insulin to oral therapy of type 2 diabetic patients. *Diabetes Care, 26*(11), 3080–3086.

Schwartz, M. W. (2008). *The 5 minute pediatric consult.* Philadelphia: Wolters/Kluwers Lippincott Williams & Wilkins.

Sinclair, A. J., Conroy, S. P., & Bayer, A. J. (2008). Impact of diabetes on physical function in older people. *Diabetes Care, 31*(2), 233–235.

Taylor, R. (2007). *Manual of family medicine* (2nd ed.). Philadelphia: Wolters/Kluwers Lippincott Williams & Wilkins.

Terpstra, T. L., & Terpstra, T. L. (2000). Sydrome of inappropriate antidiuretic hormone secretion: Recognition and management. *Medsurg Nursing, 9,* 61–70.

Weinzimer, S. A., Ternand, C., Howard, C., Chang, C. T., Becker, D. J., & Laffel, L. M. (2008). A randomized trial comparing continuous subcutaneous insulin infusion of insulin aspart versus insulin lispro in children and adolescents with type 1 diabetes. *Diabetes Care, 31*(2), 210–215.

Neurologic Disorders

Tiffany Boysen, RN, MSN, APRN-BC, CCRN,
and Deborah Gilbert-Palmer, EdD, FNP-BC

GENERAL APPROACH

For All

- Neurological disorders range from chronic to acute to lethal.
- A screening neurological exam should be done on all patients with symptoms suspicious for a neurologic disorder and would include mental status (level of consciousness, orientation, memory, cognitive function, language), motor function (body position, involuntary movement, muscle tone, strength), sensory function (light touch, pain, position sense), reflexes (deep tendon reflexes [DTRs], abdominal, Babinski), cerebellar function (gait, rapid alternating movements, point-to-point movements, Romberg), and cranial nerves (I–XII, motor and sensory components).
- Abnormalities should be further evaluated with additional assessment techniques, referred to a neurologic specialist and for diagnostic testing, or both. Additional assessment includes techniques such as the Mini Mental Status Examination (MMSE), discriminating sensory testing (stereognosis, two-point discrimination), and meningeal irritability testing.

Older Adults

- 20% decrease in blood flow to the brain with changes in autoregulation; contributes to risk of orthostatic hypotension
- No changes in thinking, behavior, or intellectual function, although response time and processing of information are slower
- The greater incidence of sensory deficits with aging and chronic illness (decreased hearing, decreased visual acuity, decreased position sense) may contribute to or mimic neurologic problems.
- Consider cardiac or metabolic etiology, or adverse medication reactions, particularly for global complaints such as syncope, weakness, or change in cognition without focal (unilateral) neurological symptoms; also consider dementia, delirium, or depression.

RED FLAGS

For All

- Refer to a neurologist if unusual presentation or no response to adequate trial of standard therapy

Adults and Older Adults

- Focal findings suggest a space-occupying lesion of the brain or spinal cord, or a peripheral compressive neuropathy; refer to neurologist or neurosurgeon
- Acute or sudden onset of symptoms, such as headache, unilateral weakness, aphasia, visual changes, or change in level of consciousness, require immediate consult, referral, or hospitalization, as do deficits resulting from head or spinal trauma.

STROKE AND TRANSIENT ISCHEMIC ATTACK

Description

- Strokes are ischemic or hemorrhagic attacks.
- Ischemic stroke is an interruption in blood flow to the brain, causing neuronal death or infarction. Hemorrhage accounts for about 20% of strokes; the bleed may be intraparenchymal or subarachnoid.
- Transient ischemic attack (TIA) is a temporary interruption in cerebral vascular blood flow; the deficit lasts less than 24 hours. *There is no infarcted tissue.*

Etiology

- Ischemic stroke
  - Lack of blood flow to brain because of hypoxia, decreased cardiac output, thrombus, or embolus
- Thrombotic stroke
  - Caused by progressive accumulation of atherosclerotic plaque that occludes an intracranial vessel
  - Most common in the posterior cerebral circulation
- Embolic stroke
  - Caused by atherosclerotic debris from the heart, aorta, or carotids that flow into the internal carotids and occlude the smaller vessels of the cerebral circulation
  - Usually affects the anterior cerebral circulation
- Lacunar infarcts
  - Less than 5 mm; occur in the internal capsule, basal ganglia, or thalamus
  - Result from slow, progressive occlusion of the penetrating arterioles
- TIAs: may be thrombotic, embolic, or lacunar in nature, but most commonly embolic hemorrhagic stroke
  - Intracerebral hemorrhage: spontaneous bleeding into parenchyma from microaneurysm of perforating vessels, which most commonly occurs in the basal ganglia; results from hypertension, hematological disorders, or anticoagulation therapy
- Subarachnoid hemorrhage
  - Bleeding from a ruptured aneurysm in the Circle of Willis or arteriovenous malformation

INCIDENCE AND DEMOGRAPHICS

- Acute stroke afflicts 600,000 Americans per year; incidence increases with age.
- One-fourth will die, making stroke the third leading cause of death.
- 50% of the survivors will have some disability; 15% to 30% will require nursing home placement.

Risk Factors

- Previous cerebrovascular disease, stroke, or TIA; 20% to 40% of ischemic strokes are preceded by TIA within days to months; highest risk is within the first month after a TIA
- Aging
- Family history of stroke
- History of carotid artery stenosis
- Alcoholism, oral contraceptive use, male gender, drug use (cocaine, amphetamines), AIDS, obesity
- Elevated blood homocysteine level
- Traditional risks for vascular disease: hypertension, diabetes, hyperlipidemia, smoking
- Traditional risks for emboli: atrial fibrillation, cardiomyopathy, coronary artery disease

Prevention and Screening

- Management of hypertension; screening for hypertension recommended at least every 2 years in the normotensive; treatment is recommended per Joint National Commission 7 guidelines
- Screening for asymptomatic carotid stenosis by auscultation of carotid bruits or carotid ultrasound remains controversial, with insufficient evidence to recommend for or against.
- High-risk patients over age 60 with other risk factors for vascular disease, who have access to vascular surgery with morbidity and mortality rates of less than 3% may benefit from screening and subsequent endarterectomy.
- Antiplatelet therapy with aspirin, or clopidogrel (Plavix) may decrease the risk of stroke in those with asymptomatic carotid artery stenosis.
- Anticoagulation is recommended for patients with atrial fibrillation, particularly those with additional risk factors.
- Evidence suggests improved glycemic control may decrease microvascular events in type 2 diabetes.
- Decreasing serum lipids may delay progression of carotid atherosclerosis and decrease cerebrovascular events.
- All patients will benefit from diet and exercise counseling and smoking cessation.

Assessment

History
- Onset, duration, and progression of symptoms most important in determining etiology and management
- Resolution of symptoms in minutes to hours is suggestive of a TIA.
- Onset during sleep with progression suggests thrombotic stroke.
- Sudden onset with activity suggests embolic or hemorrhagic stroke.
- Detailed description of symptoms or deficits, including visual changes, aphasia, motor weakness, paresthesias, may give clue to location of stroke or lesion
- Review of systems: headache, seizure, loss of consciousness, syncope, vertigo, vomiting, cardiac symptoms
  - Lack of headache excludes hemorrhagic stroke.
  - Vomiting is associated with increased intracranial pressure, usually because of hemorrhage.
  - Loss of consciousness is associated with hemorrhage or posterior circulation thrombosis.
  - Syncope is more often related to cardiac etiology than stroke.
  - Vertigo suggests vestibular disease, but may occur with vertebrobasilar insufficiency.
- Past medical history—cardiac disease; peripheral vascular disease; diabetes; IV drug abuse; or previous neurologic conditions such as seizure, head trauma, dementia, or brain tumor—gives clues to etiology and possible differential diagnosis.
- Review all medications, particularly those that can alter level of consciousness or cause bleeding.

Physical Examination
- Complete neurologic exam, including level of consciousness; cognitive ability (apraxia, agnosia, aphasia, agraphia); motor and sensory function (contralateral deficits); cranial nerve exam, including funduscopic and visual deficits; and reflexes (hyperreflexia or Babinski on affected side)

- Cardiovascular exam: hypertension, orthostatic changes, atrial fibrillation, heart murmurs, carotid bruits, and abdominal bruit from aneurysm
- Signs of carotid TIA: weakness of contralateral arm, leg, or face, individually or in combination; numbness or paraesthesia may occur alone or in combination with motor deficit; dysphagia; monocular visual loss; carotid bruit; TRS may be hyperreflexic during attack; atherosclerotic changes on funduscopic exam. Signs and symptoms disappear as attack resolves.
- Signs of vertebrobasilar TIA: vertigo, ataxia, diplopia, dysarthria, dimness or blurry vision, perioral numbness, weakness or sensory complaints on one or both sides of the body, drop attacks with bilateral leg weakness
- Lacunar infarction: contralateral pure motor or sensory deficit, ipsilateral ataxia, dysarthria, with complete symptom resolution over 1 to 2 months
- Cerebral infarction: deficit depends on vessel; any variety of focal neurological deficits may develop
- Cerebellar infarction: vertigo, ataxia, nystagmus, nausea and vomiting
- Hemorrhagic CVA: typically associated with hypertension, sudden onset, symptoms usually present during activity, initial loss of or impaired consciousness, rapidly evolving hemiplegia or paresis

Diagnostic Studies
- CT scan initially but may not reveal an ischemic stroke in the first 24 to 48 hours
- MRI is the standard diagnostic imaging tool for the diagnosis of stroke.
- Blood glucose to rule out hypoglycemia as cause of altered LOC
- Urine drug screen
- Lumbar puncture if CT negative for hemorrhage and subarachnoid hemorrhage suspected
- Carotid duplex for evaluation of symptomatic carotid stenosis, if patient is surgical candidate for endarterectomy; carotid studies are useless for evaluation of posterior circulation
- Angiography remains the "gold standard" for assessing carotid stenosis, as well as identifying aneurysms, AVM, and vasculitis.
- Electrocardiogram, chest radiograph, echocardiogram
- Transesophageal echocardiogram if intraventricular thrombus suspected
- CBC, ESR, coagulation studies, RPR, chemistry panel, and lipid profile to evaluate cause

Differential Diagnosis

- TIA, thrombotic, embolic, or lacunar stroke
- Subarachnoid or intracerebral hemorrhage
- Cerebral aneurysm or AVM
- Intracranial tumor
- Seizure
- Migraine with aura
- Encephalopathy
- Intoxication
- Hypoglycemia
- Multiple sclerosis
- Syncope
- Vertigo
- Postural hypotension

Management

Nonpharmacologic Treatment

- Airway management
- Carotid endarterectomy for surgical candidates with carotid stenosis over 70%
- Diet and exercise counseling for primary and secondary prevention; smoking cessation
- Care post-stroke is largely supportive: physical therapy, occupational therapy, and speech therapy
- Emotional support of patient and family
- Management after TIA is aimed at identifying risk factors for stroke and modifying them.
  - Diet, weight management, physical activity and exercise, smoking cessation
  - Managing diabetes, hypertension, and hyperlipidemia
  - Identifying and treating any other underlying conditions such as atrial fibrillation, arteritis, or hematologic disorders

Pharmacologic Treatment

TIA management
If caused by cardioembolic event, then:

- Aspirin 325 mg daily
- Heparin infusion to a target PTT of 1.5 times baseline (facilities now have heparin protocols for loading doses and subsequent infusion rates and changes), then start warfarin
- Warfarin (Coumadin): starting dose is 5 to 15 mg orally daily
  - Indicated for recurrent TIAs when patient already taking antiplatelet therapy, if TIA caused by prosthetic heart valve mural thrombus following a myocardial infarction
  - International Normalized Ratio (INR) is stabilized at 2 to 3 for atrial fibrillation or antiplatelet failure and 2.5 to 3.5 for prosthetic valve.
- If noncardioembolic cause:
- Aspirin 325 mg PO daily *or*
- Aspirin 325 mg daily + dipyridamole (Aggrenox) sustained release 200 mg b.i.d. (optimal stroke prevention)
- Clopidogrel (Plavix) 75 mg daily
  - Use if patient already taking aspirin at the onset of TIA or if aspirin is contraindicated
  - Recent studies have indicated that adding aspirin to clopidogrel provides no additional benefit; however, this is still being studied.

Ischemic and thromboembolic CVA management
- Tissue plasminogen activator (tPA) must be administered in a hospital **within 3 hours of onset of symptoms** of ischemic stroke (0.9 mg/kg to maximum dose of 90 mg). Contraindications to tPA:
  - Hemorrhagic stroke
  - Rapidly resolving symptoms
  - Multilobar infarct on CT scan
  - Presentation is suspiscious of subarachnoid hemorrhage, even if CT is negative
  - History of stroke or head trauma in previous 3 months
  - Arterial puncture at noncompressible site in the past 7 days
  - Use of heparin within 48 hours and PTT > 40 seconds
  - Current use of oral anticoagulants, INR > 1.7, or PT > 15
  - Systolic BP > 185 mm Hg or diastolic BP > 110 mm Hg after hypertensive treatment
  - History of intracranial hemorrhage, AVM, aneurysm, or brain tumor
  - Major surgery or serious trauma in past 14 days

- GI or urinary tract hemorrhage in last 21 days
- Platelet count < 100,000 µL
- Blood glucose < 50 or > 400 mg/dL
- Seizure at onset of stroke
- Bacterial endocarditis or suspected pericarditis
- Known or suspected pregnancy

- Hypertension should only be treated if systolic BP > 220 or diastolic > 120 mm Hg, aortic dissection, end-organ compromise, or receiving tPA
  - Use IV nicardipine drip or labetolol drip to decrease blood pressure by 15% in first 24 hours
  - Blood pressure can be lowered to < 140/90 mm Hg after 2 weeks.
  - Avoid hypotension; this may worsen deficits.
- Medical management in the post-acute phase involves anticoagulation or antiplatelet agents, and treatment of underlying heart disease, hypertension, diabetes, and hyperlipidemia.
- Nonhemorrhagic strokes
- Aspirin 325 mg each day
- Ticlopidine (Ticlid) 250 mg b.i.d.; reduce dose to daily for renal patients (monitor for agranulocytosis)
  - Not preferred agent secondary to side effects *or*
- Clopidogrel (Plavix) 75 mg each day; does not cause neutropenia but has been more effective at preventing peripheral vascular disease than stroke
- If caused by cardioembolic event
  - Warfarin (Coumadin): Used for patients with symptoms on antiplatelet medication or those with atrial fibrillation or prosthetic heart valves. Dose is individualized because of the small therapeutic window and interactions with food and other medications. International Normalized Ratio (INR) is stabilized at 2 to 3 for atrial fibrillation or antiplatelet failure and 2.5 to 3.5 for a prosthetic valve.

How Long to Treat
- As long as antiplatelet or anticoagulation treatment is not contraindicated (increase risk of GI or intracerebral bleeding)

Hemorrhagic Stroke
- Airway management if warranted
- Treatment focused on
  - Supportive care
  - Blood pressure control
- Treat hypertension: to a goal of 15% decrease in first 24 hours
  - Use IV nicardipine drip or labetalol drip
  - Avoid hypotension—may worsen deficits
- Consider fresh frozen plasma, platelet transfusion, or vitamin K if patient on anticoagulation
- Surgical evacuation if life-saving

SAH
- Airway management if warranted
- Strict bedrest and quiet environment
- Colace or other stool softeners to prevent straining
- Treat hypertension: Maintain SBP < 160 mm Hg.
  - Use IV nicardipine drip or labetolol drip.
  - Omit

- Nimodipine 60 mg p.o. every 4 hours for 21 days to prevent cerebral vasospasm
- If vasospam, treat with volume expansion and hypertensive therapy if aneurysm has been repaired
- Neurosurgery evaluation for possibility of aneurysm clipping, bypass, or coiling
- Supportive care from speech, physical, and occupational therapy

Treatment and Prevention of Increase Intracranial Pressure (ICP)

- Hypotension and hypoventilation contribute to increased ICP; avoid hypotension and provide adequate oxygenation.
- Strict bedrest and quiet environment
- Temperature regulation to promote normothermia
- Head of bed elevated (> 30°); head in midline position to promote jugular blood return
- Sedation
- Pain management
- Colace or other stool softeners/laxatives to prevent straining
- Hyperventilation to keep PCO_2 30–35 mm Hg in selective cases—no longer traditional therapy
- Maintain cerebral perfusion pressure (CPP = MAP – ICP) 50 to 70 mm Hg
- Mannitol, an osmotic diuretic, may be used to decrease ICP and maintain serum osmolality.
  - Hypertonic saline (such as 3%)

Special Considerations

- Men are at greater risk than women, although more women die of stroke because of age and population dynamics.
- Increased risk with age and poorer prognosis; increased incidence of infection, myocardial infarction, renal failure, and delirium
- Consider patient's risk of falls, ability to manage a complex medication regime, and INR monitoring when initiating warfarin therapy.
- Do not discount stroke in young people; may be hemorrhagic stroke secondary to AVM, cavernous malformations, or embolic stroke secondary to unidentified patent foramen ovale (right-to-left shunt)

When to Consult, Refer, or Hospitalize

- Consider neurosurgery consult.
- Suspected TIA will need urgent work-up and treatment to prevent stroke; if diagnosed as stroke and of less than 3 hours duration, may start tPA therapy
- Patients with sudden severe headache, decreasing level of consciousness, vomiting, or focal neurological deficits should be evaluated in a hospital setting.

Follow-up

- Patients with risk for cerebrovascular disease should be monitored every 3 to 6 months for symptoms of TIA or hypertension, and counseled regarding stroke prophylaxis, diet, exercise, and smoking cessation.

Expected Outcomes

- Variable; most stroke recovery occurs early; the longer deficits last, the less likely they are to resolve, although improvement may be seen for 6 months
- 27% of stroke patients die within 1 year, and 53% within 5 years.
- Physical therapy improves functional recovery.
- Older age, coma, and early acute CT changes are associated with a poor prognosis.

Complications

- Intracerebral hemorrhage from tPA therapy
- Myocardial infarction, infection, renal failure
- Falls, depression, dementia
- Intracerebral bleed or GI bleed from anticoagulation

MYASTHENIA GRAVIS

Description

- Mysthenia gravis is an autoimmune disorder involving antibody and cell-mediated acetycholine receptor destruction, resulting in muscle weakness and fatigability.

Etiology

- Body produces autoantibodies against the acetycholine receptors
- The cause of autoantibody production is not known.

Incidence

- Occurs in women in their 20s and 30s; men in their 60s
- 65% of patients have thymic hyperplasia.
- 10% of patients have a malignant thyoma.

Risk Factors

- Associated factors
  - Surgery
  - Infection
  - Other autoimmune disorders such as RA and SLE
  - Medications such as quinine, aminoglycosides, calcium channel blockers, magnesium sulfate

Assessment

History
- Muscle weakness and fatigue with activity, improves with rest
- Difficulty in chewing or swallowing
- Diplopia
- Intensity of symptoms fluctuates over hours to days

Physical Examination
- Muscle weakness noted on exam
- Ocular palsies
- Ptosis
- Deep tendon reflexes and sensation are normal.

Diagnostic
- Tensilon (edrophonium) test: 2 mg IV test dose given; if no reaction after 30 seconds, then give 8 mg IV. If muscle weakness improves, test is considered positive.
  - Side effects are bradycardia (have atropine on hand) and atrioventricular block.
- Serum acetycholine receptor antibodies are present in 85% to 90% of patients.
- Electromyography
- Thyroid panel
- CT scan to evaluate for thyoma

Differential Diagnosis
- Lambert-Eaton myasthenic syndrome
- Amyotrophic lateral sclerosis (Lou Gehrig's Disease)

Management

Nonpharmacologic Treatment
- Refer to neurologist
- Treat underlying triggering event if identified
- Thymectomy

Pharmacologic Treatment
- Symptomatic relief with anticholinesterase drugs such as neostigmine and pyridostigmine
- If no relief with anticholinesterase drugs and thymectomy, then patients are treated with corticosteroids.
- IVIG therapy or plasmapheresis for preoperative thymectomy or for myasthenia gravis crisis

When to Consult, Refer, or Hospitalize

- All patients should have neurology consult and referral.
- Hospitalize if in crisis.

Complications

- Myasthenia gravis crisis
- Presents as respiratory failure and airway compromise.
- Usually requires mechanical ventiliation
- Treat with plasmapheresis or IVIG therapy.

GUILLAIN-BARRÉ SYNDROME

Description

- Guillain-Barré syndrome acute inflammatory polyneuropathy, characterized by symmetrical muscle weakness.

Etiology

- Unknown
- Thought to be autoimmune in nature
- Precipitated by infection, surgery, or vaccination
- Infection is culprit in > 50% of cases
- Common pathogens: *Campylobacter jejuni*, CMV, *Mycoplasma pneumonia*

Assessment

History
- Weakness, mostly flaccid in nature
- Ascending, symmetrical paralysis
- Pain in back, hips, and thighs
- Infection caused by *Campylobacter jejuni*, CMV, *Mycoplasma pneumonia* in previous weeks to days
- Recent vaccination

Physical
- Loss of deep tendon reflexes
- Autonomic disturbances causing blood pressure and heart rate fluctuations
- Facial and oropharyngeal muscles weakness noted in approximately 50% of patients
- Respiratory muscle impairment requiring mechanical ventilation in 25% to 30% of patients

Diagnostic
- Electromyography (EMG): slowed nerve conduction and demyelination
- CSF analysis: high protein with normal cell content
- Measurement of forced vital capacity: intubation for < 15 mL/kg

Differential Diagnosis

- Myasthenia gravis
- West Nile virus
- Poliomyelitis
- Metabolic neuropathies
- Botulism
- Tick paralysis

Management

Nonpharmacologic Treatment
- Considered medical emergency
- Place in ICU setting.
- Intubation and mechanical ventilation if indicated
- Early physical therapy to avoid adverse effects of prolonged immobilization
- DVT prophylaxis
- Monitor for cardiac arrhythmias.

Pharmacologic Treatment
- Treatment of choice is plasmapheresis.
- Immune globulin is used if plasmapheresis is not available or was previously given.
- Use of corticosteroids does not affect outcome.

When to Consult, Refer, or Hospitalize

- All patients should be hospitalized.
- ICU setting
- Neurology consult

Expected Outcomes

- Disease lasts 2 to 4 weeks and recovery for several weeks to months.
- 5% mortality rate
- 3% of patients will be wheelchair-bound.
- 80% recover without any deficits or with only minor deficits.

Complications

- Aspiration pneumonia
- Decubitus ulcers
- DVT/pulmonary embolism

PARKINSON'S DISEASE

Description

- Parkinson's disease is a neurodegenerative disease characterized by slow movement (bradykinesia), rigidity, flexed posture, loss of postural reflex, freezing, and resting tremor.

Etiology

- Unknown, although genetics, endogenous toxins, and exogenous toxins have been implicated
- Destruction of the substantia nigra and nigrostriatal tract occurs, resulting in damage to dopaminergic neurons, leaving active unopposed acetylcholine neurons intact.
- Imbalance of dopamine and acetylcholine result in loss of refinement of voluntary movement
- Can be reversible in patients receiving metoclopramide, neuroleptic agents, or reserpine.

Incidence and Demographics

- Prevalence 350 per 100,000 in the United States with 50,000 new cases per year
- Greater in men than women at a 3:2 ratio; usual onset occurs during ages 45 to 65
- Less prevalent in Africans and Blacks than in Asians, Europeans, and Whites
- Affects 1% of those age > 50

Risk Factors

- Age, heredity
- Possible environmental factors

Prevention and Screening

- None, although older patients may benefit from periodic assessment of mobility, cognitive, and functional status

Assessment

History
- Focused detailed history of chief complaint, including time frame and progression, and aggravating and alleviating factors, such as stress or rest; interview family, patient, and caregiver

- Complete review of neurologic symptoms, including weakness, paresthesia, tremor, diplopia, aphasia, mood, and cognitive changes
- Past medical history, including neurological disorders, exposure to environmental toxins, illicit drugs
- Family history of Parkinson's disease, other movement disorders, or dementia
- Medications, including over-the-counter anticholinergics, antihistamines, decongestants, or cough and cold preparations that worsen condition
- Functional assessment: difficulty with functional and instrumental activities of daily living (ADLs), mobility, including stair-climbing (patients with progressive supranuclear palsy will have problems descending stairs) and rising from chair
- Falls and injuries
- Review of systems for associated autonomic dysfunction, including perspiration, incontinence, constipation, and postural hypotension
- Assess for depression and mental status—may use Geriatric Depression Scale and MMSE or other tools

Physical Examination
- General: manner, affect, and dress and hygiene; speech may be soft and monotone
- Cranial nerve exam: normal in Parkinson's, 4th cranial nerve palsy with progressive supranuclear palsy
- Motor exam: no weakness but has cogwheel rigidity (rigidity to passive movement)
  - Bradykinesia: slowness of voluntary movement and difficulty initiating movement, difficulty rising from chair, shuffling gait, problems with turns and stopping movement
  - Tremor: slow (4 to 6 cycles per second) resting tremor present in one limb, limbs on one side, four limbs, or may be absent in 20% of Parkinson's patients; tremor may be obvious at rest and exaggerated with stress; some tremor of mouth and lips
    - Tremor may increase with emotional stress, and decrease with voluntary activity.
- Gait and posture: stooped posture with knees and hips flexed, hands held in front, close to body
- "Masked facies": fixed facial expression, drooling, wide palpebral fissures, soft voice
- Myerson's sign: Repetitive tapping on the bridge of the nose produces sustained blink response.
- Incoordination of rapid alternating movements; decreased automatic movement, decreased blinking
- Deep tendon reflexes are unaffected.
- General examination: seborrhea
- Vital signs: orthostatic hypotension

Diagnostic Studies
- Consider head CT if diagnosis not clear and stroke or space-occupying lesion is suspected

Differential Diagnosis

- Benign essential tremor
- Progressive supranuclear palsy
- Depression
- Dementia
- Cerebrovascular disease
- Brain tumor
- Adverse effects of anticholinergic medications, particularly antipsychotics
- Drug-induced Parkinson's
- Carbon monoxide poisoning
- Normal pressure hydrocephalus
- Huntington's disease
- Creutzfeldt-Jakob disease

Management

- There is no cure for Parkinson's. Current therapy is aimed at managing symptoms to preserve independence and mobility.
- The Hoehn and Young Scale can be helpful for staging the disease and guiding pharmacological and supportive therapy.
  - Stage I: unilateral involvement
  - Stage II: bilateral involvement but no postural abnormalities
  - Stage III: bilateral involvement with mild postural instability; patient leads an independent life
  - Stage IV: bilateral involvement with postural instability; patient requires substantial help
  - Stage V: severe, fully developed disease; patient is restricted to bed and chair

Nonpharmacologic Treatment
- Patient and family education regarding progressive nature of disease and complex pharmacologic treatments
- Nutritional counseling regarding low-protein diet and dietary management of constipation
- Compression stockings for postural hypotension
- Physical, occupational, and speech therapy with appropriate assistive devices for ambulation and ADLs
- Fall precautions and home safety evaluation; install rails, raised toilet seats, and tub chairs
- Encourage walking, social activities, and interaction
- Emotional support
- Deep brain stimulation
- Surgical interventions: unilateral stereotaxic thalamotomy or pallidotomy, implantable high-frequency thalamic stimulation to suppress resting tremor for difficult-to-control cases

Pharmacologic Treatment (see table)

- Dopamine precursor
  - 25 mg carbidopa/100 mg levodopa t.i.d. to q.i.d.; or 10 mg carbidopa/100 mg levodopa t.i.d. to q.i.d., titrate up by 1 tablet every 2 to 7 days as needed and tolerated, not to exceed 200 mg carbidopa and 800 mg levodopa a day
    - "On–off" phenomenon occurs in 40% to 50% of patients—after 2 to 3 years, patients will experience inconsistent effect from the same dose.
    - "Wearing-off" symptoms appear before next dose is due
    - Use lowest doses possible, consider addition of dopamine agonists
- Dopamine agonists
  - Pramipexole (Mirapex) 0.125 mg t.i.d., titrate up to 1.5 mg t.i.d. over 7 weeks
  - Ropinirole (Requip) 0.25 mg t.i.d., titrate up weekly by 1.5 mg a day to a total dose of 24 mg a day. Maintenance dose is 3 to 24 mg a day. Discontinue slowly over 1 week.
- MAO-B inhibitor
  - Selegiline (Eldepryl) 5 mg b.i.d. (at low doses is a selective MAO inhibitor and can be safely administered with levodopa)
  - Nonselective MAO inhibitors are contraindicated in combination with levodopa. Their use can precipitate hyperpyrexia and hypertensive crisis and must be discontinued at least 14 days before initiating levodopa.
- Anticholinergic agent
  - Benztropine (Cogentin) 1 to 2 mg q.d.
- Catechol O-methyltransferase (COMT) inhibitor
  - Tolcapone (Tasmar) 100 to 200 mg 3 t.i.d.

Table 7–1. Treatment Algorithm for Parkinson's Disease

Stage or Problem	Therapeutic Alternatives
Mild disease (Stage I and II)	Selegiline for neuroprotection Anticholinergics if tremor predominant Amantadine (best for rigidity and bradykinesia) Group support, exercise, education, nutrition
Functionally impaired (Stage III)	Tremor predominant: anticholinergics Functional disability: sustained-release carbidopa/levodopa
Age ≤ 60 years	(lowest dose possible); dopamine agonist
Age ≥ 60 years	Sustained-release carbidopa/levodopa
Stage IV or V	Immediate-release carbidopa/levodopa Dopamine agonists
Poor symptom control	Increase carbidopa/levodopa dose Add or increase dopamine agonist dose Add COMT inhibitor

Continued

Table 7-1. Treatment Algorithm for Parkinson's Disease *(cont.)*

Stage or Problem	Therapeutic Alternatives
Suboptimal peak response	Begin combination dopaminergic therapy Add levodopa to dopamine agonist Add dopamine agonist to levodopa Increase dose of levodopa/carbidopa or dopamine agonist Add COMT inhibitor as levodopa adjunct, switch dopamine agonists
Wearing off	Begin combination of dopaminergic therapy Add levodopa to dopamine agonist Add dopamine agonist to levodopa Increase frequency of levodopa dosing Increase dose of levodopa/carbidopa (sustained or immediate release) Add COMT inhibitor and decrease levodopa dose Change to sustained-release carbidopa/levodopa Add liquid levodopa/carbidopa Add selegiline if not already taking
On-off	Begin combination dopaminergic therapy Add levodopa to dopamine agonist Add dopamine agonist to levodopa Add COMT inhibitor Modify distribution of dietary protein
Freezing	Increase or decrease carbidopa/levodopa dose Add dopamine agonist Increase or decrease dopamine agonist dose Discontinue selegiline Gait modification, assistance device
No "on" time	Manipulate time and dose of levodopa Add COMT inhibitor Avoid dietary protein Increase GI transit time

Adapted from "Antiparkinson agents" by L. R. Young, 2004, in Edmunds, M. W. & Mayhew, M. S. (Eds.), *Pharmacology for the primary care provider* (2nd ed.). St. Louis, MO: Mosby, p. 512.

How Long to Treat
- Medication combinations and dosages must be individualized and adjusted during the course of the disease; the disease is lifelong and progressive.

Special Considerations

- Prescribe Parkinson's medications with caution in older adults, particularly those with comorbidity of heart, renal, or liver disease.
- Avoid anticholinergics in older adults—they tend to be poorly tolerated and have increased risk of side effects, including confusion, agitation, arrhythmias, and urinary retention.
- Differentiate Parkinson's disease from essential tremor; may occur at any age from childhood on, but likelihood increases with age and affects the distal upper extremities and head; may be familial
  - If mild, reassurance may be only intervention needed
  - May be treated with beta-adrenergic blockers such as propranolol (Inderal) and metoprolol (Lopressor); primidone (Mysoline); benzodiazepines
  - May be disabling; refer for possible neurosurgery

When to Consult, Refer, or Hospitalize

- Refer to neurologist for confirmation of diagnosis and guidance with medical management
- Neurosurgical consultation for those with severe symptoms refractory to medications, or unable to tolerate medications

Follow-up

- Every 3 months, as well as any time a change is made in medication and/or therapy regimens
- Episodic office visit if symptoms worsen
- Annual health assessment and physical examination

Expected Outcomes
- Progressive; 30% develop coexisting dementia with poorer prognosis

Complications
- Related to immobility and falls; hip fractures are common, pneumonia may occur in Stage 5
- Aspiration of food
- Depression and social isolation occur

MULTIPLE SCLEROSIS

Description

- Multiple sclerosis (MS) is a progressive neurodegenerative disease characterized by demyelination and inflammation of the neuronal sheath in the brain and spinal cord that produces episodic neurologic symptoms such as sensory abnormalities, visual disturbances, sphincter disturbances, and weakness with or without spasticity.

Etiology

- Autoimmune disease; possible causes may be genetic, viral, immunologic, or environmental; strong association with HLA-DR2 antigen

Incidence and Demographics

- Incidence is 250,000 to 300,000 per year in the United States.
- Prevalence is higher in temperate zones, ranging from only 5 to 10/100,000 in tropical zones to 50 to 175/100,000 in cooler environments.
- Female-to-male ratio is 2 to 3:1; estrogen and progesterone may be implicated, given that symptoms often develop during the menstrual cycle and after pregnancy.
- Age of onset 15 to 55 years; greatest incidence in young adults < 55 years
- Late onset of MS in the 6th to 7th decade usually severe and rapidly progressive

Risk Factors

- Familial 1% to 3% increased risk in first-degree relatives (15 times greater than general population)
- Climate or place of residence, established by residence in the first 15 years of life
- Urban dwelling, upper socioeconomic status, Western European descent

Assessment

History
- Neurological history: paresthesias, weakness, and spasticity; ataxia fatigue; visual changes; vestibular disturbances; trigeminal neuralgia; optic neuritis; bowel and bladder dysfunction
- Time frame with exacerbations and remission

- Past medical history for differential diagnosis: systemic lupus erythematosus, Lyme disease, cerebral and spinal tumors, HIV, seizures, peripheral neuropathy, head or spinal trauma
- Triggers may be infection, trauma, pregnancy

Physical Examination
- Complete neurologic exam
  - Cranial nerve deficits
  - Optic neuritis: decreased visual acuity, abnormal pupillary response, hyperemia, and edema of optic disk
  - Internuclear ophthalmoplegia: cranial nerve 6 palsy or weakness of the medial rectus muscle with lateral gaze, nystagmus
  - Decreased strength, increased tone, clonus, positive Babinski; weakness, numbness, tingling, or unsteadiness in a limb; disequilibrium; urinary urgency, hesitancy, incontinence
  - Decreased proprioception and vibratory sensation, positive Romberg; pyramidal, sensory, or cerebellar deficits in some or all limbs
  - Lhermitte's sign: an electrical sensation down the back into the legs produced with neck flexion

Diagnostic Studies
- MRI may visualize characteristic multiple lesions of demyelinated areas with reactive gliosis
- Cerebrospinal fluid analysis for lymphocytosis, immunoglobulins, and oligoclonal bands
- Visual, auditory, and sensory evoked potentials

Differential Diagnosis

- Stroke
- Cerebral or spinal tumors
- Ischemic optic neuropathy
- Systemic lupus erythematosus
- Lyme disease
- Peripheral neuropathy
- Seizure disorder
- AIDS
- Intoxication
- Amyotrophic lateral sclerosis

Management

- Aimed at delaying progress, managing chronic symptoms, and treating acute exacerbations

Nonpharmacologic Treatment
- Physical and occupational therapy
- Mental health services for assistance with coping strategies

Pharmacologic Treatment
- Complex; treatment regimen *must* be coordinated with a neurologist
- Immunosuppressive therapy may arrest progression
  - Interferon-beta (Avonex) 30 mcg IM once a week
  - Glatiramer acetate (Copaxone) 20 mg SQ q.d.
  - Azathioprine (Imuran) unlabeled use
- Acute exacerbations: prednisone 60 to 80 mg/day for 1 week, taper over 2 to 3 weeks
- Spasticity: baclofen (Lioresal) 40 to 80 mg a day in divided doses, start with 5 mg t.i.d. and titrate up every 3 days
  - Clonazepam (Klonopin) unlabeled use
- Fatigue
  - Amantadine (Symmetrel) 100 mg b.i.d.
  - Consider tricyclic antidepressants or selective serotonin reuptake inhibitors
  - Treat underlying spastic bladder, depression

How Long to Treat
- Use corticosteroids only for acute exacerbations, not for maintenance
- Antibodies may develop to interferon
- Stop interferon if progression of disabilities continues after 6 months of treatment

Special Considerations

- New onset or exacerbations with menstrual cycle and postpartum
- Family planning and fertility should be discussed with women of childbearing age; menses may be irregular and fertility impaired because of demyelination but pregnancy is not contraindicated.
- Oral contraceptives are not contraindicated except with impaired mobility.
- Consult with obstetrician regarding medications for pregnancy and lactation.

When to Consult, Refer, or Hospitalize

- Refer all patients with suspected MS to neurologist for confirmation of diagnosis and development of management plan
- Ophthalmology referral
- Continence specialist or urologist for bladder dysfunction
- Mental health referral for coping or depression

Follow-up

- Followed closely by neurology; primary care for routine health visits

Expected Outcomes
- Progressive with exacerbations and remissions

Complications
- Hydronephrosis and renal failure secondary to urinary retention
- Falls
- Depression

HEAD TRAUMA

Description

- Head trauma can be caused by traumatic brain injury: brain injury secondary to acceleration–deceleration forces or penetrating forces
- Concussion: posttraumatic mental status alteration, which usually lasts seconds to minutes, but absolutely < 6 hours. No abnormalities noted on radiography or lasting neuro deficits
- Contusion: "bruised brain": trauma induced either from closed head injury or from penetrating trauma. Effects on brain function depend on the size of the contusion with larger contusions causing cerebral edema and increased ICP.

Etiology

- Trauma-induced: Motor vehicle accidents, sports injuries, or falls are common causes of head trauma.

Incidence

- 1.4 million people per year experience traumatic brain injuries.
- 50,000 of these will die.
- 80,000 of these will have a disability.
- Leading cause of death in trauma patients

Assessment

History
- Duration of amnesia and/or loss of consciousness
- Mechanism of injury
- Patient experienced a lucid period and then rapid decline in neuro status (this would indicate epidural bleed)
- Complaint of headache, vertigo, inability to recall events, or nausea and vomiting
- Suspect subdural hematoma in patients who are delibitated, aged, or alcoholics

Physical Examination

- Ideally assess patient before sedatives, paralytics, or opioids are administered.
- Assess for adequacy of airway and breathing.
- Glasgow Coma Scale (GCS)
- Level of consciousness, focal deficits
- Pupillary response
- Assess for area of injury.
- Raccoon eyes, mastoid ecchymosis or "battle signs," rhinorrhea or otorrhea of CSF fluid—indicates basilar skull fracture
- Posturing: decorticate or decerebrate
- Monitor for signs of increased ICP: Cushing's triad—hypertension, bradycardia, respiratory depression

Diagnostic Studies

- Non-contrast CT scan used initially to evaluate for intracranial hemorrhage
- MRI used later to evaluate for diffuse axonal injury or smaller contusions
- Angiography used only when vascular injury is suspected or when CT results do not coincide with physical findings
- Cervical films (trauma patient)

Management

- Evaluate ABCs
- Intubate and mechanically ventilate if unable to protect airway or GCS < 8
- Neurosurgical consult if indicated
- Frequent evaluation of neurologic status and vital signs
- If increased ICP
  - Head of bed elevated (> 30 degrees); head in midline position
  - Colace or other stool softeners or laxatives to prevent straining
  - Hyperventilation to keep PCO_2 30 to 35 mm Hg
  - Maintain cerebral perfusion pressure (CPP = MAP – ICP) 50 to 70 mm Hg
  - Mannitol, an osmotic diuretic, may be used to decrease ICP and maintain serum osmolality.
  - Paralytics or sedation for agitation (only if intubated)
  - Goal ICP is < 20 mm Hg
- Consider anticonvulsant such as phenytoin to prevent seizures in patients with severe head trauma.
- Rehab with physical, occupational, and speech therapy

Special Considerations

- Monroe–Kelley doctrine: Blood, brain, and CSF are contained in a closed area (skull); when there is an increase in one of these components, another must decrease to maintain a normal intracranial pressure.
- Immediate CT scan is indicated for patient experiencing neurologic deterioration, to evaluate for expanding hematoma or increasing cerebral edema
- Recent study has shown that hypertonic saline has reduced ICP and increased CPP

When to Consult, Refer, or Hospitalize

- Hospitalization and neurosurgical consult for patients who experience skull fracture, contusion, hematoma, or cervical fractures, or who have focal neurologic deficits

Expected Outcomes

Severe traumatic brain injury:
- Rapid recovery in the first 6 months post-injury and then less improvement over the next few years
- 50% of patients have a good recovery or moderate disability.
- Also experience personality or behavior changes, decreased attention span and memory

Complications

- Long-term disability
- Effects of prolonged immobility: pulmonary embolism, DVT, pressure ulcers

SPINAL CORD TRAUMA

Description

- Spinal cord trauma causes bruising, tearing, crushing, or penetration of the spinal cord.
- Complete cord transection: immediate, complete, flaccid paralysis; loss of sensation, reflex, and sphincter tone
- Partial cord injury: patient has mixed sensory and motor activity below lesion
  - *Brown-Sequard's syndrome*: unilateral cord lesion causing contralateral pain and temperature loss; ipsilateral weakness and proprioceptive loss
  - *Anterior cord syndrome*: usually caused by flexion injuries; causes bilateral pain, temperature loss, and weakness below lesion, but vibratory sensation and proprioception remain intact
  - *Cauda equine syndrome*: compression of lower lumbar and sacral roots; causes sensory loss, flaccid leg weakness, decreased reflexes, and urine/bowel incontinence
  - *Central cord syndrome*: usually as a result of a hyperextension/flexion injury; increased motor impairment in upper extremities in comparison to lower extremities; bladder dysfunction

Etiology

- Result from all types of trauma such as motor vehicle accidents, diving accidents, assaults, falls, sports injuries, etc.

    ### Mechanism of Injury
    - Hyperextension
    - Hyperflexion
    - Compression
    - Rotation
    - Penetration

Incidence

- More than 10,000 spinal cord injuries occur annually in the United States.
- Motor vehicle accidents account for 40%.
- Assaults account for 25%.
- More common in males (80%)

Assessment

History
- Time and mechanism of injury
- May complain of back pain, neck pain, numbness, paresthesia
- Prehospital treatment

Physical Examination
- Assess airway, breathing, and circulation.
- Assess neurologic function above and below suspected injury.
- Classic sign of spinal cord trauma is when neurologic function is intact above the level of injury and impaired or absent below the level of injury
- C5 or above: respiratory muscle impairment
- C4 or above: quadriplegia
- C5: quadriplegia, some gross upper extremity function possible
- C6 to C7: quadriplegia with some shoulder movement and elbow flexion possible
- C6 to T11: variable degrees of intercostal and abdominal muscle impairment
- T12 to L1: paraplegia, loss of sensation, and areflexia to lower extremities; bowel and urine retention
- L1 to L5: partial flaccid paralysis to flaccid paralysis; ankle and plantar reflexes absent

Diagnostic Data

- Plain films of suspected injured area
- CT scan
- MRI—identifies type and location of injury

Management

Nonpharmacologic Treatment
- Management of airway and breathing
- Do not hyperextend neck during intubation; use jaw-thrust.
- Complete immobilization
- Neurosurgery consult
- Log roll only
- Foley and NG tube placement
- Maintain MAP between 85 and 90 mm Hg—prevents spinal cord ischemia.
- Rehab with physical and occupational therapy
- DVT prophylaxis

Pharmacologic Treatment
- Corticosteriods are helpful if initiated within 8 hours of injury.
  - Methylprednisolone 30mg/kg IV bolus followed by an infusion of 5.4 mg/kg/hr for 23 hours

Special Considerations

- Trauma patients may be intoxicated, thus masking spinal cord injuries.
- Spinal cord injuries should be suspected in patients who present with pelvic fractures, head trauma, penetrating trauma near spinal cord, motor vehicle accidents, falls, and diving injuries.

When to Refer, Consult, or Hospitalize

- Neurosurgical consult for patients with neurologic deficits
- Patients with spinal cord injury, compression, or vertebral fracture that may compress the cord should be hospitalized.

Expected Outcomes

- Depend on severity and level of injury
- Complete transection is a permanent injury.
- Recovery is favorable in compressed nerve tissue when motor function and sensation begin to return within 1 week.

Complications

- Long-term disability
- Effects of prolonged immobility: pulmonary embolism, DVT, pressure ulcers
- Chronic pain
- Pneumonia
- Autonomic dysreflexia
  - Life-threatening situation
  - Hypertension, bradycardia, facial flushing, headache caused by noxious stimuli
  - Common causes: full bladder, fecal impaction, line insertions
  - *Treatment is to remove the stimuli* such as place a urine catheter if not present or, if present, check for occlusions and treat hypertension.

MENINGITIS

Description

- Meningitis is a central nervous system infection of the covering of the brain and spinal cord by any infectious agent, including bacteria, virus, mycobacteria, spirochetes, fungi, protozoa, and parasites.

Etiology

- Caused by virulent infectious organism in a susceptible host; local host defenses are overcome
- Viral meningitis can be caused by any of more than 70 different strains of viruses; most common are the enteroviruses (85%) and herpes simplex. It is a less serious form of meningitis and resolves spontaneously.
- Most common fungal causes are *Candida sp.*, *Aspergillus*, and *Cryptococcus neoformans*
- Candidal meningitis occurs mostly in ill premature infants and immunocompromised patients, but 30% of all patients with fungal meningitis have no underlying immunodeficiency.
- Aseptic meningitis can be caused by *Borrelia burgdorferi* (Lyme disease) or *Treponema pallidum* (syphilis).
- Meningitis can also be caused by tuberculosis.
- *N. meningitides* (meningococcal) and *S. pneumoniae* (pneumococci) cause bacterial meningitis in adults.
- *H. influenza* not as common secondary to vaccination, but can occur in immunocompromised individuals or in unvaccinated head trauma patients.
- *S. aureus*, *S. pneumoniae*, and gram-negative bacilli are common causes of postsurgical or posttraumatic meningitis.

Incidence and Demographics

- Incidence is approximately 1 per 100,000 persons per year.
- More prevalent in lower socioeconomic groups, crowded housing, urban areas
- Three times more prevalent in college students residing on campus than in those living off-campus and the general population

Risk Factors

- Poverty and lack of childhood immunizations
- Crowded living conditions
- Immunodeficiency
- College students living in campus housing and soldiers in barracks
- Infectious disease close to meninges: pneumonia, pharyngitis, otitis media, sinusitis, endocarditis
- Penetrating head trauma
- Syphilis infection
- Lyme disease

Prevention and Screening

- Routine administration of the *H. influenzae* type b (HIB) vaccine has significantly reduced the incidence of meningitis.
- The following is the CDC recommendation for administration of meningococcal vaccination for at-risk groups:
  - College first-years living in a dormitory
  - Military recruits
  - Those with damaged spleen or whose spleen has been removed
  - Those who have terminal complement deficiency
  - Microbiologists who are routinely exposed to *Neisseria meningitidis* (the causal pathogen)
  - Those who are traveling to or residing in countries in which the disease is common
- Post-exposure prophylaxis for bacterial meningitis with ciprofloxacin 500 mg oral, single dose, for household contacts, those with direct exposure to oral secretions (kissing) of infected patient, or face-to-face contact (e.g., medical staff)
- Alternative post-exposure prophylaxis
  - Rifampin 600 mg orally b.i.d. x 2 days
  - Ceftriaxone 250 mg IM once

Assessment

History
- Rapid onset within 24 to 36 hours
- Progressive, severe headache accompanied by neck and back pain with flexion
- Neurologic symptoms: drowsiness, irritability, confusion, photophobia, hearing loss, focal neurologic deficits, seizures, and nuchal rigidity
- Associated symptoms: fever, nausea, vomiting, rash

- Recent history of respiratory infection, head trauma, invasive neurosurgical procedures, or dental procedures
- Past medical history: meningitis, polio, immunodeficiency
- Social history: living in crowded environment, IV drug use, foreign travel
- Environmental exposure to bird or pigeon droppings (fungal) or tick bite (Lyme)
- Medications: immunosuppressants

Physical Examination
- General: fever, tachycardia, hypotension, rash
- Complete neurologic exam: decreased level of consciousness (drowsiness or agitation); papilledema; cranial nerve III, IV, VI, VII, and/or VIII deficits; focal motor deficits; seizure; mental status
- Meningeal irritation: nuchal rigidity
  - Positive Brudzinski's sign: adduction and flexion of legs with neck flexion
  - Positive Kernig's sign: after flexing thighs, extension is met with resistance and pain in hamstring muscles
- Complete physical exam for sites of primary infections
  - Head trauma or surgery, dental abscess or caries, otitis media, sinusitis, pneumonia, pancreatitis, genital lesions, skin rashes

Diagnostic Studies
- Cerebrospinal fluid analysis, culture (diagnosis usually made on Gram stain): gold standard diagnosis
  - Viral infection: some lymphocytes, normal glucose, moderately high protein content, normal or mildly elevated opening pressure
  - Bacterial infection: increased lymphocytes, decreased glucose, high protein content, markedly elevated opening pressure
- Brain CT prior to lumbar puncture (LP) if space-occupying lesion (brain abscess, subdural empyema, tumor, subdural hematoma) suspected with papilledema, focal neurologic findings, or both; LP is contraindicated with increased intracranial pressure
- CBC, platelet count, PT/PTT, electrolytes, BUN, creatinine, glucose, arterial blood gases (as indicated), blood cultures
- Chest x-ray, sinus x-ray, or both if exam indicates source of infection

Differential Diagnosis

- Bacterial meningitis
- Aseptic meningitis
- Encephalitis (herpes, rabies)
- Brain abscess
- Non-infectious meningeal irritation (sarcoidosis, systemic lupus erythematosus, cancer, medications, and chemical irritants)
- Bacterial sinusitis or mastoiditis
- Vertebral osteomyelitis
- Amebic meningoencephalitis

Management

Nonpharmacologic Treatment
- Medical emergency; immediate transport to hospital for IV antibiotics and supportive care
- Assurance of adequate airway, cardiac function, fluid support
- Educate family or significant others regarding illness, treatment, and prognosis
- Inform family and contacts of post-exposure prophylaxis
- Place in a private room with droplet isolation

Pharmacologic Treatment
- Needs prompt treatment
- While waiting on culture results, may start ceftriaxone 2 g IV every 12 hours and vancomycin 1 g IV every 8–12 hours. Add ampicillin, 2 g IV every 4 hours, if the patient is immunocompromised or more than 50 years old.
- *H. influenzae:* Third-generation cephalosporin or ampicillin plus chloramphenicol
- *N. meningitidis:* High-dose ceftriaxone or cefotaxime. Use chloramphenicol if patient has PCN allergy.
- *S. pneumoniae:* Penicillin IV 4 million units every 4 hours. If patient is allergic to PCN, may use chloramphenicol, or vancomycin plus rifampin. Administration of dexamethasone (10 mg IV every 6 hours) given before or during antibiotic regimen for 4 days may reduce neurologic sequelae.
- Gram-negative bacilli: Occurs mostly after head trauma or neurosurgical procedure. Treat with ceftazidime or cefepime, 2 g IV every 8 hours.
- *Listeria monocytogenes:* Seen in the elderly and in immunocompromised patients. Treat with ampicillin plus IV aminoglycoside. If patient has PCN allergy, may use bactrium.

How Long to Treat
- *H. influenzae:* 7 days
- *N. meningitidis:* 3–7 days
- *S. pneumoniae:* 10–14 days
- *Gram-negative bacilli:* 21 days
- *Listeria monocytogenes:* 3–4 weeks

Special Considerations

- Antibiotics given in doses smaller than usually used to treat meningitis for the 3 to 4 days before lumbar puncture will not significantly alter the cerebrospinal fluid (CSF) findings.
- Rifampin contraindicated for post-exposure prophylaxis in patients who are pregnant

When to Consult, Refer, or Hospitalize

- Medical emergency; immediately transfer all suspected meningitis cases to an acute care facility
- Most patient with viral meningitis can be managed at home, if stable, after physician consultation.
- Infectious disease consult

Follow-up

- Patients should be seen in follow-up a few days after hospital discharge.
- The patient and close contacts should be instructed to follow up if any new neurological sequelae present, including hearing and vision problems.

Expected Outcomes
- 90% survival with early diagnosis, treatment, and supportive care

Complications
- Mortality rate is over 50% in those who are not diagnosed early and referred; 10% for those who receive prompt diagnosis, appropriate IV antibiotics, and supportive care.
- Complications of meningitis include seizures (2% to 8%), hearing defects (10%), mental retardation (10%), visual abnormalities (3% to 7%), language delay (15%), motor abnormalities (3% to 7%), inappropriate ADH secretion (SIADH), and sixth cranial nerve palsy. Occurrence of sequelae is estimated at 25% to 50% of meningitis survivors.

SEIZURES AND EPILEPSY

GENERAL INFORMATION

- A seizure is a transient sudden, paroxysmal electrical discharge of a group of neurons in the brain that causes an alteration in neurological function.
- May involve abnormal motor activity, sensory symptoms, a change in the level of alertness, an alteration in autonomic function, or a combination of these
- A seizure is not a diagnosis, but rather a clinical symptom of an underlying neurological dysfunction.
- Seizures classified by etiology: genetic (25%), symptomatic (50%), and idiopathic (25%)
- Neonatal seizures are rarely idiopathic and immediate attention must be paid to identifying the underlying disorder.
- Febrile seizures occur in infants and children as a result of fever, not underlying neurologic disorder
- Epilepsy, or recurrent, spontaneous seizures unrelated to fever, may occur in children and adults.
  - Rolandic epilepsy, associated with a typical EEG pattern, is the most common type in children.
  - Infantile spasms are myoclonic seizures occurring in the first year of life, usually in clusters, associated with a typical EEG pattern.

SEIZURES

Description

- A transient alteration in behavior, function, or consciousness, or a combination of these that results from an abnormal electrical discharge from neurons in the brain
- Epilepsy refers to chronic recurrent seizures.

- Most older adults have partial seizures that may quickly generalize to tonic-clonic.
- The International League Against Epilepsy has classified seizures based on clinical presentation and EEG findings (see the Table 7–2).

Etiology

- A seizure is a symptom of an underlying disorder; most frequent cause of repetitive seizures is failure to take antiseizure medications
- Cause is unknown for most epilepsy, including primary epilepsy, but is believed to be related to abnormalities of neurotransmission
- Patients with primary epilepsy can continue to have seizures into old age.
- Secondary epilepsy is the result of injury to the cerebral cortex.
- Most new-onset epilepsy in older adults is secondary from tumors, hematomas, or stroke.
- Space-occupying lesions, stroke, metabolic disorders, and alcohol withdrawal can also cause seizures.
- Vascular disease is the most common cause of onset > age 60.

Incidence and Demographics

- 10% of Americans will have a seizure at some time during their lives; 1% to 2% have epilepsy.
- New-onset epilepsy is highest among those < 20 years of age.

Risk Factors

- Intracranial lesions, head trauma, hypoglycemia, or chronic illness that predisposes one to metabolic abnormality; medications that lower the seizure threshold (e.g., selective serotonin reuptake inhibitors, certain atypical antidepressants, ciprofloxacin, metronidazole, theophylline)
- Certain triggers: sleep deprivation, menses, flashing lights or television; emotional stress, fever, or hormonal imbalance
- Alcohol intoxication or alcohol withdrawal

Prevention and Screening

- Head trauma prevention: seat belt use, bicycle and motorcycle helmets
- Fall prevention for older adults; home safety counseling

Assessment

History
- Interview witness to seizure if possible. This information is most important in making a diagnosis.
- Detailed history of event; include description of seizure activity, loss of consciousness, duration, incontinence, possible triggers

- Prodromal symptoms such as aura, confusion, or focal neurological symptoms
- Postictal state: antegrade amnesia, level of consciousness
- Prior seizure history, including type, frequency, duration
- Seizure medications: any changes, missed doses, levels
- Past medical history: previous intracranial lesions or trauma, diabetes, HIV, stroke, migraines, dementia, psychiatric illness
- Medications: ciprofloxacin (Cipro), metronidazole (Flagyl), theophylline, stimulants, and antipsychotics can lower seizure threshold
- Diuretic, antihypertensives, and diabetes medicines can cause metabolic disturbances that can cause seizures.
- Family history of seizure

Physical Examination
- Assess for head trauma.
- The screening neurologic exam may be normal, even with structural lesions.
- Focal deficits may be worse immediately after a seizure.
- Evaluate cardiovascular and pulmonary status.
- Blood pressure and pulse will be elevated during and immediately after a seizure.

Diagnostic Studies
- First-time seizure: metabolic panel, toxicology if appropriate
- Brain CT scan even with a metabolic etiology because the metabolic abnormality could lower the seizure threshold in the presence of a structural lesion
- EEG for first-time patient who has seizure with identified etiology but need not be repeated
- EEG for first-time seizure without etiology, may determine seizure type and guide treatment and prognosis; if seizures continue and EEG nondiagnostic, may consider closed-circuit video EEG
- Lumbar puncture if new neurologic findings are not explained by imaging, or if fever or continued unexplained headache are present

Differential Diagnosis

Causes for Seizure
Head trauma
- Brain tumor
- Stroke
- Metabolic disorders
- Alcohol withdrawal
- Withdrawal from some medications can also cause seizure.

Disorders That May Appear to Be Seizures
Syncope
- Transient ischemic attack
- Pseudo-seizures
- Panic attacks or psychosis
- Drug intoxication
- Migraine
- Multiple sclerosis
- Postural hypotension

Table 7–2. Seizure Classification and Recommended Medication

Seizure Type	Description	Medication
Simple partial	Focal motor or sensory symptoms, reflects area of brain affected; no change in consciousness	Phenytoin, carbamazepine, valproic acid, phenobarbital, levetiracetam, topiramate, oxcarbazepine, lamotrigine, zonisamide, gabapentin
Complex partial	Characterized by an aura, followed by impaired consciousness with automatisms, usually originating from temporal lobe	Carbamazepine, phenytoin, phenobarbital, valproic acid, levetiracetam, topiramate, oxcarbazepine, lamotrigine, zonisamide, gabapentin
Secondarily generalized	Simple or complex partial seizures that progress to generalized tonic-clonic seizures	Phenytoin, carbamazepine, phenobarbital, valproic acid, levetiracetam, topiramate, oxcarbazepine, lamotrigine, zonisamide, gabapentin
Generalized tonic-clonic	Formerly "grand mal;" sudden loss of consciousness with tonic-clonic motor activity; postictal state of confusion, drowsiness, and headache	Phenytoin, carbamazepine, phenobarbital, valproic acid, levetiracetam, oxcarbazepine, topiramate, lamotrigine, zonisamide, gabapentin
Absence	Formerly "petit mal," brief (< 30 seconds) episodes of unresponsiveness characterized by staring, blinking, or facial twitching	Ethosuximide, valproic acid, clonazepam

Management

Nonpharmacologic Treatment
- Educate patient and family about seizure disorder and cause.
- Educate them about safety management, including using any aura period to prepare for seizure.
- Stress the importance of keeping an extra supply of medication readily available at all times.
- First episodes of seizures without known cause do not have to be treated with anticonvulsants.
- Educate family about acute seizure management: To protect patient from injury, place on left side to maintain airway if possible.
- Patients with known recurrent seizures do not need to go to emergency department for every seizure; only if seizure lasts more than 2 minutes or breathing is impaired (aspiration)
- Advise regarding state driving regulations
- Advise regarding swimming alone or operating dangerous equipment

- Teach about side effects and toxic effects of medications, not to discontinue seizure medicines abruptly—may precipitate seizure
- Discuss seizure triggers: sleep deprivation, alcohol, menses, stress, low-grade fever, and infection
- Advise to wear Medic Alert bracelet

Pharmacologic Treatment

- Anticonvulsants first initiated by a neurologist: phenytoin (Dilantin), phenobarbital (Luminal), carbamazepine (Tegretol), and valproic acid (Depakene) are first-line choices (see the following table)
- 40% to 50% of patients can be maintained seizure-free on a single agent.
- Phenytoin initially 100 mg 3 times a day, maintenance dose 300 to 600 mg/day divided
- Phenobarbital 60 to 100 mg/day
- Carbamazepine initially 200 mg twice a day, increase by < 200 mg/day in divided doses 3 to 4 times a day up to 1,200 mg
- Valproic acid initially 15 mg/kg/day, increase at 1-week intervals by 5 to 10 mg/kg/day until seizures are controlled or side effects prevent further increase in dose, maximum dose 60 mg/kg/day; divide totally daily doses over 250 mg. Before initiating, baseline liver enzyme levels (specifically ALT and AST) must be drawn and then monitored thereafter approximately every 3 to 6 months, to determine safe serum levels.

How Long to Treat

- Consider discontinuing seizure medications in those without seizures for more than 2 years.
- Obtain an EEG before stopping medication.
- 40% will have a reoccurrence, most within the first year.
- Must consider the risk factors of seizure reoccurrence and medications for each individual patient; consult with neurologist

Special Considerations

- For first-time seizures in patients > 50, must consider an underlying intracranial lesion or metabolic etiology
- Anticonvulsants are metabolized in the liver and involve the cytochrome P450 enzyme system; care must be used when administering these medications with any other medications.
- Patients must be counseled about the signs and symptoms of liver disease, including nausea and vomiting that seem protracted, abdominal pain, anorexia, fatigue, and dark urine and stools.
- Lower, less-frequent doses may be needed for those with hepatic and renal dysfunction.
- Must counsel all women of childbearing age regarding risks of medications during pregnancy
- Seizures may increase, decrease, or remain the same during pregnancy.
- Neurologist should be consulted before pregnancy for medical management
- Anticonvulsants except valproic acid alter the effectiveness of birth control pills
- Some anticonvulsants are excreted in breast milk and may have serious adverse effects for the nursing infant.
- There is no evidence that prophylactic anticonvulsant therapy prevents epilepsy following head trauma or brain surgery; therefore, not necessary to maintain these patients on long-term anticonvulsants
- Educate patients about specifics of state laws limiting driving for seizure patients.

When to Consult, Refer, or Hospitalize

- Referral to neurologist for first-time seizures, when considering discontinuing therapy, and with seizures refractory to adequate trials of monotherapy or pregnancy
- Refer to neurosurgeon for stereotaxic procedures for intractable seizures.

Follow-up

- Most patients should be seen every 3 months by their primary care provider and at least annually by their neurologist; more frequent visits are needed if medications or seizures change.
- Anticonvulsants have small therapeutic ranges; levels should be drawn when adjusting therapy, and with change in seizure frequency.
- Liver enzymes must be monitored.

Expected Outcomes
- Variable—one seizure to intractable seizures

Complications
- Status epilepticus, airway obstruction, injury during seizure activity
  - Status epilepticus is a medical emergency defined as two or more seizures without complete recovery or a seizure lasting more than 30 minutes
  - Management
    - Assess and manage airway; provide oxygen.
    - Telemonitoring; ensure IV access; continually monitor vital signs, including continuous pulse oximetry.
    - Give dextrose 50% IV (25–50 mL).
    - Give Lorazepam 4 mg IV or diazepam 10 mg IV over 2 minutes. Either may be repeated after 10 minutes.
    - Give Phenytoin 18–20 mg/kg loading dose over 50 mg/min or can give fosphenytoin 10 mg/kg loading dose over 150 mg/min.
    - If seizures continue after above measures, intubate patients and give phenobarbital 10–20 mg/kg.
    - If seizures continue, consider midazolam, propofol, or pentobarbital infusions.
    - Consult neurology.

HERNIATED DISK

Description

- Weakness and degeneration of annulus fibrosis and posterior longintudinal ligament can lead to a herniated disk, which can be bulging, protrusion, or extrusion of the disk
- The disk usually herniates postolaterally, and compresses neighboring nerve roots, causing radiculopathy (radiating pain along the dermatome).

Incidence

- 90% affect L5 or S1 nerve roots.
- Peak incidence at ages 35 to 45

Etiology/Risk Factors

- Heavy lifting
- Trauma
- Obesity
- Sedentary lifestyle
- Intense coughing or sneezing

Prevention and Screening

- Strengthening core muscles
- Weight reduction
- Proper lifting techniques

Assessment

History
- Onset usually associated with heavy lifting
- Increase in pain with bending, prolonged sitting, lifting, sneezing, coughing, straining.
- Lying down relieves pain.
- Numbness and weakness are indicators of radiculopathy.
- Low back pain that radiates to hips/buttocks

Physical Examination
- Lumbar herniation: positive straight leg-raise test
- Cervical herniation: neck flexion or tilting is painful.
- Abnormal gait
- Proprioception decreased
- Symptoms associate with the nerve involved.
- Decreased or absent reflexes

Diagnostic Studies
- AP and lateral plain x-rays of spine
- CT scan with and without contrast
- MRI
- Electromyelography—may help identify nerve root

Differential Diagnosis

- Spinal abccess
- Spinal tumor
- Infectious process

Management

- Restricted to light activity with lifting limited to 5 to 10 lbs
- NSAIDS used for pain relief
- Prolonged bedrest is *not* recommended
- Physical therapy for core strengthing
- Teach proper body mechanics
- Weight reduction if indicated
- Heat or cold application and massage

When to Consult, Refer, or Hospitalize

- Consult or refer to neurosurgery or spine surgeon if bowel, bladder, or sexual dysfunction occurs.
- Refer to neurosurgery if noninvasive management not effective, for possible surgical intervention

Expected Outcomes

- 95% recover without surgical intervention in about 3 months.

Complications

- Bowel, bladder, or sexual dysfunction
- Spinal cord compromise

HEADACHE: TENSION, MIGRAINE, CLUSTER

Description

- Headache or head pain may be a symptom of underlying disease or pathology or the disease process itself (cluster headache, migraine). Head pain arises from extracranial structures (muscles, skin, scalp arteries), or from the posterior fossa, the dura, intracranial arteries, and cranial nerves at the base of the brain.
  - Brain tissue itself is not sensitive to pain
- Tension, migraine, and cluster are primary headaches.

- Unusual for new-onset primary headache syndromes to occur after age 50
- Secondary headaches are a symptom of an underlying disorder.
- A sudden and severe headache is significant and warrants immediate attention.
- The pattern of a headache may suggest the etiology, such as acute recurrent headaches. A chronic nonprogressive pattern might suggest postconcussion syndrome. A chronic progressive headache is more concerning and would possibly indicate a brain tumor or other serious etiology.
- Tension headaches are described as squeezing, bandlike pain; onset is usually gradual and lasts days to years; is present when awaking; and may be associated with anxiety or depression, no aura or associated neurological symptoms
- Medication overuse headache (MOH), previously referred to as analgesic rebound headache, is a chronic headache that can develop from the frequent use of headache medications, including OTC analgesic, triptans, ergotamine, caffeine, opiates, or benzodiazepines.
- Cluster headaches have unilateral, excruciating pain lasting 20 minutes to 2 hours with several attacks a day for 4 to 8 weeks, followed by a cluster-free interval for 6 months to years; or chronic form with little cluster-free interval.
- Migraines may be preceded by a prodromal or "warning" feeling; then some have an aura of visual or somatosensory disturbance immediately prior to headache; the headache may be unilateral or bilateral, lasting hours to several days, associated with photophobia, phonophobia, and nausea and vomiting.
- Migraines are recurrent, throbbing headaches of vascular origin.
- The majority of primary pediatric headaches are migraines, MOH, and tension.
- Classified as migraines without aura (80%) or migraines with aura (focal neurologic dysfunction begins and ends prior to onset of headache)
- Migraine variants include ophthalmoplegic migraine, hemiplegic migraine, basilar migraine (vertigo, dysarthria, ataxia, tinnitus), persistent migraine, and transformed migraine (chronic).

Etiology

- Tension headache
  - Essentially unknown cause
  - Studies have not supported "muscle tension" or increased muscle contractions.
  - Depression, anxiety, or stress may play a role.
- Migraines
  - Believed to be caused by a genetically linked vascular disruption (constriction and dilation of extracranial and intracranial blood vessels), possibly triggered by neurochemical disruption
- Cluster
  - Unknown; may be related to cyclic neurochemical imbalances causing an inflammatory response; tend to be seasonal, occurring in spring or fall
- Secondary headaches
  - Are most common in older adults, often the result of disease outside the central nervous system (CNS)
  - Causes include subarachnoid hemorrhage, head trauma, brain tumors, giant cell (temporal) arteritis, meningitis, encephalitis, cervical arthritis, visual acuity problems, fever, sinusitis, intoxication (drugs, chemicals, carbon monoxide), and hypothyroidism.

Incidence and Demographics

- 18 million outpatient visits a year are for headache.
- Incidence declines in 6th to 10th decades.
- Tension
    - 70% to 90% of adults experience tension-type headache at some time.
    - 5:4 ratio of women to men; 40% have family history
- Migraines
    - Prevalence is 16% to 45% women, 10% to 21% men.
    - Most common during ages of 30 to 45, unusual to begin after age 50; unmask earlier incidence of undiagnosed migraine via focused history; rule out other causes
    - Migraine occurs in 3% to 5% of children before puberty, and increases to 10% to 20% during the second decade of life.
    - Female-to-male ratio is equal in childhood and rises to 2:1 after puberty.
    - There is a strong genetic component; family history supports the diagnosis in the child.
- Cluster
    - Rare, much more frequent in men > 30

Risk Factors

- Age, sex, stress, alcohol, caffeine (for all)
- Migraine triggers: menstruation; foods such as chocolate and aged cheese; caffeine and nicotine or withdrawal; alcohol; sunlight; too much or too little sleep; missing meals; emotional stress or relief of stress; medications, including estrogen and vasodilators

Prevention and Screening

- Because of the many causes of headache, there is no primary prevention.
- Avoid identified individual triggers.
- Keeping a headache diary helps in the identification of triggers and also in the administration of prophylactic medications.

Assessment

History
- Evaluate every headache for chronology (most important item); location, duration quality; associated activity (exertion, sleep tension, relaxation); timing of menstrual cycle; presence of associated symptoms (focal neurological deficits, vomiting, fever); presence of triggers.
- Recent falls or head injuries, trauma, previous and current medical and nonpharmacologic management, diagnostic testing and referrals
- Activities using the trapezius muscles, such as wearing heavy backpacks

- Suspect tension headaches with gradual onset over months to years, with episodes lasting days without neurological symptoms; may be associated with anxiety, depression, and stress.
- Suspect migraine with a history of aura and neurologic symptoms that resolve, then actual headache accompanied by photophobia and/or nausea and vomiting; usually follows the same pattern and precipitating events each episode.
- Suspect tension headache with constant, gradual onset, daily headaches; generalized, bilateral; common around occiput, lasts for several hours, vague symptoms, and no focal neurological deficits.
- Suspect cluster headaches by the cyclic nature of attacks.
- Headache described as the "first" or "worst" of the patient's life should be evaluated to rule out potentially serious etiology.
- Functional history: headache interferes with work, school, functional activities of daily living (ADLs) and instrumental ADLs; headaches that do not interfere with ADLs tend to be the tension type.
- History of sudden onset, change in character, associated neurologic symptoms, fever, neck pain, rash, or weight loss suggests a serious headache and potential emergency; brain tumor usually causes additional symptoms within 6 months of headache onset.
- Family history of headache
- If patient is febrile, consider meningitis, brain abscesses or other infection, encephalitis, or sinusitis.
- Review of systems
  - Neurological: aura, paresthesias, paralysis, vertigo, mood, sleep changes
  - Visual symptoms: photophobia, diplopia, scotoma, tearing
  - Any ear, nose, or throat symptoms: may indicate sinusitis
  - Gastrointestinal: nausea, vomiting, diarrhea, constipation
  - Constitutional symptoms: fever, chills, weight changes, appetite changes
- Also see brain tumor, stroke, meningitis for pertinent history of these secondary causes of headache

Physical Examination
- The screening neurological exam is usually normal with primary headaches; neurologic deficits suggest a secondary cause such as subarachnoid hemorrhage (SAH), cerebrovascular accident (CVA), tumor, or subdural hematoma.
- Funduscopic exam to rule out papilledema (signals increased intracranial pressure)
- Muscle tone, reflexes, gait, sensation, coordination, and strength for any abnormality
- Auscultate for bruits, a sign of cerebrovascular disease
- Measure head circumference, and check the fontanels and sutures in the young child.
- Cervical and suboccipital tenderness, range of motion (decreased in cervical arthritis)
- Temporal artery tenderness and visual changes, particularly in patients > 50 years; suggests giant cell arteritis
- Focused physical exam, including vital signs, to rule out secondary causes or infectious process
- Rash over facial distribution of cranial nerve V with corresponding pain indicates herpes zoster.
- Examine the teeth for obvious cavities; include an assessment of jaw movement.
- ENT exam for signs of infection of the pharynx or sinuses

Diagnostic Studies

- History consistent with primary headache with normal physical exam usually does not require further diagnostic evaluation
- Tension headaches with stress or psychogenic component—consider psychological testing
- CBC if chronic anemia or infection is suspected
- Consider brain CT if
  - Significant new type headache of few weeks' duration
  - New headache in patient over 50
- Immediate CT if
  - Sudden, severe headache
  - Progressive headache
  - Headache with exertion, straining, sexual activity, or coughing
  - Change in mental state, persistent focal neurologic deficits, or fever
- Lumbar puncture (if there is a negative CT but SAH suspected, or to rule out meningitis)
- Erythrocyte sedimentation rate (ESR) to rule out giant cell arteritis in those over 50
- Sinus CT or x-rays if sinusitis without response to adequate antibiotics, recurrent sinus pain, vague symptoms without definite physical findings
- Cervical spine x-rays or MRI if cervical arthritis or radiculopathy is suspected
- Other diagnostic testing as directed by history and physical exam to rule out infectious, metabolic, or autoimmune process
- Evaluate for cardiovascular disease with ECG and risk factors before prescribing 5-HT agonists ("triptans") or dihydroergotamine (DHE 45 or Migranal)
- Electroencephalogram not useful in screening or diagnosing headaches

Differential Diagnosis

- Subarachnoid or intracranial hemorrhage/cerebral aneurysm
- Brain tumor
- Giant cell arteritis
- Subdural hematoma
- Posttraumatic headache
- Meningitis
- Encephalitis
- Brain abscess
- Hydrocephalus
- Sinusitis or other referred pain from ear, eyes, teeth, or temperomandibular joint (TMJ)
- Viral syndrome
- Drug-induced, caffeine withdrawal, or intoxication
- Depression and anxiety
- Postconcussive syndrome
- Stress
- Cervical radiculopathy
- Trigeminal neuralgia
- Pseudotumor cerebri or benign intracranial hypertension (cause unknown)

Management

Nonpharmacologic Treatment
- Tension
  - Relaxation techniques, biofeedback, stress reduction
  - Physical therapy: TENS, massage, ultrasound
  - Headache logs
- Migraine and cluster
  - Avoid food and drugs that trigger attacks.
  - Rest and periods of exercise
  - During attack; rest in quiet, dark room with head elevated; use cold compresses
  - 100% oxygen inhaled for 10 to 15 minutes

Pharmacologic Treatment

Abortive therapy
- Tension
  - Analgesics: acetaminophen 650 to 1,000 mg q.i.d. as needed, or NSAIDs
  - Under age 10, acetaminophen 15 mg/kg/dose q4h, or ibuprofen 10 mg/kg/dose q6h
  - Children under 10 with headaches more than once per week may benefit from daily prophylactic therapy with cyproheptadine (Periactin) 0.2 to 0.4 mg/kg/d in 2 to 3 divided doses, starting with 4 mg at bedtime.
  - Older children can be managed with analgesics to control pain, including acetaminophen and ibuprofen.
  - Avoid opioids, including butalbital (Fiorinal and Fioricet) because of risk of habituation as well as rebound phenomenon.
  - If headache occurs more than once per week, preventive medications for adults and children include amitriptyline (Elavil), propranolol (Inderal), or both.
- Migraines and cluster headaches: treatment very individualized
  - Analgesics: acetaminophen, aspirin, or NSAIDs, often in combination with caffeine taken as soon as possible at onset. Avoid opioids for reasons noted above.
  - 5-HT agonists ("triptans") if nonnarcotic analgesics ineffective
  - Sumatriptan (Imitrex)—oral: 25 mg taken as soon as possible at onset, 25 to 100 mg every 2 hours up to 300 mg in 24 hours in adults; in children, maximum oral dose is 0.6 mg/kg
  - Injection: 6 mg SC adults. In children, maximum dose 0.6 mg/kg.; may be repeated once after 1 hour
  - Following initial injection, 25 to 50 mg tablets q2h up to 200 mg orally in 24 hours
  - Intranasal: single dose of 5, 10, or 20 mg administered in one nostril, may repeat once after 2 hours, not to exceed 40 mg in 24 hours in adults; dosage based on body weight in children
  - Other 5-HT agonists include zolmitriptan (Zomig), naratriptan (Amerge), and rizatriptan (Maxalt).

- Ergotamine derivatives: cafergot: 2 tablets taken as soon as possible at onset, may repeat at 30-minute intervals; do not exceed 6 tablets per day, 10 tablets per week; not recommended in children
- Injectable triptans at migraine doses more effective than oral agents for individual attacks (*Note:* 1st dose of injectable preparations should be given under medical supervision and, possibly, accompanied by monitoring with ECG.)
- Injectable or inhaled ergotamines and triptans are contraindicated in those with history of uncontrolled hypertension, Prinzmetal's angina, myocardial infarction, or symptomatic ischemic heart disease.
- Sumatriptan should not be used in conjunction with any vasoconstrictor medication, nor should it be used within 2 weeks of taking a monoamine oxidase inhibitor.
- Treat nausea or vomiting in adults and children with metoclopramide (Reglan) or phenothiazine 15–20 minutes before oral medication.
  - Prophylactic treatment for 2 or more migraine attacks per month that produce impairment lasting 3 or more days per month: daily NSAIDs, beta-blockers, calcium channel blockers, tricyclic antidepressants (limited experience with SSRIs, especially in children; see the following table)
  - Topiramate, lithium carbonate, methysergide, and valproate can also be effective. However, before initiating valproate, baseline liver enzyme levels must be drawn and then monitored thereafter approximately every 3 to 6 months.
  - Generally, prophylactic agent(s) should be tried for a minimum of 2 to 3 months before switching to another drug.
  - Neurology referral for headaches unresponsive to treatment or prophylaxis

Preventive therapy
- U.S. Headache Consortium Guidelines based on clinical efficacy, significant adverse events, safety profile, and clinical experience of the participants
  - Group 1. Medications with proven high efficacy and mild-to-moderate adverse events
  - Group 2. Medications with lower efficacy (e.g., limited number of studies or studies reporting conflicting results) or efficacy suggesting only "modest" improvement, and mild-to-moderate adverse events

Secondary Headaches
- Manage and treat the underlying cause.
- Avoid opioids if level of consciousness should be monitored.
- Acetaminophen for pain and fever if not contraindicated

How Long to Treat
- Treat acute attacks until headache resolves or maximum daily dose is reached; narcotics can be used to treat intractable pain.
- Prophylaxis: primary headache syndromes tend to decrease or resolve in late middle age or after menopause; attempt to wean periodically

Table 7–3. Pharmacologic Treatment: Preventive Therapy for Migraine

Group	Medication	Usual Daily Adult Dose	Usual Daily Peds Dose	Side Effects
1	Divalproex Na (Depakote)	Usual dose for age > 16: start with 250 mg b.i.d.; usual max 1 g/day	20–40 mg/kg	GI upset, liver disease, thrombocytopenia; therefore, need to monitor closely
	Sodium Valproate	800–1500 mg/day	—	Alopecia, rash, abdominal pain, constipation, diarrhea, pancreatitis
1	Propranolol	160–240 mg/day in divided doses	< 35kg: 10–20mg PO t.i.d. > 35kg: 20–40mg PO t.i.d.	Heart block, Raynaud's, SLE, fatigue, dizziness, constipation, hypotension
1	Timolol (Blocadren)	10–30 mg/day divided q.d.–b.i.d.	—	Heart block, Raynaud's, fatigue, dizziness, nightmares, hypotension
1	Amitriptyline (indicated for relief of symptoms of depression only)	50–100 mg/day	—	HTN, syncope, QT prolongation, seizures, extrapyramidal symptoms, leucopenia, drowsiness, dizziness, dry mouth
2	Guanfacine (Tenex)	0.5–1 mg/day	—	Hypotension, alopecia, dermatitis, constipation, loss of appetite, xerostomia
2	Gabapentin	900–2,400 mg/day	—	Peripheral edema, myalgia, ataxia, dizziness, mood swings, fatigue

Continued

Table 7-3. Pharmacologic Treatment (cont.)

Group	Medication	Usual Daily Adult Dose	Usual Daily Peds Dose	Side Effects
2	Fluoxetine	20 mg qod–40 mg/day	—	Insomnia, fatigue, tremor, stomach pain, rash, sweating, xerostomia
2	Atenolol	100 mg/day	—	Arrhythmia, diarrhea, dizziness, fatigue, insomnia
2	Verapamil	240 mg/day	—	Edema, hypotension, constipation, nausea, dizziness
2	NSAIDS: Aspirin Flurbiprofen Ketoprofen Naproxen sodium	325 mg/day 200 mg/day 150 mg/day 1,100 mg/day	—	Gastritis, occult GI bleed, tinnitus, indigestion, nausea, vomiting
2	Ergotamine+ caffeine+ butalbital+ belladonna	2 caps a day for 3 days before, during, and 2 days after menses	—	Pruritus, nausea, vomiting, muscle weakness, parasthesia, visual disturbances
2	Estradiol gel	1.5 mg/day for 7 days	—	Edema, pruritus, weight gain, nausea, amenorrhea, break-through bleeding
2	Feverfew	50–82 mg/day	—	Eczema, edema, nausea, abdominal pain, diarrhea, tachycardia

Continued

Table 7-3. *Cont.*

Group	Medication	Usual Daily Adult Dose	Usual Daily Peds Dose	Side Effects
2	Magnesium	400–600 mg/day	—	Blurred vision, diarrhea, HTN, increased bleeding times
2	Vitamin B$_2$	400 mg/day	—	Rare adverse events

HTN = hypertension

Special Considerations

- Consider cardiovascular, gastrointestinal, renal, and hepatic disease when prescribing therapy for geriatric patients.
- Increased risk of GI bleed, renal failure, edema and elevated blood pressure (BP) with NSAIDS in older adults
- There are no randomized control studies for migraine treatment in older adults.

When to Consult, Refer, or Hospitalize

- Consult with physician as needed, if narcotic analgesics needed
- Refer to neurologist if unable to manage symptoms using typical therapy or if patient develops symptoms of increased intracranial pressure (ICP), or if tumor, aneurysm, or AVM suspected
- Refer to neurologist if patient is experiencing multiple headaches/week, and/or is taking multiple doses of medication without benefit (e.g., rebound headaches due to medication effects)
- Refer to emergency department (ED) for severe unresponsive migraine or cluster headache with vomiting and need for IV hydration; sudden, severe headache; or headache with change in level of consciousness
- Refer to surgeon or ophthalmologist for temporal artery biopsy if temporal arteritis suspected
- Refer to psychologist or therapist for relaxation therapy or psychotherapy, or when depression suspected that does not respond to trial of antidepressants
- Refer to interdisciplinary pain center for chronic, intractable pain, interfering with daily life

Follow-up

- Routine annual health assessments
- Weekly to monthly when adjusting or changing medications

Expected Outcomes
- Tension headaches can be lifelong.
- Migraines get better in more than two-thirds of all children, but the prognosis of remission diminishes after age 18.
- In adults, migraines and cluster headaches usually resolve during middle age, or following completion of menopause.

Complications
- Unrecognized or mistreated serious headaches from secondary causes
- Lost wages and productivity, troubled relationships from chronic pain

ALZHEIMER'S DISEASE / MULTI-INFARCT DEMENTIA

Description

- Alzheimer's disease (AD) and multi-infract dementia (MID) involve impairment of global intellectual and cognitive function, characterized by memory loss, aphasia, agnosia, and apraxia with preservation of level of consciousness
- MID and Alzheimer's disease make up the majority of progressive, irreversible dementias.
- MID: dementing process caused by strokes characterized by stepwise decline
- AD: gradual onset and progressive decline without focal neurological deficits
  - First stage of AD manifested by short-term memory impairment. Activities of daily living become increasingly challenging. Social, occupational, and cognitive impairment manifest themselves.
  - Second stage of AD characterized by increasing loss of social and cognitive ability, with concomitant increasing behavioral changes. These can range from agitation and restlessness to outright combativeness. Eventually, the patient no longer recognizes friends and loved ones.
  - Third and last stage of AD brings disease full cycle, as cognitive disability is eventually followed by physical decline

Etiology

- AD: not fully understood
- More neuritic plaques and neurofibrillary tangles are found on autopsy compared to nondemented patients
- Three genes on different chromosomes have been identified in families with history of AD, although not all cases may be inherited.
- MID: multiple lacunar infarcts

Incidence and Demographics

- Affects 5% to 10% of those > 65 and increases with age
- AD and related dementias affect 2 to 4 million Americans.
- Often misdiagnosed or unrecognized, especially in early stages
- AD: 50% to 60% of all dementias; MID: 10% to 20% of all dementias

Risk Factors

- AD: Down syndrome
- Familial or inherited
- MID: hypertension, previous stroke, TIA

Prevention and Screening

- Routine screening is not recommended because there is no definitive treatment, and it is difficult to recognize early dementia.
- Those > 65 should have cognitive and functional evaluation at least every 3 years.
- Be aware of early symptoms to facilitate early assessment and recognition, and rule out age-related memory changes, unidentified conditions, or reversible forms of dementia (see the following table).
- Interpretation: Positive findings in any of these areas generally indicate the need for further assessment for the presence of dementia.

Assessment

History
- Detailed history of present illness, including time frame and progression, any associated neurological symptoms such as amaurosis fugax, aphasia, or unilateral weakness
- Past medical history: hypertension, strokes, head trauma
- Psychiatric history: depression, anxiety, schizophrenia
- Social history: present living situation, marital status, occupation, education, alcohol, tobacco, illicit drug use
- Medications, including over-the-counter, supplements, and home remedies
- Initial and periodic functional history and assessment
- Validate history with family member, caregiver, or both, but also be aware of potential for self-serving motives; informants may exaggerate or deny symptoms.

Table 7-4. Guide for Recognition and Initial Assessment of Dementia

Does the person have increased difficulty with any of the activities listed?

Activity	Description
Learning and retaining new information	Is repetitive; has trouble remembering recent conversations, events, appointments; frequently misplaces objects
Handling complex tasks	Has trouble following a complex train of thought or performing tasks that require many steps, such as balancing a checkbook or cooking a meal
Reasoning ability	Is unable to respond with a reasonable plan to problems at home or work, such as knowing what to do if the bathroom is flooded; shows uncharacteristic disregard for rules of social conduct
Special ability and orientation	Has trouble driving, organizing objects around the house, finding way to or around familiar places
Language	Has increasing difficulty with finding the words to express what he or she wants to say and with following conversations
Behavior	Appears more passive and less responsive; is more irritable than usual; is more suspicious than usual; misinterprets visual or auditory stimuli

Physical Examination
- Assess level of consciousness along a continuum from alert to drowsy to stupor to coma
- Perform complete mental status evaluation using instrument such as Folstein Mini-Mental State Examination (MMSE), the Short Portable Mental Status Questionnaire, or Blessed Dementia Rating Scale; test results are not diagnostic, but serve as baseline for assessing trends in cognitive impairment
  - Generally, a score of < 26 on the MMSE (which tests orientation, registration, attention and calculation, recall, and language) indicates cognitive impairment, but this is only a crude indicator of functioning.
- Complete neurologic exam with attention to focal neurologic deficits, which may indicate MID or other neurologic problem
- MID: focal motor weakness or impaired sensation, reflex asymmetry, positive Babinski
  - Assess for sensory impairments (hearing, vision) that masquerade as or worsen dementia.
  - Pulmonary and cardiac exams (murmurs, arrhythmias, heart enlargement, orthostatic hypotension)
  - Any evidence of infectious processes
  - Signs of physical and mental abuse

Diagnostic Studies

- CBC, chemistry profile, thyroid function tests, B_{12} level, folate level to rule out causes of delirium and reversible dementia; syphilis, HIV, and drug toxicity if indicated by history
- CT for early dementia of < 2 years' duration may show atrophy, infarcts, or unexpected lesions
- Other testing based on presentation
- Neuropsychological testing is recommended under certain circumstances: to differentiate depression, stroke, or delirium in unusual presentations; identify areas of preserved cognitive function to develop a care plan

Differential Diagnosis

- Delirium
- Other dementias: Lewey bodies dementia, Pick's disease
- Depression and anxiety
- Normal pressure hydrocephalus
- Tumor
- Hearing loss
- B12 and folate deficiency
- Parkinson's disease
- Trauma—consider subdural hematoma, falls (whether witnessed or not)
- Alcohol intoxication
- Infectious process: chronic infection, AIDS, tertiary syphilis
- Cardiovascular or cerebrovascular accidents
- Medications: polypharmacy, interactions

Management

- Foremost, rule out or treat any conditions that may contribute to cognitive impairment.
- Discontinue all unnecessary medications, especially sedatives and hypnotics.
- MID: nonpharmacologic and pharmacologic reduction of stroke risks (see management of TIA and stroke)

Nonpharmacologic Treatment

- Explain memory and cognitive status assessment results to the patient, putting them within the context of overall patient status.
- Educate the patient and family about the illness, treatment, and community resources.
- Assist with long-term planning, including financial, legal, and advance directives.
- Assess home and driving safety.
- Behavior therapy identifies causes of problem behaviors, and changes the environment to reduce the behavior.
- Recreational, art, and pet therapy create pleasurable experiences for the patient.
- Reminiscence therapy
- Incontinence care; supportive care

Pharmacologic Treatment

- Cognitive symptoms
  - Cholinesterase inhibitors such as donepezil (Aricept) 5 mg, may increase to 10 mg q.d.
    - Common side effects are headache, nausea, and diarrhea.
    - LFT monitoring not required as was with tacrine (Cognex), an earlier cholinesterase inhibitor
- Psychosis and agitation
  - Haloperidol (Haldol) 0.5 to 3 mg at bedtime or divided up during day
  - Risperidone (Risperdal) 0.5 to 3 mg b.i.d.
  - Lorazepam (Ativan) 0.5 to 4 mg a day in divided doses as needed for anxiety
- Depression
  - Paroxetine (Paxil) HCl 10 to 40 mg/day
  - Sertraline (Zoloft) HCl 25 to 200 mg/day
  - Nortriptyline (Pamelor) 10 to 50 mg/day for older adults, may be divided or given at bedtime
- Sleep disturbances
  - Zolpidem (Ambien) 5 to 10 mg at bedtime
  - Trazodone (Desyrel) 25 to 75 mg at bedtime

How Long to Treat

- Cholinesterase inhibitors: may be initiated for mild to moderate Alzheimer's disease and discontinued when significant cognitive decline is noted; ineffective for MID
- Use other medications PRN; if needed regularly, use the lowest effective dose and attempt to wean periodically.

Special Considerations

- Consider language and education level when administering and interpreting mental status tests.
- Integrate cultural beliefs into the management of minority patients with dementia.

When to Consult, Refer, or Hospitalize

- Consult with physician for diagnosis and long-term treatment planning
- Refer to neurologist for unusual presentation
- Refer to psychiatrist if unable to differentiate from depression; intractable behaviors
- Use social worker and multidisciplinary services for long-term care planning
- Hospitalize with deteriorating conditions such as exacerbation of chronic heart failure (CHF), chronic obstructive pulmonary disease (COPD), dehydration, pneumonia, or injury. Be aware that demented patients are likely to become more confused and delirious, and fall more when hospitalized.

Follow-up

- Generally, follow up every 60 days.

Expected Outcomes
- AD: slowly progressive
- MID: stepwise with gradual deterioration; associated with new focal deficits and decline with each additional stroke

Complications
- Depression and suicide
- Complications usually related to comorbidity or complications because of immobility with severe end-stage dementia

DELIRIUM

Description

- Delirium is an acute disorder of attention with onset of hours to days, characterized by confusion, disorientation, and fluctuation over the course of a day.

Etiology

- Functional disorder of the brain caused by organic factors
- Any number of factors can cause delirium: polypharmacy, infections, metabolic and electrolyte abnormalities, dehydration, nutritional deficiencies, cardiopulmonary disease, urinary retention, fecal impaction, trauma, anesthesia, or environmental change.

Incidence and Demographics

- 10% to 40% of hospitalized patients > 65 years old

Risk Factors

- Age, dementia, frailty, visual impairment; presence of many other chronic diseases

Prevention and Screening

- Eliminate unnecessary medications
- Adequate hydration, nutrition, and oxygenation
- Correct visual and auditory deficits
- Continuity of care and environment

Assessment

History
- Detailed history of present illness, including cognition, time frame, and progression
- Comprehensive review of systems to identify underlying etiology
- Functional history and assessment
- Validate history with family member, caregiver, or both.

Physical Examination
- Complete neurologic exam with attention to level of consciousness, focal neurologic deficits
- Hearing and visual impairments
- Pulmonary and cardiac exams (murmurs, arrhythmias, heart enlargement)
- Any evidence of infectious processes
- Signs of trauma
- Evaluate for orthostatic hypotension, urinary retention, and fecal impaction.
- Folstein Mini-Mental State Examination
- Geriatric Depression Scale

Diagnostic Studies
- CBC, chemistry profile, thyroid function tests, B_{12} level, folate level to identify a reversible cause for cognitive impairment or etiology of delirium
- Computed tomography to identify infarcts, space-occupying lesions
- Syphilis, HIV, and drug toxicity if indicated by history
- Urinalysis if urinary tract infection suspected
- Arterial oxygen or pulse oximetry if hypoxemia considered
- ECG and chest x-ray identify cardiopulmonary cause
- EEG to rule out seizure disorder
- Lumbar puncture for suspected encephalopathy or meningitis

Differential Diagnosis

- Dementia
- Depression
- See etiologies above

Management

- Identify and treat underlying cause

Nonpharmacologic Treatment
- Continuity of care
- Minimize environmental stimuli
- Provide eye glasses or hearing aids
- Clocks and calendars to maintain orientation
- Maintain hydration, nutrition, oxygenation
- Adequate bowel and bladder regimen

Pharmacologic Treatment
- Haloperidol (Haldol) 0.5 mg p.o. or IM q 2 to 6 h for agitation

How Long to Treat
Depends on etiology; often continue therapy until baseline cognitive function returns

Special Considerations

- Highest incidence in hospitalized elderly

When to Consult, Refer, or Hospitalize

- Consult physician for any primary care patient with suspected delirium.
- Hospitalize unless underlying etiology such as urinary tract infection (UTI) without sepsis can be managed at home with supervision to ensure patient safety, adequate hydration, and prescribed treatment.

Follow-up

- Regularly to monitor for recurrence

Expected Outcomes
- Usually reversible

Complications
- Injury from falls
- Associated with increased morbidity and mortality

REFERENCES

Agency for Health Care Policy and Research. (1996). *Early Alzheimer's disease: Recognition and assessment. Guideline 19.* Washington, DC: U.S. Department of Health and Human Services.

Barkley, Jr., T., & Myers, C. (2008). *Practice guidelines for acute care nurse practitioners* (2nd ed.). Philadelphia: Elsevier.

Burke, M. M., & Laramie, J. A. (2003). *Primary care of the older adult.* Philadelphia: Elsevier Health Sciences.

Buttaro, T. M., Bailey, P. P., & Trybulski, J. (2007). *Primary care: A collaborative practice.* Philadelphia: Elsevier Health Sciences.

Centers for Disease Control and Prevention. (2008). Meningococcal disease. In *Manual for the surveillance of vaccine-preventable diseases* (4th ed.). Atlanta: Author. Retrieved from http://www.cdc.gov/vaccines/pubs/surv-manual/chpt08-mening.htm

Center for Disease Control and Prevention. (2010). *Meningococcal vaccination.* Retrieved from http://www.cdc.gov/meningitis/vaccine-info.html

Downey, D. (2008). Pharmacologic management of Alzheimer disease. *Journal of Neuroscience Nursing, 40*(1), 55–59.

Edmunds, M. W., & Mayhew, M. S. (2004). *Pharmacology for the primary care provider* (2nd ed.). St. Louis, MO: Elsevier Mosby.

Foster, C., Mistry, N. F., Peddi, P. F., & Sharma, S. (2010). *The Washington manual of medical therapeutics* (33rd ed.). Philadelphia: Wolters Kluwer/Lippincott Williams & Wilkins.

Hilton, G. (1997). Seizure disorders in adults: Evaluation and management of new onset seizures. *The Nurse Practitioner, 22*(9), 42–59.

Labuguen, R. H. (2006). Initial evaluation of vertigo. *American Family Physician, 73*(2), 244–251.

Leira, E. C., & Adams, H. P. (1999). Management of acute ischemic stroke. *Clinics in Geriatric Medicine, 15*(4), 701–720.

McPhee, S. J., Tierney, L. M., & Papadakis, M. A. (2007). *Current medical diagnosis & treatment* (46th ed.). New York: McGraw-Hill.

McPhee, S. J., Papadakis, M. A., & Tierney, L. M. (2011). *Current medical diagnosis & treatment* (50th ed.). New York: Lange Medical Book/McGraw Hill.

Moloney, M. F., Matthews, K. B., Scharbo-Dehaan, M., & Strickland, O. L. (2000). Caring for the woman with migraine headaches. *The Nurse Practitioner, 25*(2), 17–36.

Morgan, G. E., Jr., Mikhail, M. S., & Murray, M. J. (2005). Pain management. In G. E. Morgan, Jr., M. S. Mikhail, & M. J. Murray, *Clinical anesthesiology* (4th ed.). New York: McGraw-Hill. Retrieved from http://www.accessmedicine.com/contentRamadan

N. M., Silberstein, S. D., Freitag, F. G., Gilbert, T. T., & Frishberg, B. M. (2000). *Evidence-based guidelines for migraine headache in the primary care setting: Pharmacological management for prevention of migraine.* Retrieved from http://www.aan.com/professionals/practice/pdfs/gl0090.pdf

Rockswold, G. L., Solid, C. A., Paredes-Andrade, E., Rockswold, S. B., Jancik, J.T., & Quickel, R. R. (2009). Hypertonic saline and its effect on intracranial pressure, cerebral perfusion pressure, and brain tissue oxygen. *Neurosurgery, 65*(6),1035–1041.

Robertson, J., & Shilkofski, N. (2005). *The Harriet Lane handbook.* Philadelphia: Elsevier Health Sciences.

Swain, S. E. (1996). Multiple sclerosis primary health care implications. *The Nurse Practitioner, 21*(7), 40–54.

Tapper, V. J. (1997). Pathophysiology, assessment, and treatment of Parkinson's disease. *The Nurse Practitioner, 22*(7), 76–95.

Uphold, C. R., & Graham, M. V. (2003). *Clinical guidelines in family practice* (4th ed). Los Angeles: Barmarrae Books.

Urden, L. D., Stacy, K. M., & Lough, M. E. (2002). *Critical care nursing: disease and management* (4th ed.). St. Louis, MO: Mosby.

U.S. Preventive Services Task Force. (2007). *Guide to clinical preventive services, 2007.* Retrieved from http://www.ahrq.gov/clinic/pocketgd.htm

Young, L. R. (2004). Antiparkinson agents. In M. W. Edmunds & M. S. Mayhew (Eds.), *Pharmacology for the primary care proviader* (2nd ed., pp. 502–515). St. Louis, MO: Mosby.

8

Renal and Urologic Disorders

Pamela Smith, MSN, RN, ACNP-BC, CCRN

GENERAL APPROACH

- Renal and urologic disorders cause kidney and related disease.
- Kidney pain is commonly located in the area of the costovertebral angle (CVA). Radiation to the umbilicus, testicle, or labia is possible.
- Pain associated with infection is typically constant.
- The normal urinary tract is sterile, and the immunocompetent patient is resistant to bacterial colonization. Urinary tract infection (UTI) is, however, the most common bacterial infection in all age groups
- Urinary tract infection is also the most common nosocomial infection.
- Limit antibiotics to category B if patient is pregnant or lactating; most antibiotics enter breast milk.
- In patients with gross or microscopic hematuria and upper tract source (kidney and ureters) is identified in about 10% of cases—stone disease accounts for about 40%, medical renal disease 20%, renal cell carcinoma 10%, and urothelial cell carcinoma of the ureter or renal pelvis 5%.
- Gross hematuria may occur from a lower tract source without evidence of infection.
- Obtain a urology consult for unusual presentations or those that do not respond to treatment.
- Kidney disease may be acute or chronic.
- Acute kidney injury is worsening of renal function over hours to days.
- Fluid, electrolyte and acid–base disorders may develop quickly with acute kidney injury.
- Chronic kidney disease is an abnormal loss of function over months to years.
- Differentiating between acute and chronic disease is important for diagnosis, treatment, and outcome.

RED FLAGS

- Gross hematuria without evidence of acute UTI should include a differential of malignancy until proven otherwise.
- Patients with UTI and hemodynamic instability or with severe dehydration who are unable to take oral medications, or both require hospitalization.
- Up to 80% of acute kidney injury has been attributed to decreased renal perfusion, major surgery, aminoglyocides, and contrast administration.
- The development of in-hospital acute renal failure is associated with increased length of stay and poor clinical outcomes.
- Although a 0.5 mg/dL rise in creatinine may seem small, it reflects a large fall in glomerular filtration rate (GFR) when the baseline creatinine is below 2 mg/dL.
- Signifcant decrements in GFR can occur while creatinine levels remain in normal range.

UROLOGIC DISORDERS

URINARY TRACT INFECTIONS

Description

- The term *urinary tract infection* (UTI) describes a wide variety of clinical entities that includes asymptomatic bacteriuria cystitis, prostatitis, and pyelonephritis. UTIs are classified according to where they occur along the urinary tract. Lower UTIs involve the urethra (urethritis) and the bladder (cystitis). Upper UTIs involve the kidneys (pyelonephritis). An infection can affect one or both kidneys. In practice, differentiating between sites may be difficult. UTIs may be further characterized as uncomplicated (without an anatomical or predisposing reason) or complicated (presence of structural abnormalities of the urinary tract and/or kidneys), and as community-acquired or nosocomial (usually as the result of catheterization).

Etiology

- In acute uncomplicated cystitis, *E. coli* causes 75% to 90% of infections; *Klebsiella* species, *Proteus* species, enteroccoci, *Citrobacter* species, and others account for 5% to 10%; and *Staphylococcus* saprophyticus for 5% to 15%, especially in young, sexually active women.
- In complicated UTIs, *E. coli* is also the most common organism; however, other aerobic gram-negative rods such as *Klebsiella, Proteus, Citrobacter, Acinetobacter* species, *Morganella* species, and *Pseudomonas aeruginosa* are also frequently identified.
- Gram-positive bacteria (enterococci, *S. aureus*, and *S. epidermis*) and yeast are also important pathogens in a complicated UTI.

- The most common mechanism of infection is ascending infection from the urethra.
- Women who are symptomatic with pyuria and have urine that is sterile (even when collected with suprapubic aspiration) may have an infection with sexually transmitted organisms such as *Chlamydia trachomatis, Neisseria gonorrhoeae,* or herpes simplex virus. These organisms are found most frequently in young, sexually active women with new sexual partners.

Incidence and Demographics

- It is estimated that 50% to 80% of women in the general population will experience a UTI at least once in their lifetimes, with most of these being uncomplicated cystitis.
  - In males
    - UTIs are rare in young men and are usually the result of a urologic abnormality.
    - Require prompt consideration of sexually transmitted disease
- Recurrent episodes occur in 20% to 30% of women.
- The urethra is longer in males, which makes it more difficult for the bacteria to ascend and cause an infection.
- Asymptomatic bacteriuria is more common among elderly men and women.
- After age 50, UTIs are more common in both sexes because of the frequency of prostate disease.
- Women with diabetes are 2 to 3 times more likely to have a UTI or asymptomatic bacteriuria; however, this is not seen in men with diabetes.
- In hospitalized patients with diabetes, especially those with multiple organ complications, the rate of infection and pyelonephritis may be increased.

Risk Factors

- Female gender because the urethra is in close proximity to the anus, is short (approximately 4 cm), and terminates beneath the labia
- Sexual intercourse may cause introduction of bacteria into the bladder and appears to be an important factor in UTIs in both pre- and postmenopausal women.
- Diabetes mellitus
- Pregnancy
- Use of spermicides, a diaphragm, or oral contraceptives
- Structural urinary tract abnormalities—strictures, stones, tumors, neuropathic bladder
- Insertion of an indwelling catheter or manipulation by instrumentation
- In men, prostatitis, anal intercourse, lack of circumcision, or intercourse with a partner who has vaginal colonization with uropathogens
- Dysfunctional voiding pattern or infrequent voiding

Prevention and Screening

- Women who experience three or more UTIs in 1 year are candidates for long-term, low-dose antibiotics to prevent recurrence, should avoid spermicides, and should void immediately after intercourse.
- Postmenopausal women not taking an oral estrogen replacement therapy can prevent recurrent UTIs with topical intravaginal cream.
- Prophylaxis may be considered in men with chronic prostatitis, men undergoing prostatectomy (intra- and postoperatively), and pregnant women with asymptomatic bacteriuria.
- All pregnant women should be screened for bacteriuria in the first trimester and treated if it is present.

Assessment

History
- Complaints of dysuria, urinary frequency, and urgency
- Nocturia, suprapubic or back discomfort
- In the elderly, mental status change may be the only symptom.
- Fever, chills, flank pain, nausea and vomiting, and malaise may be associated with pyelonephritis.
- Sexual history

Physical Examination
- Fever
- Costovertebral tenderness with pyelonephritis
- Urine is grossly cloudy, malodorous, and with hematuria in about 30% of cases.
- Tenderness of urethra and/or suprapubic area
- Pelvic examination may be indicated when vaginal or urethral discharge is present.

Diagnostic Studies
- Clean-catch urine specimen for urinalysis and culture and sensitivity
- Urinalysis reveals pyuria, bacteriuria, and varying levels of hematuria.
- Dipstick testing may be considered as an alternative to microscopy in women with classic signs and symptoms of acute uncomplicated UTI and, if positive, empirical therapy is instituted.
- Urologic evaluations are recommended for a select patient group—women with recurrent infections, a history of childhood infections, stones, painless hematuria, or recurrent pyelonephritis and both sexes with suspected anatomic abnormalities. Most men with UTIs are considered to have a complicated infection and should undergo a urological evaluation.
- For systemic symptoms—complete blood count, blood urea nitrogen, and creatinine

Differential Diagnosis

- Urethritis
- Vulvovaginitis
- Prostatitis
- Female urethral syndrome
- Sexually transmitted disease
- Pyelonephritis
- Renal calculi
- Bladder carcinoma

Management

Nonpharmacologic Treatment
- Hygiene measures
  - Female: front to back wiping
  - Male: cleansing of uncircumcised penis
- Frequent and complete voiding
- Voiding after sexual intercourse
- Hydration, cranberry juice (helps to prevent E. coli from adhering to bladder)

Pharmacologic Treatment
- Single-dose regimen
  - Trimethoprim-sulfamethoxazole 160/800 mg two tablets orally
  - Fosfomycin 3 grams orally one dose
- 3-day course
  - Trimethoprim-sulfamethoxazole 160/800 mg one tablet twice daily
- Trimethoprim 100 mg orally twice daily for 7 to 10 days
- Nitrofurantoin 100 mg orally every 6 hours for 7 days
- Cephalexin 250 to 500 mg orally every 6 hours for 7 to 10 days
- Ciprofloxacin 250 to 500 mg orally every 12 hours for 3 days
- Norfloxacin 400 mg orally every 12 hours for 3 days
- Ofloxacin 200 mg orally every 12 hours for 7 to 10 days
- Males: If no complicating factors—trimethoprim-sulfamethoxazole 160/800 orally twice daily for 7 days

Special Considerations

- Geriatric patients may not demonstrate signs/symptoms other than mental status change.
- Consult obstetrics for management in the pregnant population, which may need prophylactic antibiotics for the duration of the pregnancy in certain situations (history of acute pyelonephritis during pregnancy, bacteriuria during pregnancy with recurrence after treatment, history of recurrent UTI before pregnancy requiring prophylaxis).
- Catheter-associated UTI (CAUTI) develops in 10%–15% of hospitalized patients with short-term indwelling catheters.
  - E. coli, Proteus, Pseudomonas, Klebsiella, Serrtia, staphylococci, and Candida are the usual cause of CAUTI.

- Many of these infecting strains have broader antimicrobial resistance profiles than community-acquired UTIs.
- Usually cause minimal symptoms without fever and often resolve after catheter removal

When to Consult, Refer, or Hospitalize

- Consult urology for recurrent infections with suspected anatomic abnormality.
- Urosepsis, or hemodynamic instability requires hospitalization with intravenous antibiotics.

Follow-up

Expected Outcomes
- Signs and symptoms should resolve in 48 to 72 hours.
- Repeat urinalysis with culture and sensitivity after therapy.

Complications
- Pyelonephritis
- Urosepsis
- Renal abscess

ACUTE PYELONEPHRITIS

Description

- Acute pyelonephritis is an infectious inflammatory disease that involves the renal parenchyma and renal pelvis.

Etiology

- Most common causative organisms are gram-negative bacteria such as *E. coli*, *Proteus*, *Klebsiella*, *Enterbacter*, and *Pseudomonas*. Gram-positive organisms such as *Enterococcus faecalis* and *Staphylococcus aureus* are less common.
- The infection usually ascends from the bladder with the exception of *S. aureus*, which is usually spread by the hematogenous route.

Incidence and Demographics

- Occurs frequently in women age 18 to 40
- 250,000 cases occur annually in the United States; approximately 200,000 require hospitalization.
- Acute pyelonephritis occurs in 20% to 30% of pregnant women with untreated asymptomatic bacteriuria—most often during the late second and early third trimesters.

Risk Factors

- Alteration/function of the urinary tract
  - Obstruction—urinary stones, strictures, bladder/renal abscesses, urinary stents, indwelling catheter, neurogenic bladder
  - Special patient groups
    - Age > 65 years old
    - Nosocomial infections
    - Nursing home patients
  - Metabolic
    - Diabetes
    - Pregancy
    - Renal impairment
    - Sickle cell disease
    - Analgesic abuse
  - Patients who are immunocompromised
    - Renal transplant
    - Neutropenia
    - Congenital/acquired immunodeficiency syndromes
    - Other transplants
    - Special pathogens
      - Tuberculosis
      - Yeasts/fungi
      - *Pseudomonas aeruginosa*
      - Resistant bacteria

Prevention and Screening

- Proper hygiene
- Hydration
- Voiding after sexual intercourse
- Remove indwelling catheters when no longer medically necessary.
- Prompt diagnosis and treatment of urinary stones, bladder/renal abscesses
- Screening pregnant women for asymptomatic bacteriuria

Assessment

History
- Fever, flank pain, shaking, chills, nausea, vomiting, diarrhea
- Hematuria, dysuria, urgency, frequency

Physical Examination
- Costrovertebral angle tenderness—usually pronounced
- Fever, tachycardia

Diagnostic Studies

- Urinalysis
  - Bacteria and white blood cells visible on microscopy
  - May see casts
  - Positive leukocyte esterase
  - Positive nitrites
  - Possible proteinuria
  - Pyuria
- Complete blood count
  - Elevated white blood cell count
- Urine culture and sensitivity
- Gram stain prior to starting antibiotic therapy
- Voiding cystourethrogram, intravenous pylorogram, renal scan, cystoscopy if structural abnormality present or suspected
- Abdominal/pelvic CT if renal abscess is suspected

Differential Diagnosis

- Kidney stones
- Prostatitis
- Renal tuberculosis
- Acute low back pain
- Tumor

Management

Nonpharmacologic Treatment
- Fluids

Pharmacologic Treatment
- Oral regimen
  - Trimethoprim-sulfamethoxazole 160 to 180 mg twice daily for 14 days
  - Ciprofloxacin 500 mg twice daily or 1 gram extended release orally once daily for 14 days
  - Ofloxacin 400 mg orally every 12 hours for 14 days
- Intravenous regimen
  - Ampicillin 1 gram every 6 hours and gentamycin 1 mg/kg every 8 hours for 21 days
  - Cefazolin 250 to 1500 mg every 6 hours for 14 days
  - Levofoxacin 750 mg every 24 hrs for 5 days
  - Ceftriaxone 1 gram every 24 hours

Special Considerations

- Geriatric patients should be hospitalized with aminoglycoside coverage—weight and renal dose adjusted.
- Aseptic technique with indwelling catheters will reduce incidence.
- Consider silver-impregnated catheters.
- Quninolones and sulfonamides should be avoided in pregnancy. Consider cephalexin.

When to Consult, Refer, or Hospitalize

- Patients with bacteremia or urosepsis, the elderly, those with hemodynamic instability, patients who are immunocompromised or pregnant, and those with an inability to tolerate oral antibiotics should be hospitalized.
- If a patient is febrile for more than 3 days, a renal abscess should be considered and urology consulted.

Follow-up

- After completion of therapy
  - Repeat culture 2 weeks after end of treatment cycle
  - If patient was treated as an outpatient for pyelonephritis, a follow-up should occur in 24 hours.
  - Posthospitalization, patient should be followed up at 2 weeks and again at 3 months.

  ### Expected Outcomes
  - Symptoms should resolve after 72 hours.

  ### Complications
  - Sepsis, preterm labor, chronic kidney disease, chronic pyelonephritis, renal abscess, death

ASYMPTOMATIC BACTERIURIA

Description

- Asymptomatic bacteriuria can be found by isolation of a specified quantitative count of bacteria in a specimen that has been appropriately obtained from a patient without symptoms or signs of a urinary tract infection.
  - For women: two consecutive voided specimens with isolation of the same bacterial strain in quantitative counts > 105 cfu/mL
  - For men: a single, clean-catch voided urine specimen with one bacterial species isolated in a quantitative count > 105 cfu/mL
  - For men and women: a single catheterized urine specimen with one bacterial species isolated in a quantitative count > 105 cfu/mL

Etiology

- *E. coli* is the most common organism in women.
- Other common organisms are *Klebsiella pneumonia, Enterococcus* species, group B streptococci, and *Gardnerella vaginalis.*
- For men: coagulase-negative staphylococci, gram-negative bacilli, *Enterococcus* species
- Men and women with indwelling catheters usually have polymicrobial bacteria.

Incidence and Demographics

- Prevalence in populations varies with age, sex, and presence of genitourinary abnormalities.
- For healthy women, the incidence increases with advancing age; in young women, it correlates with sexual activity.
- Women who are pregnant and nonpregnant have a similar incidence (2% to 7%).
- More common in women with diabetes and is correlated with the duration of the diabetes and presence of long-term complications
- Rare in healthy young men
- Incidence in men increases significantly after the age of 60. The prevalence is that 6% to 15% of men > 75 years of age are bacteriuric.
- Men with diabetes do not have an increased prevalance.

Risk Factors

- Indwelling catheters
- Advancing age
- Diabetes mellitus in women
- Spinal cord injury

Prevention and Screening

- Pregnant women should be screened by urine culture at least once in early pregnancy and treated if positive.
- In men, prior to transurethral resection of the prostate
- Screen and treat prior to urological procedures when mucosal bleeding is anticipated.
- Screening or treatment not recommended for
  - Women who are premenopausal and not pregnant
  - Women with diabetes
  - Older persons living in the community
  - Persons with spinal cord injury
  - Patients who are catheterized, while the catheter remains in place
- Encourage fluid intake
- Empty bladder fully and frequently

Assessment

- Urinalysis and culture as described under Description
- No signs or symptoms of urinary tract infection
- Pyuria may be present, but its presence is not an indication of a need for treatment.

Differential Diagnosis

- Cystitis
- Urethritis
- Acute pyelonephritis

Management

- Women who are premenopausal and are not pregnant: treatment and screening are not indicated.
- Women who are pregnant, if positive:
  - Antimicrobial therapy should be given for 3 to 7 days.
  - Periodic screening should occur after therapy.
- Women with diabetes: Treatment and screening are not indicated.
- Older persons in the community: Treatment and screening are not indicated.
- Older patients who are institutionalized patients: Treatment and screening are not indicated.
- Patients with spinal cord injury: Treatment and screening are not indicated.
- Patients who are immunocompromised and other patients: no recommendations per the Infectious Diseases Society of America for or against screening treatment in this population
- Patients with indwelling urethral catheters: Treatment and screening are not indicated.
- Treatment may be considered of women with catheter-acquired bacteriuria that persists 48 hours after catheter removal.

Special Considerations

- No recommendation is made for or against repeated screening of culture-negative women later in pregnancy.
- The diagnosis must be made with a urine culture that is collected in such a way as to minimize contamination.

When to Consult, Refer, or Hospitalize

- Urology consult for frequent recurrence or resistance to antibiotic therapy if treated
- Hospitalize for urosepsis.

Follow-up

- If a patient is treated, repeat urinalysis and culture 1 to 2 weeks after completion of therapy.

UROLITHIASIS/NEPHROLITHIASIS

Description

- Urolithiasis is a condition in which urinary calculi are formed in the urinary tract.
- Nephrolithiasis is a condition in which a patient has kidney stones.
- Urinary calculi are polycrystallin aggregates composed of varying amounts of crystalloid and a small amount of organic matrix.
- The five major types of urinary stones are calcium oxalate (85%), calcium phosphate, struvite, uric acid, and cystine.
- Up to 98% of stones < 0.5 cm in diameter will pass spontaneously.

Etiology

- Supersaturation of urine with stone-forming salts
- Calcium stones are the most common.
- Diet and fluid intake are important factors in stone formation.
  - Patients with recurrent stones are placed on a diet restricted in sodium and protein.
  - Sodium is restricted to 100 mEq/d; protein is limited to 1g/kg/d.
  - Only type II absorptive hypercalciuric patients benefit from a low-calcium diet.
- Low serum levels of magnesium and citrate
- Genetic factors
  - Cystinuria is an autosomal recessive disorder.
  - Distal renal tubular acidosis may be transmitted as a hereditary trait, and urolithiasis occurs in up to 75% of these patients.

Incidence and Demographics

- The lifetime prevalence of urinary tract stones in the United States is 10%.
- Stones in the upper urinary tract are more prevalent in the United States.
- About 2 million patients will present as outpatients for stone disease each year.
- The male to female ratio is 3:1.
- Most occur between the ages of 30 and 50.

Risk Factors

- Middle age
- Genetic defects
- Renal tubular acidiosis
- Low water intake
- High-protein diet
- Excessive oxalate intake
- Sedentary lifestyle
- Caucasian ethnicity
- Family history

- Obesity
- Diabetes mellitus
- Malabsorption syndrome
- History of bowel or bariatric surgery
- Medications
  - Vitamins A, C, D
  - Loop diuretics
  - Ammonium chloride
  - Acetazolamide
  - Alkali, antacids

Prevention and Screening

- Adequate fluid intake—most important
- If the patient has a history of recurrent stones, restrict protein, sodium, and dairy products and other oxalate-rich foods.
- If the patient is prone to uric acid stones, alkalization of urine may be beneficial.

Assessment

History
- The patient may not exhibit symptoms even with severe obstruction.
- Acute intermittent back/flank pain
- With ureteral obstruction, acute, colic-type flank pain may be episodic with anterior radiation of pain, nausea, vomiting, and diaphoresis. The patient may frequently change position to relieve pain.
- Stone progression: Pain is referred to ipsilateral testis or labia, urinary urgency or hesitancy
- High-volume fluid intake or diuretic use may precipitate pain.
- Associated symptoms include dysuria, frequency, hematuria, diaphoresis, restlessness, chills, fever, nausea, and vomiting.

Physical Examination
- Obvious discomfort, acute onset of pain, pacing, facial grimacing, unable to find a position of comfort
- Fever, tachycardia, tachypnea, diaphoresis, restlessness, costovertebral tenderness

Diagnostic Studies
- Urinalysis, culture, complete blood count, blood urea nitrogen, creatinine
- Urinalysis that shows hematuria with or without proteinuria suggests calculus or tumor.
- Plain film of the abdomen will show renal calculi, stones in the ureter and bladder, or both (85% to 90% of stones are radiopaque).
  - Limitation: Overlying bowel gas and rib cartilage calcification may hamper interpretation.
- Ultrasound is preferred when an obstruction is suspected because of ultrasound's high sensitivity for detecting hydronephrosis. It is also used in pregnancy to detect renal colic. However, the image cannot reveal if an obstruction is present.
- Spiral CT is now the preferred imaging technique because it can identify both radiopaque and radiolucent stones.

Differential Diagnosis

- Acute pyelonephritis
- Lower urinary tract infection

Management

Nonpharmacoligic Treatment
- Increase fluid intake to maintain urinary output at 2 to 3 liters per day.
- Increase dietary fiber.
- Decrease animal fat.
- For ureteral stones < 0.6 cm, observe and provide pain management.
- Strain urine to collect stones and sediment as they pass; if found, the stone must be analyzed.
- Renal calculi < 2 cm should be treated with lithotripsy, those > 2cm are best treated with percutaneous nephrolithotomy.
- For distal ureteral stones > than 0.6 cm, perform lithotripsy, ureteroscopy, percutaneous nephrolithotomy, or open surgery to remove the stone.
- Intervention may also be required for patients with refractory pain.

Pharmacologic Treatment
- Calcium nephrolithiasis—hypercalciuric calcium nephrolithiasis (> 200 mg/24 hr or 4 mg/kg/24 hr
  - Absorptive hypercalciuria—type I, II, III
    - Type I
      - Cellulose phosphate 10 to 15 g orally in three divided doses with meals
      - Use with caution in postmenopausal women.
      - Follow up every 6 to 8 months.
      - Monitor for hypomagnesuria and secondary hyperoxaluria.
      - Alternative: thiazide therapy—decrease renal calcium—therapy time is limited; after 5 years may lose its hypocalciuric effect
    - Type II
      - Diet-dependent
      - Decrease calcium intake by 50% (about 400 mg/day); this will reduce the hypercalciuria to within normal limits (150 to 200 mg/24).
      - No specific medical therapy
    - Type III
      - The result of renal phosphate leak
      - Orthophosphates 250 mg orally 3 to 4 times per day
  - Resorptive hypercalciuria
    - Result of hyperparathyroidism
    - Surgical resection of parathyroid adenoma
  - Renal hypercalciuria
    - Result of renal tubules, inability to efficiently reabsorb filtered calcium
    - Thiazides are an effective long-term therapy.
- Hyperuricosuric
  - Result of dietary excess of uric acid or alterations in uric acid metabolism
  - Purine dietary restrictions

- Hyperoxaluric
  - Encourage increased fluid intake
  - Result of primary intestinal disorders
- If diarrhea or steatorrhea cannot be controlled, use oral calcium supplements with meals.
- Hypocitraturic
  - Seen in conditions causing metabolic acidosis
  - Potassium citrate supplement 20 mEq orally three times daily
- Uric acid calculi
  - Uric acid stone formers have a pH < 5.5
  - Potassium citrate 10 mEq orally 3 or 4 times per day—liquid or crystals that need to be taken with fluid will increase pH of the urine
  - If hyperuricemia is present: allopurinol 300 mg orally once daily
- Struvite calculi
  - Same as magnesium-ammonium-phosphate stones
  - Seen in women with recurrent urinary tract infections that have not responded to antibiotics
  - Target underlying organism with appropriate antibiotics.
  - Percutaneous nephrolithotomy
- Cystine calculi
  - Alkalinization of the urine
  - Penicillamine
  - Tiopronin
- Ureteral stones
  - Oral corticosteroids, alpha-blockers, and calcium channel blockers may help to pass stones.
    - Tamsulosin 0.4 mg orally once daily
    - Terazosin 5 mg orally once daily
    - Doxazosin 4 mg orally once daily
- Pain management
  - NSAIDS and opioids
    - Hydrocodone/acetaminophen 1 to 2 tablets every 4 hours as needed
    - Acetaminophen/codeine 1 to 2 tablets every 4 hours as needed
    - Oxycodone/acetaminophen 1 to 2 tablets every 4 hours as needed
    - Ketorolac 30 to 60 mg IM, then 30 mg orally every 6 hours as needed
    - Morphine 5 to 10 mg IM every 4 hours as needed

Special Considerations

- For prevention of all stone recurrence, instruct patient to drink 2 to 3 liters of water per day, dividing intake evenly throughout the day to keep the urine dilute.
- Avoid apple and grapefruit juices.
- Avoid long periods of immobilization.
- Patients with alkalinizing medications should be given Nitrazine pH paper to monitor effectiveness.
- Geographic factors contribute to stone formation. High humidity and elevated temperatures are contributing factors; occurrence of symptomatic ureteral stones is highest during hot summer months.
- For oxalate stones, restrict dietary oxalate—tea, rhubarb, leafy green vegetables, peanuts.

When to Consult, Refer, or Hospitalize

- Obtain urology consult if obstruction is suspected or symptoms persist for more than 3 to 4 days.
- Patient will need hospitalization if an infection is present (pyelonephritis), the stone is > 6 mm in diameter, or patient has excessive nausea and vomiting, intractable pain, or gross hematuria.
- Solitary kidney

Follow-up

- Strain urine until stone has passed.
- After surgical intervention: abdominal plain film radiography after stone procedure every 6 to 12 months
- After medical therapy
  - > 40 years of age with single stone that passed spontaneously or easily treated: may not require follow-up care—low incidence of recurrence if patient stays well-hydrated
  - Other patients: plain abdominal radiography or renal ultrasound with radiolucent stones every 6 to 12 months
  - A 24-hour urinalysis 3 months after starting new therapy; once stable regimen is established, annual 24-hour urinalysis

Expecte Outcomes
- 98% of stones will pass spontaneously.
- Usually resolve in 4 weeks
- In 50% of patients, reoccurrence happens within 5 years.

Complications
- Urinary obstruction
- Hydronephrosis
- Renal failure
- Infection

BENIGN PROSTATIC HYPERTROPHY

Description

- Benign prostatic hypertrophy is a nonmalignant adenomatous overgrowth of the periurethral prostate gland.
- Hyperplastic process that is the result of an increase in cell numbers

Etiology

- Mostly unknown, but may be the result of hormonal changes associated with aging
- Multiple fibroadenomatous nodules develop in the periurethral glands.
- As the lumen of the prostatic urethra narrows and lengthens, urine outflow is progressively obstructed.
- Urinary retention may be precipitated by attempts to retain urine, exposure to cold, use of anesthestics, anticholinergics, sympathomeimetics, or alcohol ingestion.

Incidence and Demographics

- Most common tumor in men and is age-related
  - 20% of men age 41 to 50 years, 50% in men aged 51 to 60, and over 90% in men over 80 years of age
- Symptoms are also age-related: At age 55, 25% of men report obstructive symptoms; at age 75, 50% report a decrease in the force and caliber of the urinary stream.

Risk Factors

- Poorly understood
- May be a genetic predisposition
- Approximately 50% of men under the age of 60 who have surgery are diagnosed with an inherited form of the disease.
  - Autosomal-domininant
  - First-degree relatives of these patients have an increased relative risk of about fourfold.

Prevention and Screening

- Digital rectal examination
- Prostate-specific antigen (PSA)
- Transrectal ultrasound
- Scoring with the American Urological Association (AUA) symptom index
- Avoid medications that increase obstructive symptoms.
  - Decongestants
  - Anticholinergics

Assessment

History
- Obstructive and irritative complaints
  - Obstructive
    - Hesitancy
    - Diminished stream
    - Sensation of incomplete bladder emptying
    - Postvoiding dribbling
    - Urinary retention
    - Double voiding
      - Voiding a second time within 2 hours
  - Irritative
    - Urgency
    - Frequency
    - Nocturia
    - Incontinence
    - Dysuria

Physical Examination
- On digital rectal examination: smooth, firm, elastic enlargement
- Palpate for distended bladder.

Diagnostic Studies
- Urinalysis
- Serum creatinine
- PSA is optional, but most clinicians include it in the initial evaluation.
- Computerized tomography or renal ultrasound if urinary tract disease or complications (hematuria, urinary tract infection, history of stone disease, chronic kidney disease) are present
- Transrectal ultrasound if palpable nodule present or PSA is elevated

Differential Diagnosis

- Urethral stricture
- Bladder neck contracture
- Bladder stones
- Prostate cancer
- Urinary tract infection

Management

Nonpharmacologic Treatment

- Mild symptoms: watchful waiting—patient may recover spontaneously
- Severe symptoms—gross hematuria, recurrent infection, high postvoiding residuals, nonresponsiveness to medication—surgical intervention
  - Uroflometry, pressure-flow studies, cystoscopy and upper tract imaging are done prior to surgical intervention.
  - Transurethral resection of the prostate (TURP)
    - 95% can be performed endoscopically
    - Symptom scores and flow rates superior to minimally invasive procedures
    - Complications
      - Bleeding
      - Urethral stricture
      - Bladder neck contracture
      - Perforation of prostate capusule
      - Incontinence
    - Risks
      - Retrograde ejaculation: 75%
      - Erectile dysfunction: 5% to10%
      - Urinary incontinence: < 1%
  - Transurethral incision of the prostate (TUIP)
    - More rapid and less morbidity than TURP
    - Lower rate of retrograde ejaculation
  - Open simple prostatectomy
    - When the prostate is too large to removed endoscopically
    - Suprapubic or retropubic approach
  - Laser therapy
    - Visually directed laser techniques used most often
    - Advantages: minimal blood loss, outpatient procedure, patient may remain on anti-coagulation, rare occurrence of transurethral resection syndrome
    - Disadvantages: lack of tissue for pathology, more frequent irritative voiding complaints, expense
  - Transurethral needle ablation of the prostate (TUNA)
    - Radiofrequencies used to heat tissue that results in coagulative necrosis
  - Transurethral electrovaporization of the prostate (TUVP)
    - Heat vaporization of tissue creating a cavity in the prostatic urethra
  - Transurethral microwave therapy (TUMT)—hyperthermia
  - Urethral stents

Pharmacologic Treatment

- Alpha-blockers
- Side effects: hypotension, dizziness, fatigue, headache, retrograde ejaculation
  - Prazosin 1 to 5 mg twice daily
  - Terazosin 1 mg at bedtime, may increase up to 10 mg as needed or as tolerated
  - Doxazosin 1 to 8 mg daily
  - Tamsulosin 0.4 or 0.8 mg daily

- 5α-reductase inhibitors
- Side effects: decreased libido, decrease in ejaculate, erectile dysfunction
  - Finasteride 5 mg daily
  - Dutasteride 0.5 mg orally daily
- Combination therapy
- Alpha-blockers and 5α-reductase inhibitors
- Phytotherapy
  - Use of plants or plant extracts for medicinal purposes
  - Saw palmetto berry
  - Bark of *Pygeum africanum*
  - Roots of *Echinacea purpurea*
  - Roots of *Hypoxis rooperi*
  - Pollen extract
  - Leaves of the trembling poplar

Special Considerations

- BPH and prostate cancer may coexist and cause similar signs and symptoms.
- Patients with symptoms or palpable prostate abnormalities should be tested to rule out malignancy and infection, and to estimate the degree of obstruction.

When to Consult, Refer, or Hospitalize

- Refer to urologist for hematuria, presence of urinary tract infection, or need for surgical intervention

Follow-up

Expected Outcomes
- Improved AUA symptom index scores
- Increased flow rates
- Decreased residual urine

Complications
- Urinary retention
- Erectile dysfunction
- Retrograde ejaculation
- Total incontinence

RENAL DISORDERS

ACUTE KIDNEY INJURY/ACUTE RENAL FAILURE

Description

- Acute kidney injury (AKI) or acute renal failure (ARF) is the decline of renal function over hours to days with the resultant increase of nitrogenous wastes, such as urea and creatinine, in the blood.
- Signs and symptoms depend on the etiology.
- The RIFLE criteria provide a clinically applicable definition.
  - Risk: increased creatinine x 1.5 or GFR decrease > 25%, urine output < 0.5 ml/kg/hr x 6 hours
  - Injury: increased creatinine x 2 or GFR decrease > 50%, urine output < 0.5 ml/kg/hr x 12 hours
  - Failure: increased creatinine x 3 ot GFR decrease > 75%, urine output <0.5 ml/kg/hr x 24 hours or anuria x 12 hours
  - Loss: persistent ARF = complete loss of kidney function > 4 weeks
  - ESKD: end-stage kidney disease > 3 months

Etiology

- Prerenal disease (60% to 70% of cases)
  - Volume depletion from gastrointestinal, renal, or third-space losses
  - Congestive heart failure or valvular heart disease
  - Hepatorenal syndrome
  - Bilateral renal artery stenosis, especially with use of angiotensin-converting enzyme inhibitor (ACE-I) or angiotension receptor blocker (ARB)
  - Use of nonsteroidal antiinflammatory medications (NSAIDS)
  - Shock from volume loss, sepsis, cardiac failure—often progresses to acute tubular necrosis
- Intrinsic renal disease (25% to 40% of cases)
  - Glomerular diseases
    - Acute glomerulonephritis, including postinfectious glomerulonephritis and lupus nephritis
    - Crescentic or rapidly progressive glomerulonephritis
    - Microangiopathic hemolytic anemias, including hemolytic-uremic syndrome and thrombotic thrombocytopenic purpura
  - Tubulointerstitial disease
    - Acute tubular necrosis (ATN)
      - Postischemic: from any cause of severe renal ischemia

- Toxic: aminoglycosides, radiocontrast media, cisplatin, rhabdomyolysis
  - Acute (often medication induced) interstitial nephritis
  - Intratubular obstruction—seen in multiple myeloma (immunoglobulin light chains), hypercalcemia, antiviral drug acyclovir, chemotherapy and radiation therapy (release of uric acid crystals and purines) for hemotologic malignancies
- Vascular disease
  - Vasculitis
  - Atheroemboli to the kidney, usually after surgical or radiologic procedures through an atheromatous aorta
- Urinary tract obstruction (postrenal disease; 5% to 10% of cases)
  - Prostatic disease
  - Pelvic or retoperitoneal malignancy
  - Calculi
  - Tumors
  - Occluded indwelling urinary catheter
  - Neurogenic bladder or spinal cord disease
  - Diabetic neuropathy

Incidence and Demographics

- Acute renal failure is seen in about 5% to 7% of hospital admissions and up to 30% in intensive care unit admissions.
- An association exists between low birth weight and the development of albuminuria and nephropathy in diabetic and nondiabetic kidney disease.
- The annual incidence of community-acquired ARF is approximately 100 cases per 1 million people.

Risk Factors

- Prerenal
  - Hypovolemia
  - NSAIDS
  - ACE-I or ARB medications
  - Heart failure
  - Preexisting kidney disease
  - Elderly
- Intrinsic
  - Atrial fibrillation
  - Vascular disease
  - Pulmonary embolism
  - History of nephritic syndrome
  - Liver disease
  - Systemic lupus erythematosus
  - Infection
  - Hypertension
  - Severe hypotension
  - Nephrotoxic medications

- Radiocontrast medium exposure
- Rhabdomyolyisis
- Tumor lysis, chemotherapy
- Postrenal
  - History of renal stones
  - Prostate disease
  - Spinal cord injury
  - Diabetes

Prevention and Screening

- Prerenal
  - Maintain euvolemia.
  - Optimize cardiac function.
- Intrinsic
  - Renal adjustment of nephrotoxic medications by calculated GFR
  - Diuretics, NSAIDS, ACE-Is, ARBs, and vasodilators should be used with caution in patients with hypovolemia or renovascular disease.
  - Allopurinol and forced alkaline diuresis as prophylactic measures for acute urate nephropathy (cancer chemotherapy)
  - Hydration with bicarbonate containing intravenous fluid and the use of N-acetylcysteine prior to radiocontrast medium exposure
- Postrenal
  - Prostate examinations
  - Maintenance of indwelling urinary catheters
  - Control of diabetes

Assessment

History
- Prerenal
  - Thirst
  - Orthostatic dizziness
  - Nausea, vomiting
- Intrinsic
  - Fever
  - Arthralgias
- Postrenal
  - Suprapubic and flank pain
  - Colicky flank pain radiating to the groin indicates acute ureteric obstruction.

Physical Examination
- Prerenal
  - Orthostatic hypotension
  - Tachycardia
  - Reduced jugular venous pressure
  - Decreased skin turgor
  - Dry mucous membranes

- Intrinisic
  - Fever, arthralgias, and pruritic erythematous rash after new medication exposure may indicate allergic interstitial nephritis—systemic signs of hypersensitivity may be absent.
  - Flank pain
  - Subcutaneous nodules, livedo reticularis, bright-orange retinal arteriolar plaques, and digital ischemia (purple toes) indicate atheroembolization.
  - Oliguria, edema, hypertension, and active urine sediment indicate acute glomerulonephritis of vasculitis.
  - Papilledema, neurologic dysfunction, and left ventricular hypertrophy associated with malignant hypertension leading to ARF
- Postrenal
  - Suprapubic and flank pain from bladder distention
  - Colicky flank pain
  - Nocturia, frequency, hesistancy, which may indicate enlarged prostate
  - Neurogenica bladder in patients receiving anticholinergic medications or who have autonomic dysfunction

Diagnostic Studies
- Urinalysis
  - Prerenal
    - Normal or hyaline casts
    - Specific gravity > 1.020
  - Intrinsic
    - Diseases of large vessels
      - Renal artery thrombosis
        - Mild proteinuria
        - Occasional hematuria
      - Atheroembolic disease
        - Esoinophiluria
      - Renal vein thrombosis
        - Granular casts
    - Diseases of small vessels
      - Glomerulonephritis/vasculitis
        - Hematuria
        - Red cell casts
        - Dysmorphic red blood cells
        - Granular casts
        - Proteinuria < 1 g/d
    - Hemolytic
      - Hematuria
      - Mild proteinuria
      - Red cell casts (rare)
    - ATN
      - Muddy brown granular or tubular epithelial cell casts
      - FENA > 1%
      - UNA > 20 mmol/L
      - Specific gravity < 1.015

- Exogenous toxins
  - Nephrotoxic antibiotics, chemotherapy
    - Muddy brown granular or tubular epithelial cell casts
    - FENA >1%
    - UNA > 20 mmol/L
    - Specific gravity < 1.015
  - Recent contrast exposure
    - Muddy brown granular or tubular epithelial cell casts
    - Urinalysis may be normal.
    - FENA often < 1%
    - UNA often < 20 mmol/L
  - Rhabdomyolosis
    - UA positive for heme but no hematuria
  - Hemolysis—recent transfusion
    - Pink, heme-positive urine without hematuria
  - Tumor lysis, recent chemotherapy
    - Urate crystals
  - Multiple myeloma
    - Dipstick negative proteinuria
    - Monoclonal spike on electrophoresis
  - Ethylene glycol ingestion
    - Oxalate crystals
- Diseases of tubulointerstitium
  - Allergic interstitial nephritis
    - White cell casts
    - Eosinophiluria
  - Acute bilateral pyelonephritis
    - Leukocytes
    - Proteinuria
    - Positive urine culture
- Postrenal
  - Usually normal
  - Hematuria if stones are present
- Urine and blood biochemistry
  - Prerenal
    - FENA < 1%
    - UNA < 20 mmol/L
    - High BUN/CR ratio > 10:1
    - Urine osmolality > 500 mOsm/L
    - Urine creatinine/plasma creatinine > 40
    - UNA/creatinine clearance < 1
  - Intrinsic
    - FE_{NA} > 1%
      - Exceptions FE_{NA} < 1%
        - Acute glomerulonephritis
        - Hepatorenal syndrome
        - Contrast induced ATN
        - Myoglobinuric and hemoglobinuric renal failure
        - Renal allograft rejection
        - Drug-related alterations in renal hemodynamics

- U_{NA} > 40 mEq/L
- BUN/CR ratio of about 10:1
- Urine osmolality < 300–400 mOsm/L
- Urine creatinine/plasma creatinine < 20
- UNA/creatinine clearance > 2

- Serial serum creatinine measurements
  - Fluctuating serum creatinine levels that follow changes in hemodynamic status point to prerenal acute renal failure
  - Creatinine rises quickly with renal ischemia, atheroembolization, and radiocontrast exposure.
    - Peak serum creatinine levels are seen after 3 to 5 days with contrast exposure.
    - Peak serum creatinine levels are seen after 7 to 10 days with ATN.
    - The initial rise of creatinine is usually delayed until the second week of therapy with many tubular epithelial cell toxins (aminoglycosides, cisplatin).
- Serial serum electrolytes
  - Prerenal
    - BUN: increased 10:1 greater than creatinine
    - Creatinine: normal to moderate increase
    - Potassium: normal to moderate increase
    - Phosphorus: normal to moderate increase
    - Calcium: normal
  - Intrinsic
    - BUN increased by 20 to 40/day
    - Creatinine: increased by 2 to 4/day
    - Potassium: large increase (especially when patient oliguric) and with rhabdomyolysis
    - Phosphorus: increased—poor correlation with duration of renal disease
    - Calcium: decreased—poor correlation with duration of renal failure
    - Creatinine kinase elevated in rhabdoymyolysis
- Renal ultrasound
  - Test of choice—excellent sensitivity and specificity for detecting hydronephrosis resulting from obstruction
  - Kidneys smaller that 9 cm suggest chronic kidney disease.
  - Hyperechogenicity indicates diffuse parenchymal disease.
  - Color Doppler allows assessment of renal perfusion and can diagnose large-vessel etiologies of ARF.
  - Bedside ultrasound in the critically ill patient can quickly diagnose treatable etiologies and give guidance for fluid resuscitation.
- Plain radiologic film of abdomen or helical CT if nephrolithiasis is suspected
- Renal biopsy
  - Reserved for evaluation of ARF when cause cannot be determined
  - Important when glomerular causes are suspected

Differential Diagnosis

- Urinary tract infection
- Hemolytic uremic syndrome
- Metabolic acidosis
- Renal calculi

Management

Nonpharmacologic Treatment
- Identify underlying cause.
- Daily weights
- Monitor intake and output.
- Monitor serial serum and urinary indices.
- Remove offending medications.
- Urinary catheter placement with obstruction
- Hemodialysis for electrolyte and volume control if needed
- Intraaortic balloon pump for cardiogenic shock
- Optimize nutrition: Intake should be 30 to 45 kcal/day.
  - Combination of carbohydrates and lipids
  - In patients not receiving dialysis, protein should be restricted to 0.6 g/kg/day.
  - In patients receiving dialysis, protein should be restricted to1 to 1.5 g/kg/day.

Pharmacologic Treatment
- Prerenal
  - Replacement of volume
    - A fluid challenge of 15 to 30 mL/kg of isotonic crystalloid unless there are signs of intravascular congestion
  - Inotropes, preload and afterload reducing agents for cardiac failure
  - Vasoactive medications in the hypotensive oliguric patient
- Intrinsic
  - Renal dose medications
  - Low-dose dopamine (< 5 mcg/kg/min) for the prevention or reduction of severity in ATN is not indicated.
  - Diuretics for volume overload: Lasix 20 to 100 mg IV every 8 to 12 hours
    - Higher doses will be required for patients with elevated serum creatinine.
  - Oral phosphate binders
  - Avoid magnesium-containing products.
  - Hyperkalemia
    - Kayexalate
    - Regular insulin 10 units, glucose 50 g, β2-adrenergic agonist and/or sodium bicarbonate 50 mEq intravenous as a transient therapy
    - Calcium gluconate for life-threatening hyperkalemia

Special Considerations

- Males and females are affected equally.
- Mortality rates are generally lower for nonoliguric ARF (> 400 mL/d) than for oliguric (< 400 ml/d) ARF.
- Patients with acute kidney injury of any type are at higher risk for all-cause mortality whether or not there is renal recovery.
- FENA values are distorted with the use of diuretics because of excess UNA.

- The major tool for distinguishing between prerenal disease and ATN is the response to intravenous fluids.
  - An improvement in renal function (over 1 to 2 days) back to baseline serum creatinine levels is diagnostic of prerenal disease; a continued elevation in serum creatinine points toward ATN.

When to Consult, Refer, or Hospitalize

- Refer to nephrology for elevated serum creatinine that does not respond to fluids and for patients who require hemodialysis.
- Refer the patient to a urologist for persistent urinary tract obstruction.
- Hospitalize for sudden loss of kidney function resulting in abnormalities such as hyperkalemia or volume overload.
- Hospitalize if urgent interventional procedures are required—hemodialysis, relief of obstruction.

Follow-up

Expected Outcomes
- Return of renal function to baseline

Complications
- Metabolic
- Metabolic acidosis
- Hyperkalemia
- Hypocalcemia
- Hyperphosphatemia
- Hyperuricemia
- Cardiovascular
  - Fluid overload
  - Hypertension
  - Arrythmias
  - Pericarditis
- Neurological
  - Neuropathy
  - Dementia
  - Seizures
- Hematologic
- Anemia
- Coagulopathy
- Gastrointestinal
  - Nausea and vomiting
  - GI bleeding
- Infectious
  - Urinary tract
  - IV-catheter sepsis
  - Pneumonia

CHRONIC KIDNEY DISEASE/CHRONIC RENAL FAILURE

Description

- Chronic kidney disease (CKD) or chronic renal failure (CRF) is associated with a progressive decline in the glomerular filtration rate and renal function.
- It is defined by means of one of two criteria set forth by the National Kidney Foundation and

  ### International Society of Nephrology
  - Kidney damage for > 3 months with structural or functional abnormalities of the kidney, with or without decreased GFR
    - Kidney damage is evidenced by pathological abnormalities, abnormalities in the composition of the blood or urine, and abnormal imaging studies.
  - CKD is suspected when the GFR is < 60 mL/min/1.73 m2 for > 3 months, with or without kidney damage.
  - CKD is divided into five stages on the basis of GFR and presence of proteinuria, hematuria, or both.

Table 8-1. Stages of CKD

Stage Description	GFR (mL/min/1.73 m²)	Related Terms
1 – Kidney damage with normal or increased GFR	> 90	Albuminuria, proteinuria, hematuria
2 – Kidney damage with mild decreased GFR	60–89	Alluminuria, proteinuria, hematuria
3 – Moderate decreased GFR	30–59	Early renal insufficiency
4 – Severe decreased GFR	15–29	Late renal insufficiency
5 – Kidney failure	< 15 (dialysis)	

Adapted from *Hospital Medicine* by S. McKean, A. Bennett, & L. Halasyamani, (Eds.), 2008, Philadelphia: Wolters Kluwer/Lippincott Williams & Wilkins.

Etiology

- CKD is a consequence of systemic disease
- Diabetic nephropathy
- Hypertensive nephropathy
- Glomerular disease
- Vasculitis
- Polycystic kidney disease
- Renal artery stenosis
- Tubulointerstitial nephritis

Incidence and Demographics

- Chronic kidney disease affects 50 million people worldwide.
- About 11% of the U.S. population is affected, and the numbers are increasing.
- The prevalence of stage 1 CKD was about 6% of the adult population and stage 3 and 4 CKD among U.S. adults age 20 and over was 4.5%.
- The number of patients with kidney failure requiring treatment with dialysis or transplantation in the United States was projected to increase from 450,000 in 2003 to 650,000 in 2010.

Risk Factors

- Hypertension
- Diabetes mellitus
- Dyslipidemia
- Autoimmune disease
- Older age
- African ancestry
- Family history of renal disease
- Previous episode of acute renal failure
- Presence of proteinuria
- Abnormal urinary sediment
- Structural abnormalities of the urinary tract
- Chronic NSAID use
- Exposure to radiocontrast material
- Neoplasm

Prevention and Screening

- Once CKD is present, it is usually irreversible.
- Major focus is to minimize further kidney damage and halt progression
- Control blood pressure
- Manage diabetes
- Reduce proteinuria
- Optimize nutrition
- Identify and treat cardiovascular risk factors
- Stage 1 and 2 CKD: urine and blood indices every 12 months
- Stage 3 and 4 CKD: urine and blood indices every 6 months

Assessment

History
- Patient may remain asymptomatic and renal dysfunction is only detectable by lab values
- Even with elevated BUN and creatinine with mild to moderate CKD, the patient may have no symptoms.
- Nocturia from failure to concentrate the urine
- Earliest manifestations include diminished energy, anorexia, and decreased mental acuity.
- Late manifestations include pruritus, metallic taste in mouth, inability to concentrate, nausea, vomiting, shortness of breath, dyspnea on exertion, irritability, impotence, decreased libido, and bone pain.

Physical Examination
- Pruritus
- Easy bruising
- Pallor, yellow-brown skin
- Edema
- Pale conjunctiva
- Epistaxis
- Urinous breath
- Pleural effusion
- Pericarditis
- Cardiomegaly
- Stupor
- Asterixis
- Myoclonus/hyperreflexia
- Restless leg syndrome/loss of vibratory sense
- Seizures (rare)
- Anemia
- Reversible hair loss, nail changes

Diagnostic Studies
- Estimate GFR
- Two equations
  - Cockcroft-Gault equation
    - GFR (mL/min) = (140 − age) × weight (0.85 weight if female) ÷ 72 × SCr
  - Modification of Diet in Renal Disease equation
    - (mL/min = 175 × (SCr) $^{-1.154}$ × (age)$^{-0.203}$ × (0.742 if female)
    - If patient is African American, multiply by 1.21.
- Serum/urine chemistry: serial creatinine
- Screen patients with a urinary dipstick and sediment.
- Screen urine for protein.
- 24-hour urine collections for GFR and protein
  - When measuring CrCl to estimate GFR, it is important to assess for completeness of the urine specimen.
  - Under age 50, creatinine excretion should be 20 to 25 mg/kg lean body weight for men and 15 to 20 mg/kg for women.
  - Over age 50, there is a decline in excretion to about 50% by age 90.
  - CrCl = (uCr x uv)/(sCr x 1440)
  - CrCl should be adjusted for body surface area
    - Adjusted CrCl (mL/min per 1.72 m^2) = CrCl x 1.73 ÷ BSA
- Renal imaging
  - Can identify a reversible process, such as kidney stones and hydronephrosis
  - May identify the cause—cysts, renal artery stenosis
  - Can determine the chronicity of the disease by kidney size, atrophy, and absence of kidney

Differential Diagnosis

- Acute renal failure

Management

Nonpharmacologic Treatment
- Save nondominant arm from blood draws, intravenous puncture
- Monitor intake and output.
- Daily weight
- Avoid gadolinium because of risk for nephrogenic fibrosing dermopathy (NSF).
- Be aware of subtle changes in GFR, reflecting loss of renal function.
- Maintain adequate blood pressure and diabetes management.
- Manage protein catabolism.
  - Avoid stresses of trauma, infection, and immobilization.
  - Physical activity in moderation
- Optimize nutrition
  - Maintain adequate caloric intake.
  - Avoid hypoalbuminemia.

- Dietary protein for CKD stages 1 to 4: 0.8 to 1 g/kg body weight/day
- Patients with nephritic syndrome should receive supplemental protein to replace urinary protein losses.
- Avoid high-potassium foods.
- Restrict phosphorus to 800 to 1,000 mg/day (colas, eggs, dairy products, meat).
- Renal replacement therapy for stage 5 CKD
  - Hemodialysis
  - Peritoneal dialysis
  - Renal transplantation

Pharmacologic Treatment

- Control of blood pressure
  - Goal of < 130/80 mm Hg for all patients with CKD or < 120/80 mm Hg for patients with CKD with proteinuria
  - Low-sodium diet
  - If proteinuria present: ACE-I (if k+ and creatinine permit) and calcium channel blockers (CCB) may be helpful in decreasing proteinuria and reducing glomerular hypertension.
  - Other antihypertensives
    - Direct vasodilators
      - Hydralazine
      - Minoxidil
    - Peripheral alpha-blockers
      - Doxazosin
      - Prazosin
    - Beta-blockers
      - Metoprolol
      - Propranolol
      - Carvedilol
    - Central alpha-blockers
      - Clonidine
    - Diuretics
      - Lasix
      - Bumex
- Diabetes management
  - Aim for a target HbAIC < 7%.
  - Most oral hypoglycemic agents and insulin have increased half-lives in CKD, and doses may need to be adjusted.
  - Rosiglitazone is mostly excreted hepatically and is, therefore, used in first-line management.
  - Use metformin with caution—discontinue with deterioration of renal function.
- Management of cardiovascular risk factors
  - Target LDL < 100 mg/dL in patients with stage 1 to 4 CKD
  - Antilipid therapy with statins may also decrease protein when used with ACE-Is.
- Hyperkalemia
  - If potassium is > 7
    - Administer hypertonic glucose, insulin, and HCO_3.
    - Hemodialysis
    - Kayexalate
    - Monitor electrocardiogram for flat P waves, peaked T waves, PR interval > 0.20 seconds, QRS > 0.10 seconds, and bradycardia.

- Consider use of loop diuretics to decrease serum K^+.
- Lower or discontinue ACE-I/ARB when serum K^+ is > 5.5 mEq/L.
- Potassium-binding resins are well tolerated and effective in reducing potassium levels.
  - Kayexalate 30 to 60 g/day (1 g resin = 1 mEq K^+ out = 1 mEq Na^+ in)
- Anemia
  - Supplemental iron
  - Vitamin supplements
  - Erythropoetin 2 to 3 injections per week subcutaneously or intravenously
- Calcium/vitamin D
  - Maintain phosphorus level < 6 mg/dL.
  - Calcium carbonate supplements
  - 1,25-OH vitamin D in severe cases of hypocalcemia
- Phosphorus
  - GFR < 20 to 30 mL/min usually requires phosphate-binding agent
  - Calcium acetate, 667 mg (2 to 6 tablets) 3 times daily with meals
  - Aluminum hydroxide
- Magnesium
  - Avoid magnesium containing laxatives/antacids.
- Renal osteodystrophy
  - Prevent acidosis, hypocalcemia, and hyperphosphatemia, and control hyperparathyroidism.
  - Correct low Ca (less than 6.5 mg/dl).
  - Correct a high phosphorus level > 5 mg/dl.
  - Correct acidosis: $NaHCO_3$, 2 to 5 mEq/kg as a 4 to 8–hour infusion (emergency) or 650 mg orally 3 times daily—titrate as needed
  - Administer vitamin D if Ca stays < 6 mg/dl (calcitrol, hexitrol), for bone pain, for increased alkaline phosphatase levels, or if x-rays reveal osteomalacia.
  - Treat secondary hyperparathyroidism.
    - Limit foods high in phosphorus.
    - Phosphate binders such as Tums, Oscal with meals
    - Sevelamer hydrochloride
- Fluid overload
  - Lasix: 20 to 80 mg/day initially
  - Bumex: 0.5 to 2 mg once daily
  - Tosemide: 10 to 20 mg orally by IV daily
- Acidosis
  - Treat when plasma HCO_3 < 20 mEq/L
  - $NaHCO_3$: 1 g = 13 mEq of Na, used in emergencies
  - Sodium citrate
  - Sodium and potassium citrate and citric acid (Polycitra): Monitor K+ levels.
- Neurologic manifestations
  - Anticonvulsants
    · Dilantin
    · Phenobarbitol
  - Sedatives
    · Benadryl

Special Considerations

- Signs and symptoms develop late—maintain a high index of suspicion for patients at increased risk, and diagnose early for best outcomes
- A reduction in renal mass from an isolated injury may lead to a progressive decline in renal function over many years.

When to Consult, Refer, or Hospitalize

- Refer a patient with stage 3 to 5 CKD to a nephrologist.
- Patients with stage 1 to 2 CKD should have an initial visit with a nephrologist to discuss future management.
- Hospitalize for worsening acid–base status, electrolyte abnormalities, or volume overload that cannot be treated as an outpatient.
- Hospitalize for renal replacement therapy when patient is not stable for outpatient initiation.

Follow-up

Expected Outcomes
- Progressive disease: management aimed at slowing progression

Complications
- Hyperkalemia
- Acid–base disorders
- Hypertension
- Pericarditis
- Congestive heart failure
- Anemia
- Coagulopathy
- Neurological complications
- Osteomalacia
- Adynamic bone disease
- Decreased libido and impotence

END-STAGE RENAL DISEASE/DIALYSIS

Description

- Chronic renal failure that requires dialysis or transplantation is called end-stage renal disease (ESRD).
- CKD stage V5: GFR < 15 ml/min/1.73m^2

Etiology

- Progressive chronic renal failure
- Diabetic neuropathy (most common cause)
- Hypertension (second-most common cause)
- Glomerulonephritis
- HIV nephropathy
- Polycystic kidney disease

Incidence and Demographics

- Approximately 520,240 patients are receiving hemodialysis in the United States.
- Approximately 178,806 patients have functioning transplants, and 95,550 patients are on the waiting list.
- Etiology differs among racial groups because of the predisposing conditions.
- In the United States, Black and Native American populations have a 3.6 and a 1.8 times higher incidence, respectively, than the White population.
- Hispanics have a 1.5 time higher incidence than non-Hispanics.

Risk Factors

- See CKD

Prevention and Screening

- Avoid dehydration in patients with renal transplants.
- Avoid nephrotoxic agents in patients with renal transplants.
- Treatment of underlying disease can delay progression to end-stage renal disease.

Assessment

History
- Malaise
- Weakness
- Fatigue
- Anorexia
- Nausea and vomiting
- Hiccups
- Malnutrition
- Peripheral neuropathy
- Restless leg syndrome
- Pruritis
- Uremia
- Electrolyte abnormalities
- Postural hypotension
- Peritonitis

- Infection at access site
- Myocardial ischemia
- Dialysis disequilibrium syndrome
  - Weaknesss
  - Dizziness
  - Headache
  - Mental status changes
  - Nonfocal neurological changes
- Vascular access problems
  - Bleeding
  - Clotting
- See CKD

Physical Examination
- Patients with arteriovenous fistulas or grafts should have the sites examined regularly.
- Continuous abdominal peritoneal dialysis (CAPD) associated peritonitis
  - Abdominal pain and tenderness—generalized and mild
  - Localized pain and tenderness suggest a local process—incarcerated hernia or appendicitis
  - Severe generalized peritonitis may be result of perforated viscus
- Transplant-related problems
  - Pain and tenderness over a transplanted kidney may indicate infection, obstruction, or graft rejection.
- Vascular access problems
  - Aneurysms
  - Pseudoaneurysms
  - Localized swelling
  - May be chronic
  - A rapid increase in size may indicate active bleeding.
- See CKD

Diagnostic Studies
- See CKD
- Platelet count
  - Abnormal platelet function can lead to abnormal bleeding.
- Amylase, lipase
  - Pancreatitis occurs with increased frequency with ESRD.
  - CKD can falsely elevate serum amylase.
  - Serum lipase is preferable to amylase for diagnosing pancreatitis.
- Total creatine phosphokinase (CPK)
  - May be falsely elevated in ESRD
- Troponin
  - May be falsely elevated in ESRD
  - Monitor trends and clinical correlation for cardiovascular etiology.
- ESRD is a relative contraindication for MRI studies using gadolinium.
  - Risk of developing nephrogenic systemic fibrosis (NSF)
  - NSF occurrence is 2.4% per radiologic study.
  - Risk/benefit ratio for the MRI must be carefully evaluated.
- Electrocardiogram
  - Hyperkalemia
  - Rule out acute coronary syndrome.

Differential Diagnosis

• See CKD

Management

Nonpharmacologic Treatment
• Hemodialysis
  • Offers more efficient clearance of solutes that peritoneal dialysis
  • Blood is pumped into a dialyzer containing two fluid compartments.
    · Blood in the first compartment is pumped along one side of a semipermeable membrane while a crystalloid solution (dialysate) is pumped along the other side in a separate compartment, flowing in the opposite direction.
    · Concentration gradients of solute between blood and dialysate lead to therapeutic changes in the patient's serum solutes.
    · The dialysis compartment is under negative pressure relative to the blood compartment to prevent filtration of dialysate into the blood stream and to remove excess fluid from the patient.
• Requires vascular access
• Electrolyte and fluid shifts
• Intermittent—most patients are treated 3 to 5 days per week
• Indications
  · Use in emergency situations for volume and uremic control
  · May be done in the home or in a dialysis center
  · Fluid overload
  · Acidosis
  · Hyperkalemia
  · Hypernatremia
  · Uremic signs and symptoms
• Complications
  · All patients are at risk of hepatitis B and C.
  · Mechanical
    - Thrombosis
    - Hemorrhage
    - Stenosis of subclavian vein or superior vena cava
      · Recurrent use of subclavian and internal jugular vein catheters
• Infectious
  · Vascular access cellulitis or abscess
  · Colonization of temporary central venous catheters
  · Bacteremia, meningitis, endocarditis, osteomyelitis
• Cardiovascular
  · Hypotension from excessive ultrafiltration
  · Arrythmia
  · Air embolism
  · Cardiac tamponade
• Metabolic
  · Electrolyte imbalance

- Miscellanous
  - Fever
  - Muscle cramps
  - Insomnia
  - Amyloid deposits
- Hemodialysis disequilibrium
  - Results from brain edema and osmolar shifts with rapid dialysis and hemodynamic instability from rapid fluctuations in potassium, calcium, and body osmoles and rapid fluid removal
- Continuous hemofiltration and hemodialysis/continuous veno-venous hemodialysis (CVVHD)
  - Continuous filtration and dialysis without interruption
  - Able to remove large volumes of fluid without hypotensive episodes
  - Indicated for patients in acute renal failure who require large volumes of fluid (sepsis) and/or are hemodynamically unstable (requiring vasopressors, multiorgan system failure)
  - Useful for the neurological patient with labile increased intracranial pressure
- Peritoneal dialysis
  - May done in the home
  - May be continued in the hospital setting if patient admitted for reasons other than renal ones
  - Risk of abdominal infection
  - Less effective than hemodialysis
  - Complications
    - Peritonitis
    - Exit site infections
    - Catheter tunnel infection
    - Catheter leak
    - Obesity
    - Protein malnutrition
    - Hyperlipidemia
    - Hyperglycemia
- Kidney transplant
- Medications to avoid using in patients receiving dialysis
  - Tetracycline
  - Nitrofurantoin
  - Probenecid
  - Neomycin
  - Bacitracin
  - Methenamine
  - Nalidixic acid
  - Clofibrate
  - Lovastatin

Pharmacologic Treatment
- See CKD
- Diuretics not indicated if patient is anuric or in advanced ESRD

Special Considerations

- The most common cause of sudden death in patients with ESRD is hyperkalemia.
- Iatrogenic complications related to fluid administration or medications are often encountered in patients with ESRD.
- Cardiovascular mortality is 10 to 20 times higher in dialysis patients.
- Anemia results in fatigue, reduced exercise capacity, decreased cognition, and impaired immunity.
- Renal transplant patients are prone to infection.
- More than 30% of patients who begin dialysis die within the first year of the initiation of treatment.
- All-cause mortality in dialysis patients older than 65 years is more than six times that of the general population.

When to Consult, Refer, or Hospitalize

- Patients receiving hemodialysis are managed by a nephrologist.
- Hospitalize for volume overload or life-threatening electrolyte abnormalities.

Follow-up

Expected Outcomes
- Progressive disease
- Management of underlying disorders

Complications
- Anemia or renal failure
- Increased coronary artery disease risk
- Hyperphosphatemia
- Hypocalcemia and secondary hyperparathyroidism
- Renal osteodystrophy
- Vitamin deficiencies
- Calciphylaxis
- Constipation

RENAL ARTERY STENOSIS (RAS)

Description
- The renal artery and its branches are potential sites for plaque formation, which can lead to ischemic renal disease and hypertension.
- Bilateral involvement is present in half of affected patients.
- Established plaques progress in > 50% of cases over 5 years (15% to total occlusion).
- Renal hypertrophy occurs in 20% of affected kidneys.

Etiology

- Atherosclerosis
- Fibromuscular dysplasia
- Elevated urinary albumin excretion

Incidence and Demographics

- Approximately 5% of hypertension is caused by renal artery stenosis.
- A > 60% stenosis is found in 9.1% of men and 5.5% of women over 65 years of age.
- The incidence is higher in patients with coronary (19%) or peripheral vascular disease (35% to 50%).
- Autopsy in patients dying of stroke revealed that at least one renal artery was > 75% stenosed in 10% of the patients studied.
- In younger women, 15 to 50, stenosis is the result of fibromuscular dysplasia.

Risk Factors

- Atherosclerotic disease
- Cardiac disease
- Peripheral vascular disease
- Carotid disease
- Chronic kidney disease
- Diabetes mellitus
- Smoking
- Hypertension

Prevention and Screening

- Control of diabetes, hypertension, hyperlipidemia
- Maintenance of normal body mass index (BMI)
- Smoking cessation
- Unexplained hypertension in a woman younger than 40 years of age is reason to screen.

Assessment

History
- Refractory hypertension
- Acute kidney injury with initiation of ACE-I

Physical Examination
- Refractory hypertension
- New-onset hypertension
- Pulmonary edema
- Audible abdominal bruit on the affected side

Diagnostic Studies
- Serum chemistry—may have elevated BUN and creatinine if renal ischemia is severe
- Abdominal ultrasound
  - Highly sensitive and specific
  - Dependent on the operator and patient for optimal results
  - Poor choice if patient is obese, unable to lie supine, or has interfering bowel gas patterns
- CT angiography
  - Intravenous digital subtraction angiography with arteriography and is noninvasive
  - Spiral CT with IV contrast
  - Sensitivity 77% to 98%, specificity 90% to 94%
- MRA
  - Expensive
  - Sensitivity is 77% to 100%; specificity is 71% to 96%.
  - Turbulent flow can cause false-positive results.
  - Gadolinium has been associated with nephrogenic systemic fibrosis, which occurs mostly in patients with GFR < 20 mL/min/1.732, acute kidney injury, or a kidney transplant.
- Renal angiography
  - Gold standard for diagnosis
  - CO_2 subtraction angiography can be used in place of contrast if risk of contrast-induced nephropathy exists.
  - Lesions are most commonly found in the proximal third or ostial region of the renal artery.
  - Risk of atherembolic phenomena after angiography is 5% to 10%.
  - Fibromuscular dysplasia has a "beads-on-a-string" appearance.
- Radionuclide scanning
  - Radionuclide scanning following a single dose of captopril is used often when fibromuscular dysplasia is suspected.

Differential Diagnosis

- Hypertension
- Acute kidney injury
- Nephrosclerosis
- Azotemia
- Chronic glomerulonephritis

Management

Nonpharmacologic Treatment
- All patients with significant (> 80%) bilateral stenosis and stenosis in a solitary functioning kidney are candidates for revascularization with or without renal insufficiency.

- When renal function is normal (or nearly normal), revascularize for stenosis > 80% to 85% or stenosis 50% to 80% with captopril-enhanced scintigraphy findings indicate renal artery stenosis.
- Observation: Stenosis is 50% to 80% with negative scintigraphy.
- CKD is present and the objective is renal recovery, revascularize for the following:
  - Serum creatinine < 4 mg/dl
  - Serum creatinine > 4 mg/dl but with possible recent renal artery thrombosis
  - Degree of stenosis > 80%
  - Serum creatinine increased after ACE-I administered
  - Stenosis 50% to 80% with positive scintigraphy
- Angioplasty with or without stenting
- Surgical bypass
- Treatment of fibromuscular dysplasia with angioplasty is often curative.

Pharmacologic Treatment
- ACE-I if tolerated
- ARB if tolerated
- Calcium channel blockers
- Statin

Special Considerations

- Renal artery stenosis is being increasingly recognized as an important cause of CKD and ESRD.
- In older individuals, atherosclerosis is the most common etiology of renal artery stenosis.

When to Consult, Refer, or Hospitalize

- Refer to nephrology for management of CKD.
- Hospitalize for malignant hypertension and management.

Follow-up

Expected Outcomes
- Improvement in hypertension and renal function with revascularization
- Delayed progression of observed RAS with medically managed hypertension, lipids

Complications
- Acute kidney injury
- CKD
- Malignant hypertension
- Nephrosclerosis

ACUTE TUBULAR NECROSIS

Description

- Acute tubular necrosis (ATN) is acute kidney injury due to tubular damage.
- May be from ischemic or nephrotoxic insults
- Tubular damage results from states of low perfusion and is often preceded by prerenal azotemia.
- In the most severe form, ischemia leads to bilateral renal cortical necrosis and irreversible renal failure.
- The course of ATN is characterized by four phases
  - Initiation
    · Lasts hours to days
    · GFR declines
  - Extension
    · Continued ischemic injury and inflammation
    · Endothelial damage resulting in vascular congestion
  - Maintenance
    · 1 to 2 weeks
    · GFR stabilizes at lowest point—usually 5 to 10 mL/minute
    · Urine output is the lowest at this time.
    · Uremic symptoms may appear.
  - Recovery
    · Tubular epithelial cell repair and regeneration
    · Gradual return of GFR toward baseline
    · May be complicated by a diuretic phase because of delayed recovery of epithelial cell function relative to GFR

Etiology

- Prerenal AKI
- Ischemic or toxic insult
- Postoperatively from major cardiovascular surgery
- Severe trauma
- Hemorrhage
- Sepsis
- Volume depletion
- Exposure to nephrotoxins—medications, contrast media
- Preexisting CKD

Incidence and Demographics

- Accounts for approximately 85% of intrinsic kidney injury
- It is the second-most common cause of all categories of AKI in the hospital setting with only prerenal azotemia occurring more frequently

Risk Factors

- Hypotension
- Volume depletion
- Preexisting renal disease

Prevention and Screening

- Avoid hypotensive states
- Volume repletion
- Identify patients at risk prior to contrast administration, surgery
- Avoid nephrotoxic medications—renal dose in patients with preexisting kidney disease

Assessment

History
- Recent exposure to nephrotoxins
- Recent hypotensive episode
- Known chronic kidney disease

Physical Examination
- Similar examination findings as seen in patients with acute kidney injury and CKD

Diagnostic Studies
- Serum chemistry
- Complete blood count
- Differentiation from prerenal azotemia

Table 8–2. Prerenal Azotemia vs. Acute Tubular Necrosis

Finding	Prerenal Azotemia	ATN and/or Intrinsic Renal Disease
Urine osmolarity (mOsm/kg)	> 500	< 350
Urine sodium	< 20	> 40
Fractional excretion of Na	< 1%	> 2%
Fractional excretion of urea	< 35%	> 50%
Urine sediment	Bland and/or nonspecific	May show muddy-brown granular casts

Adapted from *Current Medical Diagnosis and Treatment* by S. McPhee & M. Papadakis, 2011, New York: McGraw-Hill, p. 873.

- Abdominal ultrasound
- CT of the abdomen
- MRI
- Biopsy is rarely necessary—used only when the exact renal cause is unknown or the course is prolonged

Differential Diagnosis

- Acute renal failure
- Azotemia
- Chronic renal failure
- Acute glomerular nephritis
- Interstitial nephritis

Management

Nonpharmacologic Treatment
- Prevent further renal damage.
- Monitor intake and output.
- Daily weight
- Avoid nephrotoxic agents.
- Early hemodialysis in severe ATN
- Optimize nutrition—adequate protein and caloric intake.

Pharmacologic Treatment
- Replace intravascular volume—crystalloid, packed cells for hemorrhage
- If oliguria is present, may attempt to increase urine output with loop diuretics
- Aggressively treat any complications.
  - Hyperkalemia
  - Metabolic acidosis
  - Anemia
- Aggressive treatment of sepsis—source control
- Renal dose all medications
- Maintain fluid and electrolyte balance.

Special Considerations

- Can distinguish between prerenal disease and ATN by the response to intravenous fluid (IV) administration
- An improvement in renal function over 1 to 2 days back to baseline creatinine levels after IV fluids is diagnostic of prerenal disease; a continued elevation of creatinine points toward ATN.
- Mortality rate of ATN is about 50%.
- Mortality rate after sepsis or severe trauma is much higher (about 60%) than the mortality rate in ATN that is nephrotoxin-related (about 30%).
- Patients with oliguric ATN have a worse prognosis than patients with nonoliguric ATN.
- A rapid increase in serum creatinine > 3 mg/dL also indicates a poorer prognosis.
- About 50% of ATN survivors have some impairment of renal function.
- About 5% never recover kidney function and require dialysis.

When to Consult, Refer, or Hospitalize

- Same as AKI

Follow-up

Expected Outcomes
- Recovery of renal function
- Recovery from underlying cause

Complications

- Electrolyte abnormalities—see AKI section
- Intravascular volume overload
- Hypertension
- Uremic syndrome
- Anemia
- Polyuric phase of ATN leading to hypovolemia
- Infections

ACUTE GLOMERULONEPHRITIS

Description

- Acute glomerulonephritis (AGN) is glomerular injury and inflammation causing renal dysfunction over days to weeks.
- Rapidly progressive glomerulonephritis may lead to > 50% loss of nephron function over the course of days to weeks.
- Prolonged inflammatory changes can lead to persistent renal dysfunction that can progress to ESRD.
- Infectious AGN commonly appears after pharyngitis or impetigo—onset is 1 to 3 weeks after infection.
- ANCA (antineutrophil cytoplasmic antibodies)-associated—more than 95% of pauci-immune glomerulonephritis is associated with antineutrophil cytoplasmic antibodies
- Antiglomerular basement membrane (GBM) and Goodpasture syndrome: defined by the presence of glomerulonephritis and pulmonary hemorrhage; up to one-third of patients do not have lung injury
- Cyroglobulin-associated—because of cold-precipitable immunoglobulins (cryoglobulins)

Etiology

- Postinfectious GN
  - Nephritogenic group A β-hemolytic streptococci, especially type 12
  - Systemic S. *aureus*
  - Infective endocarditis
  - Shunt infections
  - Viral, fungal, parasitic causes of peri-infectious AGN
    - Hepatitis B, C
    - Cytomegalovirus (CMV)
    - Mononucleosis
    - Coccidioidomycosis
    - Malaria
    - Toxoplasmosis

- IgA nephropathy GN
  - Berger disease—IgA deposition in the glomerular mesangium—inciting cause unkown
  - ANCA-associated GN
  - Seen with Wegener granulomatosis, Churg-Strauss disease, and microscopic polyangiitis
- Antiglomerular basement membrane and Goodpasture syndrome
  - Injury mediated by anti-GBM antibodies
- Cryoglobulin-associated GN disease is the result of the precipitation of cryoglobulins in glomerular capillaries and the result of an underlying infection.

Incidence and Demographics

- Infectious AGN can occur sporadically or in clusters and during epidemics and can account for up to 10% of known streptococcal infections.
  - A rapidly progressive glomerulonephritis will develop in < 5% of cases, and a smaller percentage will go on to develop ESRD.
- IgA nephropathy is seen in patients with hepatic cirrhosis, celiac disease, immunodeficiency virus (HIV), and (CMV).
  - Most common form of AGN in the United States and worldwide
  - Males affected 2 to 3 times more often than females
  - One-third of patients will have a clinical remission.
  - 40% to 50% will have progressive CKD.
- ANCA-associated GN is seen in patients with small-vessel vasculitis.
  - Seen in patients with Wegener granulomatosis, Churg-Strauss disease, and microscopic polyangiitis
- Antiglomerular basement membrane and Goodpasture syndrome
  - The incidence in males is six times that in females.
  - Occurs in the second and third decades of life but has a wide range
- Cryoglobulin-associated GN
  - Seen in those with an underlying infection

Risk Factors

- Infectious AGN
  - Exposure to infection
- IgA GN
  - Liver disease, immunocompromised
- ANCA-associated GN
  - Asthma
  - Vasculitis
- Cryoglobulin-associated GN
  - Exposure to infection

Prevention and Screening

- Identification of at-risk populations
- Treat underlying cause.

Assessment

History
- Infectious AGN
  - Recent infection
  - Decreased urine output
- IgA GN
  - Flulike symptoms
  - Gastrointestinal (GI) symptoms
  - Upper respiratory infection
- ANCA-associated GN
  - Fever
  - Malaise
  - Weight loss
- Anti-GBM/Goodpasture syndrome
  - Upper respiratory tract infection
  - Dyspnea
- Cryoglobulin-associated GN
  - Arthralgias
  - Fever

Physical Examination
- Infectious AGN
  - Edema
  - Hypertension
  - Cola-colored urine
- IgA GN
  - Gross hematuria
  - Urine that is red or cola-colored 1 to 2 days after onset
  - Proteinuria
  - Hypertension
- ANCA-associated GN
  - Hematuria
  - Proteinuria
  - Purpura from dermal capillary involvement
  - Mononeuritis multiplex from nerve arteriolar involvement
  - 90% of patients with Wegener granulomatosis will have upper or lower respiratory tract symptoms with nodular lesions that can cavitate and bleed.

- Anti-GBM/Goodpasture syndrome
  - Upper respiratory infection in 20% to 60% of cases
  - Hemoptysis
  - Respiratory failure in some cases
  - Hypertension
  - Oliguria
- Edema
- Cryoglobulin-associated GN
  - Necrotizing skin lesions in dependent areas
  - Hepatosplenomegaly

Diagnostic Studies
- Infectious AGN
  - Serum complement levels are low because of group A streptococcal infection
  - ASO titers can be high unless immune response is blunted because of antibiotics
  - Urinary red blood cells
  - Red cell casts
  - Proteinuria < 3.5 g/d
  - Electron microscopy shows large, dense, subepithelial deposits or "humps"
  - Throat and skin cultures may be positive for streptococcal organisms
- IgA GN
  - Urine that is red or cola-colored
  - Asymptomatic microscopic hematuria
  - May have proteinuria > 1 g/d
- ANCA-associated GN
  - ANCA subtype analysis
  - C-ANCA is specific for antiproteinase-3 antibodies.
  - P-ANCA is specific for antimyeloperoxidase antibodies.
  - 80% of patients with Wegener syndrome have C-ANCA.
- Anti-GBM/Goodpasture syndrome
  - Iron deficiency anemia
  - Sputum contains hemosiderin-laden macrophages.
  - Chest x-ray can show shifting pulmonary infiltrates from pulmonary hemorrhage.
  - Circulating anti-GBM antibodies are positive in over 90% of patients.
  - Renal biopsy
  - 15% of patients will have positive ANCAs as well.
- Cryoglobulin-associated GN
  - Serum complement levels are low.
  - Rheumatoid factor is often elevated when cryoglobulins are present.
  - Rapidly progressive glomerulonephritis is seen on pathological examination, with the presence of crescents.

Differential Diagnosis

- Nephrotic syndrome
- Nephritic syndrome
- Systemic lupus erythematosus (SLE)
- Subacute bacterial endocarditis

Management

Nonpharmacologic Treatment
- Infectious AGN
  - Salt restriction
  - Supportive care
- IgA GN
  - Kidney transplant in those with ESRD
- ANCA-associated GN
  - Plasmapheresis
  - Monitor ANCA levels.
- Anti-GBM/Goodpasture syndrome
  - Plasma exchange therapy
- Cryoglobulin-associated GN
  - Plasma exchange

Pharmacologic Treatment
- Infectious AGN
  - Antihypertensives
  - Diuretics
  - Appropriate antibiotics
- IgA GN
  - In patients with significant proteinuria (> 1 g/d): ACE-I, ARBs
  - Target blood pressure is < 130/80
  - Corticosteroid therapy for proteinuria 1.0–3.5 g/d
  - Fish oil
- ANCA-associated
  - High doses of corticosteroids—methylprednisolone
  - Cytotoxic agents
    - Cyclophosphamide
    - Azathioprine
    - Mycophenolate moefetil
    - Patients receiving cyclophosphamide should receive prophylaxis for *Pneumocystis jiroveci.*
  - With combination of corticosteroids and cytotoxic agents: 75% remission
- Anti-GBM/Goodpasture syndrome
  - Combination of plasma exchange therapy and immunosuppressive drugs
- Cryoglobulin-associated GN
  - Treat underlying infection
  - Corticosteroids
  - Plasma exchange
  - Interferon-α when associated with hepatitis C

Special Considerations

- Acute glomerulonephritis may have several etiologies; therefore, at-risk patients require a detailed history and serology testing to determine etiology.

When to Consult, Refer, or Hospitalize

- Any patient with a diagnosis of glomerulonephritis should have a nephrology consult.
- Hospitalize for severe symptoms and intravenous therapy.

Follow-up

Expected Outcomes
- Remission
- Avoid ESRD

Complications
- Hypertension
- Anemia
- Acute renal failure
- Chronic kidney disease
- ESRD

NEPHROTIC SYNDROME

Description

- Nephrotic syndrome refers to a disorder in which there is increased glomerular permeability to macromolecules, leading to heavy proteinuria (> 3.5 g/d), hypoalbuminemia, and edema.

Etiology

- One-third of patients have a systemic renal disease such as diabetes mellitus, amlyoidosis, or SLE.
- Two-thirds have a primary renal lesion.
  - Minimal change disease
    - Associated with allergy, Hodgkin's disease, NSAID use
  - Focal glomerular sclerosis
    - Associated with heroin use, HIV infection, reflux nephropathy, obesity
  - Membranous nephropathy
    - Associated with non-Hodgkin's lymphoma, carcinoma (GI, renal, bronchgenic, thyroid), gold therapy, penicillamine, lupus erythematosus
  - Membranoproliferative glomerulonephritis
    - Idiopathic: associated with upper respiratory infection

Incidence and Demographics

- Diabetic nephropathy with nephrotic syndrome occurs in 50 cases/million population
- Male predominance
- Native Americans, Hispanics, and Blacks have higher occurrence rates.

Risk Factors

- Diabetes mellitus
- NSAID use
- Administration of gold and penicillamine
- Anticancer agents
- Cancer
- Obesity

Prevention and Screening

- Control of underlying disease
- Avoidance of nephrotoxic medications
- Identify at-risk populations.

Assessment

History
- Dyspnea
- Abdominal fullness
- Sign/symptoms of infection

Physical Examination
- Peripheral edema
- Pulmonary edema
- Pleural effusions
- Diaphragmatic compromise with ascites

Diagnostic Studies

- Urinalysis
  - Proteinuria
  - Spot urine protein to urine creatinine ration
  - Urinary sediment has few cellular elements or casts.
  - If hyperlipidemia is present, patient may have oval fat bodies in the urine.
- Blood chemistry
  - Decreased serum albumin (< 3 g/dL)
  - Total serum protein < 6 g/dL

- Hyperlipidemia occurs in over 50% of those with early nephritic syndrome.
- Elevated erythrocyte sedimentation rate (ESR)
- Renal biopsy
  - Performed in adults with new-onset idiopathic nephrotic syndrome if a primary renal disease that may require drug therapy is suspected

Differential Diagnosis

- Diabetic nephropathy
- Acute glomerulonephritis
- Focal segmental glomerulosclerosis
- Membranous glomerulonephritis

Management

Nonpharmacologic Treatment
- Protein restriction 0.6 to 0.8 g/kg/d in patients with a GFR < 25 mL/minute
  - Total dietary protein should equal losses.
- Avoid malnutrition.
- Salt restriction

Pharmacologic Treatment
- Edema
  - Thiazide and loop diuretics
- Hyperlipidemia
  - Statin therapy
  - Rhabdomyolysis is more common in patients with chronic kidney disease who take gemfibrozil in combination with statins.
- Hypercoagulable state
  - Patients with a serum albumin < 2 g/dL can become hypercoagulable.
  - Nephrotic patients have urinary losses of antithrombin, protein C, and protein S as well as increased platelet activation.
- Anticoagulation is recommended for at least 3 to 6 months in patients with evidence of thrombosis in any location.

Special Considerations

- Patients may show symptoms and signs of infection more frequently than the general population because of loss of immunoglobulins and certain complementary moieties in the urine.

When to Consult, Refer, or Hospitalize

- Any patient with nephrotic syndrome should have a nephrology consult for aggressive volume and blood pressure management, assessment for renal biopsy, and treatment of the underlying disease.
- Hospitalize for treatment of edema refractory to outpatient therapy or rapidly worsening kidney function.

Follow-Up

Expected Outcomes
- Remission

Complications
- Infection
- Atherosclerotic vascular disease
- Hypocalcemia
- Osteomalacia
- Venous thrombosis
- Pulmonary embolism
- Hypertension

POLYCYSTIC KIDNEY DISEASE

Description

- Polycystic kideny disease is the progressive expansion of many fluid-filled cysts resulting in massive enlargement of the kidneys and frequently causes renal failure.
- Autosomal dominant polycystic kidney disease (ADPKD) is seen predominantly in adults.
- Autosomal recessive polycystic kidney disease (ARPKD) is primarily seen in childhood.
- Two genes account for the disorder: ADPKD1 and ADPKD2.
  - ADPKD1: short arm of chromosome 16 (85% to 95% of patients)
  - ADPKD2: on chromosome 4 (10% to 15% of patients)
- Patients with PKD2 have a slower progression of the disease and a longer life span.

Etiology

- ADPKD is a disorder that results from mutations of either the PKD1 or PKD2 gene.
- Both are transmembrane proteins present in all segments of the nephrin.
- Proteins function to regulate fetal and adult epithelial cell gene transcription, apoptosis, and differentiation and cell-matrix interactions.

- Disruption of these processes leads to cyst formation in utero; as the cysts accumulate fluid, they enlarge, separate from the nephron, compress the parenchyma, and progressively compromise renal function.

Incidence and Demographics

- One of the most common hereditary diseases in the United States
- Affects 1 in 800 live births
- 50% of patients will have ESRD by 60 years of age.
- Accounts for approximately 10% of dialysis patients in the United States
- 90% of cases are inherited; 10% may be the result of spontaneous mutations.

Risk Factors

- Genetic predisposition
- Autosomal dominant trait—patient has one copy of the mutant gene and one normal gene on the autosomal chromosome
- Affected persons have a 50–50 chance of passing it on to each of their children.

Prevention and Screening

- Genetic counseling and screening renal ultrasound with family history

Assessment

History
- Often asymptomatic until the fourth or fifth decade of life
- Abdominal discomfort
- Hematuria
- The diagnosis is often made prior to the onset of symptoms from requested screening by affected families.
- Nephrolithiasis
- Family history positive in 75% of cases

Physical Examination
- Hematuria
- Urinary tract infection
- Hypertension
- Abdominal mass
- Large palpable kidneys on examination

Diagnostic Studies

- Serum chemistry
- May have elevated creatinine
- Complete blood count
  - Normal hemoglobin and hematocrit
  - Cysts produce erythropoietin
- Urinalysis
  - Hematuria
  - Mild proteinuria
- Renal ultrasound
  - Confirms diagnosis in patients with PKD1
  - Two or more cysts in patients under age 30 years (sensitivity 88.5%)
  - Two or more cysts in patients aged 30 to 59 years (sensitivity 100%)
  - Four or more cysts in each kidney in patients aged 60 or more
- Abdominal CT if ultrasound is inconclusive—highly sensitive
- Blood cultures
  - May be positive with negative urine as infected cysts do not communicate with the urinary tract

Differential Diagnosis

- Medullary cystic disease
- Renal dysplasia
- Simple renal cysts
- Acquired renal cystic disease
- Tuberous sclerosis

Management

Nonpharmacologic Treatment

- Bedrest for abdominal/flank pain
- Cyst decompression for pain control
- Hydration 2 to 3 L/day to prevent nephrolithiasis

Pharmacologic Treatment

- Pain control
  - Analgesics
- Kidney infection
  - Antibiotics with cystic penetration
  - Fluoroquinolones
  - Trimethoprim-sulfamethoxazole
  - Chloramphenicol
  - Treatment may require 2 weeks of parenteral therapy followed by long-term oral therapy.

- Hypertension
  - Target blood pressure: 130/85 or less
  - Multidrug approach to inhibit the renin-angiotensin system

Special Considerations

- Patients with ADPKD seem to survive longer on peritoneal or hemodialysis compared to patients with other causes of ESRD.
- Kidney transplantation may require bilateral nephrectomy if the kidneys are massively enlarged or have been the site of infected cysts.

When to Consult, Refer, or Hospitalize

- Patient should receive a nephrology consult when diagnosis is made.
- Genetic counseling
- Hospitalize for infection not responsive to outpatient therapy, transplant surgery

Follow-up

Expected Outcomes
- Progressive disease; goal is to slow progression to ESRD

Complications
- Infection
- Hypertension
- Cerebral aneurysms
  - 10% to 15% of patients have arterial aneurysm in the Circle of Willis.
  - Vascular complications
  - Seen in up to 25% of patients
    - Mitral valve prolapse
    - Aortic aneurysms
    - Aortic valve abnormalities
- Colonic diverticula

REFERENCES

Barkley, T., & Myers, C. (2008). *Practice guidelines for acute care nurse practitioners.* St. Louis, MO: Saunders.

Beers, M., Porter, R., Jones, T., Kaplan, J., & Berkwits, M. (Eds.). (2006). *The Merck manual of diagnosis and therapy.* Whitehouse Station, NJ: Merck Research Laboratories.

Centers for Disease Control and Prevention. (2006). Sexually transmitted diseases treatment guidelines. *MMWR: Morbidity and Mortality Weekly Report, 55*(RR-11), 1–93.

Donders, G. (2006). Management of genital infections in pregnant women. *Current Opinion in Infectious Disease, 19*(1), 55–61.

Habermann, T., & Ghosh, A. (Eds.). (2008). *Mayo Clinic internal medicine concise textbook.* Rochester, MN: Mayo Clinic Scientific Press.

Fauci, A., Braunwald, E., Kasper, D., Hauser, S., Longo, D., Jameson, J., & Loscalzo, J. (Eds.). *Harrison's principles of internal medicine.* New York: McGraw Hill.

Marini, J., & Wheeler, A. (2010). *Critical care medicine: The essentials.* Philadelphia: Wolters Kluwer/Lippincott Williams & Wilkins.

McKean, S., Bennett, A., & Halasyamani, L. (Eds.). (2008). *Hospital medicine: Just the facts.* Philadelphia: Wolters Kluwer/Lippincott Williams & Wilkins.

McPhee, S., & Papadakis, M. (Eds.). (2011). *Current medical diagnosis and treatment, 2011.* New York: McGraw Hill.

National Guidelines Clearinghouse. (2007). *Gonococcal and chlamydial infections.* Retrieved from http://www.guideline.gov/content.aspx?id=12570&search=gonococcal+and+chlamydial+infections

Rennke, H., & Denker, B. (2007). *Renal pathophysiology: The essentials.* Philadelphia: Lippincott Williams & Wilkins.

9

Gastrointestinal Disorders

Pamela Smith, MSN, RN, ACNP-BC, CCRN

GENERAL APPROACH

- Patients who are elderly may not feel pain with abdominal conditions or present with classic symptoms of gastrointestinal disorders; they are more likely to have vague diffuse pain with a less acute presentation.
- Antidiarrheals should never be given to patients with bloody diarrhea, fever, fecal leukocytes, or abdominal pain because of a systemic infection from retained toxins—refer to a gastroenterologist.
- Examine the tender area last to avoid referred pain.
- When caring for patients with acute abdominal disorders
  - Assume the most life-threatening condition is causing the problem.
  - Avoid excessive analgesics and sedation.
  - Involve surgical and specialty consultants early in the course of the condition.
  - Carefully select diagnostic studies.
- The patient's age, gender, and comorbid conditions can give valuable clues to a diagnosis in the absence of a detailed history.

RED FLAGS

- Patients with fever, chills, leukocytosis, and rebound tenderness need rapid assessment and surgical referral.
- Abdominal pain lasting > 6 hours or that wakes the patient up in the middle of the night requires evaluation.
- Signs and symptoms of peritonitis may indicate peforation in the acute abdomen.
- Patients in the intensive care unit rarely have typical presentations of acute abdominal conditions—low-grade fever, mild agitation, or inability to tolerate tube feedings may be the only signs.
- Thoracic diseases causing diaphragmatic distention can imitate acute abdominal conditions.

APPENDICITIS

Description

- Appendicitis is inflammation of the appendix from an obstruction of the appendiceal lumen that leads to increased intraluminal pressure, venous congestion, infection, and thrombosis of intramural vessels.
- If left untreated, gangrene and perforation can develop within 36 hours.
- It was once thought the appendix served no purpose for the body, but it is now thought to aid the immune system of the intestinal tract.

Etiology

- Obstruction by a fecalith, inflammatory process, foreign body, neoplasm
- Usually a polymicrobial process
  - Enterobacteriaceae
  - Anarobes
  - Enterococcus

Incidence and Demographics

- Most common abdominal surgical emergency—affects about 10% of the population
- Occurs most commonly between the ages of 10 and 30
- The incidence is about 1.4 times greater in men than women.
- The incidence of primary appendectomy is equal in both sexes.

Risk Factors

- Low dietary fiber intake
- Refined carbohydrate diet
- Bacterial gastroenteritis
- Mumps
- Coxsackie virus B
- Adenovirus
- Amebiasis
- Family history—position of the appendix can make a person more vulnerable to infection

Prevention and Screening

- Increase dietary intake of fiber and decrease refined carbohydrates.
- Include green, leafy vegetables in diet.
- Maintain adequate hydration.
- Monitor for the presence of appendicitis post gastrointestinal infection.

Assessment

History
- Vague, colicky periumbilical, or epigastric pain
- Within 12 hours, pain shifts to right lower quadrant (RLQ)—a steady ache that is worsened by walking or coughing
- Almost all patients will have nausea; about 50% will have vomiting.
- Some patients sense a feeling of constipation while others report diarrhea.
- Low-grade fever
- Dysuria
- Right flank pain

Physical Examination
- RLQ pain is present in 96% of patients.
- Rebound tenderness, pain on percussion, rigidity, guarding
- Rovsing sign
  - RLQ pain with palpation of the left lower quadrant (LLQ)
  - Peritoneal irritation in the RLQ
- Obturator sign
  - RLQ pain with internal and external rotation of the flexed right hip
  - Suggests that the inflamed appendix is deep in the right hemipelvis
- Psoas sign
  - RLQ pain with extension of the right hip or with flexion of the right hip against resistance
  - Suggests that the inflamed appendix is located along the right psoas muscle
- Dunphy's sign
  - Sharp pain in the RLQ elicited by a voluntary cough
  - May be helpful in making the clinical diagnosis of localized peritonitis

- If the appendix is retrocecal, even deep pressure in the RLQ may not elicit tenderness.
- If the appendix lies entirely within the pelvis, there may be complete absence of abdominal rigidity.
- For the preceding two situations, a digital rectal examination will elicit tenderness in the rectovesical pouch.

Diagnostic Studies

- Complete blood count
  - Leukocytosis 10,000 to 20,000/mcL with neutrophilia
- C-reactive protein (CRP)
  - An acute phase reactant synthesized by the liver in response to infection or inflammation
  - Several studies have shown that, in adults who have had symptoms longer than 24 hours, a normal CRP has a negative predictive value of 97% to 100%.
- Urinalysis
  - Microscopic hematuria and pyuria are seen in 25% of patients.
- Abdominal ultrasound
  - The normal appendix is not seen.
  - An outer diameter > 6 mm, noncompressibility, and lack of peristalsis or periappendiceal fluid collection identifies an inflamed appendix.
  - Sensitivity of 85% to 90%, specificity of 92% to 95%
- Abdominal CT
  - Has become the most important imaging study to identify patients with atypical presentations
  - The addition of contrast enhances image quality.
  - Sensitivity 94%, specificity 95%
- Abdominal MRI may be considered for the patient who is pregnant.

Differential Diagnosis

- Abdominal abscess
- Cholecystitis and biliary colic
- Constipation
- Crohn's disease
- Diverticular disease
- Ectopic pregnancy
- Endometriosis
- Gastroenteritis
- Inflammatory bowel disease
- Mesenteric ischemia
- Omental torsion
- Ovarian cysts
- Ovarian torsion
- Pelvic inflammatory disease
- Renal calculi
- Urinary tract infection

Management

Nonpharmacologic Treatment
- Nothing by mouth until after surgery
- Treatment of perforated appendicitis with generalized peritonitis is emergency surgery.
- Appendectomy is the only curative treatment
  - Laparotomy
  - Laparoscopy
- Treatment of patients with perforated appendicitis and a contained abscess is controversial.
  - Surgery is an option but may be difficult to perform.
  - Percutaneous CT-guided drainage of the abscess, with IV fluids and antibiotics, to allow the inflammation to subside is an option.
    - An interval appendectomy may be performed after 6 weeks to prevent recurrent appendicitis.

Pharmacologic Treatment
- Prior to surgery, broad-spectrum antibiotics with gram-negative and anaerobic coverage
  - Cefoxitin or cefotetan 1–2 g every 8 hours IV
  - Ampicillin-sulbactam 3 g every 6 hours IV
  - Ertapenem 1 g as a single-dose IV

Special Considerations

- With pelvic appendicitis, pain is the lower abdomen, often on the left side, with an urge to urinate or defecate.
  - Abdominal tenderness is absent; tenderness is present on rectal or vaginal examination.
  - Obuturator sign may be present
- In older adults, the diagnosis is often delayed because patients present with minimal, vague symptoms, and mild abdominal tenderness.
- Appendicitis in pregnancy may present with mild pain in the RLQ, periumbilical area, or right subcostal area because of displacement of the appendix by the uretus.
- Perforation rates are higher among patients younger than 18 and older than 50, perhaps because of a delay in diagnosis.
- Appendical perforation is associated with an increase in morbidity and mortality.

When to Refer, Consult, or Hospitalize

- Upon diagnosis, a general surgeon should be consulted and the patient hospitalized for IV antibiotic therapy and preparation for surgery.

Follow-up

Expected Outcomes
- Mortality rate from uncomplicated appendicitis is very low.
- Perforated appendicitis has a mortality for most groups of 0.2%; in older adults, it approaches 15%.

Complications
- Perforation in 20% of patients
- Septic thrombophlebitis
- Wound infection
- Bowel obstruction
- Abdominal/pelvic abscess
- Stump appendicitis (rare)

ACUTE CHOLECYSTITIS

Description

- Acute cholecystitis is an inflammation of the gallbladder.

Etiology

- Occurs most commonly as the result of an obstruction of the cystic duct from cholelithiasis
- 99% of cases involve stones in the cystic duct; the other 10% are cases of acalculous cholecystitis.
- Bile cultures are positive for bacteria in 50% to 75% of cases, but may be a result of the cholecystitis and not the cause.
- Usually inflammatory and non-infectious but, if infection present, frequently polymicrobial
  - *E. coli*
  - *Klebisella* species
  - *Enterbacter* species
  - *Enterococcus*
- Acalculous cholecystitis is associated with biliary stasis, major surgery, severe trauma, sepsis, long-term parenteral nutrition (TPN), prolonged fasting, cardiac events, sickle cell disease, *Salmonella* infections, diabetes mellitus, cytomegalovirus, cryptosporidiosis, or microsporidiosis infections in patients with AIDS.

Incidence and Demographics

- An estimated 10% to 20% of people in the United States have gallstones and about one-third will develop cholecystitis.
- Incidence increases with age.
- In the United States, Whites have a higher incidence than Blacks.

- Gallstones are 2 to 3 times more frequent in females than males, which results in a higher incidence of calculous cholecystitis in females.
- Elevated progesterone levels during pregnancy predispose women who are pregnant to gallbladder disease.
- Acalculous cholecystitis is seen more often in older men.

Risk Factors

- Cholelithiasis
- Increasing age
- Ethnicity
  - Pima Indian, Scandinavian
- Obesity or rapid weight loss
- Medications
  - Hormone replacement therapy
  - Birth control pills
- Pregnancy

Prevention and Screening

- High-fiber diet associated with a lower risk for gallstones
- Avoid a diet high in saturated fats.
- Fish oil may be beneficial because it improves emptying of the gallbladder.
- Maintain normal weight and avoid rapid weight loss.
- Regular exercise can decrease risk of forming gallstones.

Assessment

History
- Appearance of a steady pain localized to the epigastrum or right hypochondrium after a large or fatty meal
  - May gradually subside over a period of 12 to 18 hours
  - Often radiates to the tip of the right scapula
- Vomiting in about 75% of patients
  - In about one-half of patients, vomiting provides some relief of the pain.
- Fever
  - If persistent or very high, suggests choledocholithiasis
- In older adults, pain and fever may be absent, and localized tenderness may be the only presenting sign.
- Acalculous cholecystitis occurs suddenly in ill patients without biliary colic.

Physical Examination

- Right upper quadrant (RUQ) tenderness is nearly always present and associated with guarding and rebound tenderness.
  - Murphy's sign—tenderness and an inpiratory pause elicited during palpation of the RUQ
- Palpable gallbladder is present in about 15% of cases.
- Jaundice occurs in about 25% of patients.
- May present with diffuse epigastric pain without localization to the RUQ
- Patients with chronic cholecystitis often do not have a palpable RUQ mass because of fibrosis of the gallbladder.

Diagnostic Studies

- Complete blood count
  - WBC elevated 12,000 to 15, 000/mcL
  - Liver function studies
  - Total serum bilirubin may be 1 to 4 mg/dL (even without bile duct obstruction).
  - Alanine aminotransferse (ALT) and aspartate aminotransferase (AST) levels are used to evaluate the presence of hepatitis and may be elevated in cholecystitis with/without common bile duct obstruction.
- Amylase/lipase
  - To determine the presence of pancreatitis
  - May be elevated if a biliary duct obstruction is present near the pancreatic duct
- Urinalysis
  - To rule out renal calculi
- Pregnancy testing in women of childbearing age
- Plain film of the abdomen
  - May show radiopaque gallstones in about 15% of cases
  - Subdiaphragmatic free air cannot originate in the biliary tract—if present, another etiology should be investigated.
  - Gas limited to the gallbladder wall or lumen indicates emphysematous cholecystitis because of gas-forming bacteria (*E. coli*, clostridial, and anaerobic streptococci species).
    - Associated with increased mortality and occurs most frequently in men with diabetes and acalculous cholecystitis
- Hepatoiminodiacetic acid (HIDA) scan
  - Up to 95% accurate in the diagnosis of cholecysitis
  - Tracks the production and flow of bile from the liver to the small intestine with a radioactive tracer administered intravenously
  - In the absence of disease, the gallbladder is usually visualized in 1 hour.
  - If the gallbladder is not visualized in 4 hours, this indicates cholecysitis or cystic duct obstruction.
- Ultrasound
  - 95% sensitivity and specificity for diagnosis of gallstones > 2 mm in diameter
  - 90% to 95% sensitive for cholecystitis and 78% to 80% specific
  - Best results if patient fasts for at least 8 hours—gallstones are seen best in a distended, bile-filled gallbladder
  - Findings suggestive of cholecystitis
    - Pericholecystic fluid
    - Gallbladder wall thickening > 4 mm and a sonographic Murphy sign
    - Presence of gallstones

- Abdominal CT
- Abdominal MRI
  - The sensitivity and specificity of CT scan and MRI for predicting acute cholecystitis are > than 95%
  - Findings suggestive of cholecystitis
    - Wall thickening > 4 mm
    - Pericholecystic fluid
    - Subserosal edema in the absence of ascites
    - Intramural gas
    - Sloughed mucosa

Differential Diagnosis

- Angina
- Appendicitis
- Bowel obstruction
- Irritable bowel disease
- Pancreatitis
- Hepatitis
- Peptic ulcer disease
- Gastroesophageal reflux disease (GERD)
- Cholangiocarcinoma
- Right renal disease
- Acute mesenteric ischemia
- Abdominal aortic aneurysm
- Bacterial pneumonia
- Gastric ulcers

Management

Nonpharmacologic Treatment
- Bowel rest
- Nasogastric suction
- Procedures
  - Endoscopic retrograde cholangiopancreatography (ERCP)
    - Combines the use of endoscopy and fluoroscopy to diagnose and treat problems in the biliary or pancreatic ducts
      - Placement of stents or dilation of strictures
      - Removal of stones
      - Sphincterotomy
    - Useful in patients at high risk for common duct gallstones if signs of common bile duct obstruction are present

- Surgery
  - Laparoscopic cholecystectomy
    - Immediate cholecystectomy or cholecystostomy is recommended for complicated cases with gangrene or perforation.
    - Early surgical intervention within 72 hours of admission has both medical and socioenconomic benefits.
    - High surgical risk—placement of sonographically guided, percutaneous, transhepatic cholecystostomy drainage tube and antibiotics may be effective
  - Rate of conversion from laparoscopy to open cholecystectomy is about 5%
  - Patients with acalulous cholecystitis may be treated with percutaneous drainage alone.
  - Contraindications for laparoscopic cholecystectomy
    - High risk for general anesthesia
    - Morbid obesity
    - Gallbladder perforation
    - Giant gallstones or malignancy
    - End-stage liver disease with portal hypertension and severe coagulopathy

Pharmacologic Treatment

- IV hydration
- Uncomplicated cholecystitis is treated with surgery and antibiotics for 24 to 48 hours.
- If surgery is delayed, use antibiotics for 3 to 5 days.
- Mild to moderate infection
  - Ticarcillin-clavulanate 3.1 grams IV every 6 hours
  - Ertapenen 1 gram IV once daily
  - Ciprofoxacin 400 mg IV every 12 hours
  - Levofloxacin 500 mg IV daily
  - Moxifloxacin 400 mg IV daily
  - Ceftriaxone 1 to 2 grams IV daily
  - Cefoxitin 1 to 2 grams IV every 6 hours
  - Tigecycline 100 mg IV × 1 dose, then 50 mg IV every 12 hours
- Severe, nosocomial, or prior antibiotics
  - Pipercillin-tazobactoam 3.375 grams IV every 6 hours or 4/5 grams IV every 8 hours
  - Meropenem 1 gram IV every 8 hours
  - Imipenem 0.5 gram IV every 6 hours
  - Doripenem 500 mg IV every 8 hours

Special Considerations

- In patients who are obese, diabetic, older, or immunocompromised, severe inflammation of the gallbladder with gangrene and necrosis may occur without obvious signs and symptoms.
- High risk for malignancy of the gallbladder
  - Pima Indians
  - Calcified gallbladder
  - Gallbladder polyps > 10 mm
  - Gallstones > 2.5 cm
  - Anomalous pancreaticobiliary duct junction

When to Consult, Refer, or Hospitalize

- All patients with acute cholecystitis require hospitalization.
- Refer patient to a general surgeon for surgery, procedural therapy
- Gastroenterology for assistance with management pre- and postsurgery

Follow-up

Expected Outcomes
- Correction of fluid and electrolyte abnormalities
- Afebrile with stable vital signs
- No evidence of obstruction
- Overall mortality rate of cholecystectomy is < 0.2%
  - Mortality rates higher in older adults
    - Usual resolution of symptoms with surgery and antibiotics

Complications
- Empyema of the gallbladder from bacterial proliferation
- Erosion of large gallstone through the gallbladder into adjacent viscus (rare)
- Emphysematous cholecystitis
  - Occurs in about 1% of cases—note by presence of gas in the gallbladder wall from invasion of gas-producing organisms (*E. coli, Clostridia perfringens, Klebsiella* species)
- Sepsis
- Pancreatitis
- Perforation occurs in up to 15% of patients

CIRRHOSIS/CHRONIC LIVER DISEASE

Description

- Cirrhosis or chronic liver disease is fibrosis of the liver that progresses to produce diffuse organization of the normal hepatic structure, characterized by nodular regeneration throughout the liver surrounded by dense fibrotic tissue.
- Hepatic scarring leads to increased stiffness and portal hypertension.
- Portal hypertension causes changes in the mesenteric vasculature and in the rennin-angiotension-aldosterone system.

Etiology

- Can be the result of any long-term, persistent injury to the liver
- Common etiologies in the United States (listed in order of occurrence—highest to lowest)
  - Hepatitis C
  - Alcohol
  - Non-classified
  - Primary biliary cirrhosis/primary sclerosing cholangitis
  - Crytogenic (unknown)
  - Hepatitis C and alcohol
  - Miscellaneous
    - Chronic right-sided heart failure
  - Autoimmune hepatitis
  - Hepatitis B
  - Non-alcoholic fatty disease of the liver
  - Congenital
    - Hemochromatosis
    - Wilson's disease
    - Cystic fibrosis
  - Metabolic
  - Hepatocellular carcinoma
  - Vascular

Incidence and Demographics

- 12th leading cause of death in the United States
- Mexican Americans and Blacks have a higher frequency rate.
- Accounts for approximately 400,000 hospital admissions and 30,000 deaths per year in the United States

Risk Factors

- Chronic hepatitis infections
- Heavy and chronic alcohol use
- Obesity
- Iron overload
- Non-alcoholic liver disease (NAFD)
- Severe excesses of vitamin A

Prevention and Screening

- Avoid excessive drinking.
  - Treatment for alcoholism
- Avoid infection with hepatitis B and C.
  - Use safe sexual practices.
  - Personal protective equipment for healthcare workers
- Phlebotomy at routine intervals for hemochromatosis
- Chelating agents to rid the body of copper in Wilson's disease
- Immunization against hepatitis A and B
- Wear protective covering when working with toxic chemicals
- Maintain healthy weight and diet—plant-based, low-fat.
- Currently there are no screening guidelines for cirrhosis

Assessment

History
- No symptoms for long periods of time
- Onset may be insidious or, less often, abrupt.
- Weakness
- Fatigue
- Disturbed sleep
- Muscle cramps
- Weight loss
- Malnutrition
- Fever
- Peripheral neuropathy
- Vague right upper quadrant pain
- Advance cirrhosis
  - Anorexia
  - Nausea
  - Vomiting
- Amenorrhea
- Men
  - Impotence
  - Loss of libido
  - Sterility
  - Gynecomastia

Physical Examination
- Hepatic enlargement in 70% of cases—firm, palpable, sharp, or nodular edges; left lobe may predominate
- Palmar erythema (mottled redness on the palm of the hand)
- Dupuytren contractures
- Glossitis
- Inflammation, cracking at the corners of the mouth
- Jaundice—not an initial sign
  - Mild initially, increasing in severity during the later stages of the disease
  - Scleral icterus
- Splenomegaly is present in 30% to 50% of cases.
- Superficial veins of the abdomen and thorax are dilated.
- Abdominal wall veins fill from below when compressed.
- Esophageal varices
- Parotid gland enlargement
- Late findings:
  - Ascites
    - Shifting dullness
    - Fluid wave on examination
  - Pleural effusions
  - Peripheral edema
  - Ecchymoses
- Encephalopathy
  - Day–night reversal
  - Asterixis
  - Tremor
  - Dysarthria
  - Delirium
  - Drowsiness
  - Coma

Diagnostic Studies
- Laboratory abnormalities may not be evident in early or compensated cirrhosis.
- Liver function studies
  - Modest elevation of AST, alkaline phosphate
  - Progressive elevation of bilirubin
  - Serum albumin is low.
  - Serum ammonia level
- Complete chemistry panel
  - Elevated blood glucose
- CBC
  - Anemia
  - Macrocytic
  - Leukopenia (hypersplenism) or leukocytosis (infection)
  - Thrombocytopenia

- Coagulation studies
  - Prolonged prothrombin time
- CT/MRI of the abdomen (contast-enhanced)
  - Reveals hepatic nodules
  - Nodules may be biopsied with CT guidance
- Abdominal ultrasound with Doppler
  - Assesses liver size
  - Presence of ascites
  - Identifies hepatic nodules
  - Patency of splenic, portal, hepatic veins
  - Nodules may be biopsied with ultrasound guidance.
- Liver scan
  - Nuclear imaging
  - May show irregular liver uptake and increased spleen and bone marrow uptake
- Esophagogastroduodenosocopy
  - Confirms the presence of varices
  - Detects the specific causes of bleeding in the esophagus, stomach, and proximal duodenum
- Liver biopsy
  - May show inactive cirrhosis (fibrosis with regenerative nodules)
  - May be performed by laparascopy
  - In patients with coagulapathy, transjugular approach
  - Wedged hepatic vein measurement can diagnose the presence and cause of portal hypertension
- Diagnostic studies for specific etiologies
  - Chronic hepatitis B
    - Hepatitis B surface antigen positive
    - Hepatitis B DNA testing
  - Hepatitis C
    - Presence of hepatitis C antibody and hepatitis C RNA
  - Alcohol-related liver disease
    - 80 g of alcohol for 10 to 20 years
  - NAFD
    - History consistent with insulin resistance
  - Autoimmune hepatitis
    - Presence of autoantibodies (antinuclear and anti-smooth-muscle antibody)
    - Gamma globulin spike on serum protein electrophoresis
  - Primary sclerosing cholangitis
    - Biliary tract strictures on ERCP
  - Primary biliary cirrhosis
    - Positive antimitochondrial antibodies
- Scoring systems to evaluate progression of cirrhosis/chronic liver disease

Table 9–1. Child-Turcotte-Pugh Scoring System

Clinical/Laboratory Measurements Points for Increasing Abnormality

	1	2	3
Encephalopathy	None	Slight to Moderate	Moderate to Severe
Ascites	None	Slight	Moderate to Severe
Bilirubin	< 2.0	2–3	> 3.0
Albumin	> 3.5	2.8–3.5	< 2.8
Protime (seconds increased)	1–3	4–6	> 6.0

Numerical score and corresponding Child class

Score:	5–6	Class: A
	7– 9	Class: B
	10–15	Class: C

Model for End-Stage Liver Disease (MELD)

Also assesses the severity of chronic liver disease and is used for determining prognosis and prioritizing patients for liver transplant:

$$3.78 \log_e (\text{bilirubin [mg/dL]}) + 11.2 \log_e (\text{INR}) + 9.57 \log e + 6.43$$

Range: 6–40

Adapted from *Current medical diagnosis and treatment* by S. McPhee & M. Papadakis (Eds.), 2011, New York: McGraw-Hill, p. 667.

Differential Diagnosis
- Congestive heart failure
- Secondary biliary cirrhosis
- Hemorrhagic telangiectasia
- NAFD
- Constrictive pericarditis
- Hemochromatosis
- Wilson's disease
- α_1 –antitrypsin deficiency

Management

Nonpharmacologic Treatment
- Treat the underlying disease.
- If alcoholic etiology: abstinence from alcohol
- Dietary modifications
  - 25 to 35 kcal/kg body weight per day in patients with compensated cirrhosis
  - 35 to 40 kcal/kg/d in those with malnutrition
  - Protein 1 to 1.2 g/kg/d in patients with compensated cirrhosis
  - Protein 1.5 g/kg/d in patients with malnutrition
  - Sodium restriction if fluid retention present
  - If hepatic encephalopathy present: limit protein to < 60 to 80 g/d
- Vitamin supplementation
- Paracentesis for ascites
- Transjugular intrahepatic portosystemic shunt (TIPS)
  - For treatment of varices refractory to standard therapy
- Liver transplantation
  - For selected cases of irreversible, progressive chronic liver disease
  - Consider for transplant candidacy:
    · Child-Turcotte-Pugh score of 7
    · MELD score of 10
  - Absolute contraindications
    · Malignancy (except relatively small hepatocellular carcinomas in a cirrhotic liver)
    · Advanced cardiopulmonary disease (except hepatopulmonary syndrome)
    · Sepsis
      - Relative contraindications
    · Age over > 70 years
    · Morbid obesity
    · Portal and mesenteric vein thrombosis
    · Active alcohol or drug abuse
    · Severe malnutrition
    · Lack of patient understanding
    · Patients with alcoholism need to abstain for at least 6 months.

Pharmacologic Treatment
- Dose medications according to patient's hepatic clearance.
- Acetominophen should not be used on a daily basis and no more than 2 g/day.
- Patients should be vaccinated for hepatitis A and B.

Special Considerations

- Patients with compensated cirrhosis may decompensate after surgical procedures.
- May be reversible if cause identified early and treated
- Patients with compensated cirrhosis may be identified on the basis of laboratory abnormalities or abnormal imaging, or incidentally at the time of surgery, before becoming symptomatic.

When to Consult, Refer, or Hospitalize

- Refer to gastroenterologist for
  - Liver biopsy
  - Child-Turcotte-Pugh score > 7
  - For upper endoscopy to screen for gastroesophageal varices
- Admit for
  - Gastrointestinal bleeding
  - Stage 3 to 4 hepatic encephalopathy
  - Worsening renal function
  - Severe hyponatremia
  - Profound hypoxia

Follow-up

Expected Outcomes
- With treatment or behavior modification, cure or delayed progression of cirrhosis

Complications
- Ascites
- Edema
- Spontaneous bacterial peritonitis
- Hepatorenal syndrome
- Hepatic encephalopathy
  - Stage 1: mild confusion
  - Stage 2: drowsiness
  - Stage 3: stupor
  - Stage 4: coma
- Anemia
- Coagulopathy
- Bleeding from esophageal varices
- Hepatopulmonary syndrome
- Portopulmonary hypertension

CROHN'S DISEASE

Description

- Crohn's disease is chronic inflammatory disease from an exaggerated immune response that usually affects all layers of the distal ileum and colon, but may occur in any part of the GI tract.
- May result in mucosal inflammation and ulceration, structuring, fistula development, and abscesses
- One-third of cases involve the small bowel only (distal ileum/ileitis).

- Half of cases involve the small bowel and colon, most commonly the distal ileum and adjacent proximal ascending colon (ileocolitis).
- In about 20% of cases, only the colon is affected.
- One-third of patients have associated perianal disease—fistulas, fissures, abscesses.
- Relapsing and remitting

Etiology

- Unknown
- Hyperimmune response in the intestinal tract

Incidence and Demographics

- Relatively rare
- Affects approximately 6 to 7.1 people in 100,000
- There has been a steady increase in the United States between 1950 and 1985.
- Can present at any age—peak ages for diagnosis are from ages 15 to 30 and 50 to 80
- Risk for Crohn's disease is equal for both sexes

Risk Factors

- Increased incidence in first-degree relatives
  - Crohn's disease susceptibility gene NOD2/CARD 15 was recently identified.
- Higher incidence among the Jewish population of northern European descent
- Lower incidence in the Black and Hispanic populations compared to Whites
- Use of NSAIDS
- Environmental triggers in genetically susceptible patients
  - Smoking
  - Oral contraceptives
  - Nutritional deficiencies
  - Infection

Prevention and Screening

- Screen for genetic susceptibility in high-risk patients
- Smoking cessation
- Cautious use of oral contraceptives
- Maintain healthy diet—small frequent meals; restrict dairy if flatulence or diarrhea is present.
- Patients with obstructive symptoms: low-roughage diet

Assessment

History
- Fever
- Weight loss
- Crampy or steady abdominal pain
- Number of liquid bowel movements
- Fecal urgency
- Prior surgery
- Anorexia
- Fatigue
- Family history

Physical Examination
- Chronic inflammatory disease
  - Most common
  - Ileitis or ileocolitis
    - Diarrhea—nonbloody, intermittent
  - Colitis
    - Bloody diarrhea
  - Focal tenderness, usually in the right lower quadrant
  - Palpable, tender mass that represents thickened or matted loops of inflamed intestine in the lower abdomen may be present
- Intestinal obstruction
  - Loud stomach rumbling
  - Postprandial bloating
- Penetrating disease and fistulae
  - Penetration through the bowel
    - Intra-abdominal abscess
    - Retroperitoneal inflammation with exudates, purulent material
  - Fistula between the small intestine and colon
    - Often asymptomatic
    - Diarrhea
  - Fistula to the bladder
    - Recurrent infections
  - Fistula to the vagina
    - Malodorous drainage
  - Fistula to the skin
    - Usually occurs at site of surgical scars
- Perianal disease
  - Large, painful skin tags
  - Anal fissures
  - Perianal abscesses
  - Fistulas

- Extraintestinal manifestations
  - Arthralgias
  - Arthritis
  - Iritis
  - Uveitis
  - Pyoderma gangrenosum
  - Erythema nodosum
  - Oral canker sores
  - Gallstones because of malabsorption of bile salts from the terminal ileum
  - Nephrolithiasis with urate or calcium oxalate stones
  - Venous and arterial thrombembolic disease
  - Sclerosing cholangitis

Diagnostic Studies
- Complete blood count
- Serum albumin level
- Anti-*Saccharomyces cerevisiae* antibodies (ASCA)—present in about 60% of patients
- Perinuclear antineutrophil cytoplasmic antibodies (p-ANCA)—present in about 10% of patients
- Acute abdomen
  - Plain film flat and upright abdominal x-rays
  - Abdominal CT scan
- Less-acute presentation
  - Upper GI series
  - Barium enema
    - Useful to document length and location of strictures; may reach places not accessible by endoscopy
- Endoscopy
  - Focal ulcerations
  - Cobblestone appearance
  - Skip lesions
    - Normal segments of bowel interrupted by large areas of disease
- Biopsy
  - Confirmatory
  - Noncaseating granulomas are found in 30% of patients

Differential Diagnosis

- Lactose intolerance
- Irritable bowel syndrome
- Ulcerative colitis
- Appendicitis
- Diverticulitis
- Diverticular colitis
- Ischemic colitis
- Infection

Management

Nonpharmacologic Treatment
- Cessation of smoking
- Limit use of NSAIDs
- Diet modifications according to severity of disease
- Avoid dehydration
- Surgery
  - Over 50% of patients will require at least one surgical procedure.
  - Indications
    - Intractability to medical therapy
    - Intra-abdominal abscess
    - Massive bleeding
    - Symptomatic refractory internal or perianal fistulas
    - Intestinal obstruction
- Total parenteral nutrition
  - Short-term use in active disease and progressive weight loss
  - Those patients awaiting surgery with malnutrition who cannot tolerate enteral feedings because of high-grade obstruction, high-output fistulas, severe diarrhea, or abdominal pain
  - Long-term in patients with extensive intestinal resections leading to short bowel syndrome

Pharmacologic Treatment
- Symptomatic medications
  - Secretory diarrhea because of reduced absorption of bile acids
  - Cholestyramine 2 to 4 grams
  - Colesevelam 625 mg
  - Both are given 1 to 2 times daily before meals to bind malabsorbed bile salts
- Specific drug therapy
  - 5-aminosalicylic acid agents
    - Mesalamine 2.4 to 4.8 grams/day po
    - Pentasa 4 grams/day po
    - Initial therapy for mild to moderate disease
    - Controversy in recent studies regarding efficacy of these agents
- Antibiotics
  - Metronidazole 10 mg/kg/day
  - Ciprofloxacin 500 mg 2 times daily
  - Rifaximin 400 mg 3 times daily
  - Administered for 6 to 12 weeks
  - Used for treatment of active luminal disease
  - May reduce inflammation by altering gut flora
  - Controversy in recent studies regarding efficacy

- Corticosteroids
  - Entocort 9 mg once daily for 8 to 16 weeks
    - After initial treatment: taper over 2 to 4 weeks in 3 mg increments
    - May be used as maintenance therapy in low doses—6 mg/day for up to 1 year
  - About one-half of patients will require corticosteroids at some point in their illness.
  - Prednisone or methylprednisolone 40 to 60 mg/day for 8 to 16 weeks
    - After improvement at 2 weeks, taper at 5 mg/wk until a dose of 20 mg/day is reached; thereafter, slow taper at 2.5 mg/wk.
    - Remission or significant improvement is seen in > 80% of patients.
    - About 20% of patients cannot be completely withdrawn without experiencing a flare-up.
    - More than 50% who experience remission initially will have a relapse in 1 year.
    - Long-term therapy with corticosteroids should be avoided.
- Immunomodulating drugs
  - Mercaptopurine 75 to 125 mg p.o. daily
  - Azathioprine 100 to 250 mg p.o. daily
  - Methotrexate 25 mg IM or subq weekly for 12 weeks, followed by 12.5 to 15 mg once weekly
    - Used for patients who are unresponsive to or intolerant of mercaptopurine or azathioprine
  - Mean time to response is 2 to 4 months
  - Not used for acute exacerbations
  - Once patients achieve remission, these medications reduce the 3-year relapse rate from > 60% to < 25%.
- Anti-TNF therapies
  - Infliximab
  - Adalimumab
  - Certolizumab
  - Used for the treatment of patients with moderate to severe Crohn's disease with an inadequate response to mesalamine, antibiotics, corticosteroids, or immunomodulators

Special Considerations

- Must be differentiated from ulcerative colitis
- Crohn's disease is a lifelong illness with no specific therapy; therefore, current treatment is aimed at symptom improvement and controlling the progression of the disease.
- Because of the variation in the location of involvement and severity of inflammation, the patient may present with a variety of signs and symptoms.

When to Consult, Refer, or Hospitalize

- Refer for the following
  - Endoscopic procedures
  - Patients with moderate or severe disease for whom therapy immunomodulators or biological agents are being considered
  - When surgery is being considered
- Hospitalize
  - When intestinal obstruction is suspected
  - When intra-abdominal or perirectal abscess is suspected
  - For infection, especially in the patient who is immunocompromised, because of the use of corticosteroids, immunomodulators, or anti-TNF agents
  - Patients with severe diarrhea, dehydration, weight loss, or abdominal pain
  - Patients with severe or persisting symptoms despite corticosteroids

Follow-up

Expected Outcomes
- Initial remission
- Control of symptoms and complications
- Ability to live a productive life with the disease

Complications
- Abscess formation
- Small bowel obstruction
- Abdominal and rectovaginal fistulas
- Perianal disease
- Colon cancer
- Hemorrhage
- Malabsorption

DIVERTICULITIS/DIVERTICULOSIS

Description

- Intestinal diverticula are saclike mucosal outpouchings that occur in the colon.
- True diverticula contain all layers of the bowel wall.
- Pseudodiverticula are mucosal projections through the muscular layer and are the most common type in the colon.
- Diverticulitis is the inflammation of a diverticulum.
- Infection can vary from a small abscess to peritonitis.
- The size of the inflamed diverticula vary from a few millimeters to several centimers, and they can number from one to several dozen.
- Diverticula are more common in the sigmoid colon (left colon).

Etiology

- In most patients, diverticula develop from increased intraluminal pressure that results from a low-fiber diet.
- Over time, the contracted colonic musculature working against greater pressure develop hypertrophy, thickening, rigidity, and fibrosis.
- Diverticula may develop more commonly in the sigmoid because of higher intraluminal pressures in this area.
- Perforation of a colonic diverticulum causes an intra-abdominal infection that can vary from microperforation with localized inflammation (most common) to macroperforation with either abscess or generalized peritonitis.

Incidence and Demographics

- In Western societies, the incidence of colonic diverticulosis increases with age.
- Affects nearly one-half of individuals over age 60
- Only 20% develop symptomatic disease.
- In the United States, it accounts for > 200,000 hospitalizations per year.
- The mean age at presentation is 59.
- Males tend to present at a younger age.

Risk Factors

- Low-fiber diet
- Increased age

Prevention and Screening

- High-fiber diet
- Fiber supplements

Assessment

History
- Diverticulosis
  - Often asymptomatic
  - Left lower quadrant pain exacerbated by eating
  - Increased pain before defecation
  - Relief of pain after defecation (often incomplete)
  - Constipation

- Diverticulitis
  - Left lower quadrant pain
  - Fever
  - Nausea
  - Vomiting
  - Abdominal muscle spasm
  - Constipation
  - 50% of patients will report experiencing an episode of pain

Physical Examination
- Diverticulosis
  - Passage of pencil-thin stools
  - Loose stools
  - Passage of mucus
  - Left lower quadrant pain
- Diverticulitis
  - Left lower quadrant pain
  - 3 to 4 times more frequent in the left than right side of the colon
  - Focal tenderness, and about 20% will have a palpable tender mass
  - Guarding
  - Rebound tenderness
  - Rectal examination may reveal a palpable mass

Diagnostic Studies
- CBC
  - Leukocytosis
- Abdominal CT scan
  - Usual method of confirming presence of acute diverticulitis
  - Sensitivity and specificity > 95%
  - Bowel wall thickening of > 4 mm
  - Increased soft tissue density
  - Masses
  - Pericolic fluid collections
  - Fat stranding
  - Extraluminal air
- Amylase may be elevated in perforation or peritonitis.
- Barium enema
  - Diverticula best seen with barium enema
  - May reveal whether a contained perforation is communicating with the bowel lumen
  - Should not be performed in the acute phase because of the risk of perforation

Differential Diagnosis

- Appendicitis
- Ruptured ovarian cyst
- Endometriosis
- Ruptured ectopic pregnancy

- Pelvic inflammatory disease
- Crohn's disease
- Ischemic colitis
- Perforated colonic carcinoma
- C. *difficile*-associated colitis

Management

Nonpharmacologic Treatment
- Diverticulosis
  - Increase dietary fiber
- Diverticulitis
  - Bowel rest
  - Clear liquid diet—advancing slowly after clinical improvement, usually in 2 to 3 days
  - Uncomplicated cases may be treated on an outpatient basis.
  - Inpatient
    - Bowel rest
    - NPO with IV hydration

Pharmacologic Treatment
- Diverticulitis
  - Outpatient
    - Oral antibiotics for 7 to 10 days
    - Ciprofloxacin 500 mg p.o. twice daily plus metronidazole 500 mg 3 times daily or
    - Amoxicillin/clavulanate 875/125 mg twice daily or
    - Trimethoprim/sulfamethoxazole 160/800 mg twice daily plus metronidazole 500 mg 3 times daily
- Inpatient
  - Metronidazole 500 mg every 8 hours plus ciprofloxacin 400 mg every 12 hours or another fluoroquinolone *or*
  - Metronidazole 500 mg every 8 hours plus cefotaxime 1 to 2 grams every 6 hours or another third-generation cephalosporin *or*
  - Ampicillin-sulbactam 3 grams every 6 hours or other beta-lactamase inhibitor combination *or*
  - Imipenem 500 mg every 6 hours or other carbapenem

Special Considerations

- If a mass or stricture is found, a colonoscopy should be performed to rule out malignancy after the acute episode is resolved.
- Avoid alcohol with metronidazole—will induce vomiting
- Older adults less likely to have classic symptoms—pursue evaluation even with minimal symptoms

When to Consult, Refer, or Hospitalize

- Refer to gastroenterologist for:
  - Failure to improve within 72 hours of medical management
  - Presence of peridiverticular abscesses > 4 cm that may require percutaneous or surgical drainage
  - Recurrent attacks
  - Chronic complications, including colonic stricture or fistulas
- Admit for
  - Severe pain or inability to tolerate oral intake
  - Signs of sepsis or peritonitis
  - CT scan reveals complicated disease (abscess, perforation)
  - Failure to improve with outpatient management
  - Immunocompromised patient
  - Frail, elderly

Follow-up

Expected Outcomes
- Symptoms should resolve in 72 hours.

Complications
- Fistula formation
  - May involve bladder, ureter, vagina, uterus, bowel, and abdominal wall
- Perforation
- Peritonitis
- Hemorrhage
- Bowel obstruction

GASTROINTESTINAL BLEEDING

Description

- Gastrointestinal bleeding (GIB) has four levels.
  - Acute upper GIB (UGIB)
    - Most common presentation is hematemesis or melena
    - Hematemesis may be bright-red or brown ("coffee ground") material.
    - Melana develops after as little as 50 to 100 mL of blood loss in the upper GI tract
  - Acute lower GIB (LGIB)
    - Defined as bleeding that originates below the ligament of Treitz—the small intestine or colon
    - 95% of cases come from the colon.

- Obscure/occult GIB (OGIB)
  - Obscure
    - Bleeding of unknown origin that persists or recurs after initial endoscopy
    - Obscure-overt bleeding is persistent or recurrent visible evidence of GI bleeding
  - Occult
    - Bleeding that is not apparent to the patient
    - Chronic GIB loss of < 100 mL/d may not change stool appearance.
    - Identified by a positive fecal occult blood test (FOBT), fecal immunochemical test (FIT), or iron deficiency anemia
- Esophageal varices (EV)
  - Dilated submucosal veins that develop in patients with portal hypertension and may result in serious upper GIB

Etiology

- Acute upper GIB
  - Peptic ulcer disease (PUD)
  - Portal hypertension
  - Mallory-Weiss tear
  - Vascular abnormalities
  - Gastric malignancy
  - Erosive esophagitis
  - Aortoenteric fistula
- Acute lower GIB
  - Depends on the age of the patient and bleeding severity
  - In 20% of cases, no cause can be found
  - < 50 years
    - Infectious colitis
    - Anorectal disease
    - Inflammatory bowel disease
  - > 50 years
    - Diverticulosis
    - Vascular abnormalities
    - Malignancy
    - Ischemia
    - Colonic polyps
- Obscure/occult GIB
  - Obscure
    - Cause not identified
  - Occult
    - May arise from anywhere in the GI tract
    - Malignancy
    - PUD
    - Esophagitis
    - Erosion with hiatal hernia
    - Infections
    - Medications (NSAIDS, anticoagulation)
    - Inflammatory bowel disease

- Esophageal varices
  - Portal hypertension
    - Causes
      - Cirrhosis of the liver—most common
      - Portal thrombosis
      - Splenic vein thrombosis
      - Septic thrombophlebitis of the portal vein
      - Nodular regenerative hyperplasia
  - Develops when gradient between the portal vein and inferior venal cava is > 10 to 12 mm Hg

Incidence and Demographics

- Acute UGIB
  - 250,000 hospitalizations for UGIB occur each year in the United States.
  - Mortality rate of 4% to 10%
  - About one-half of patients are > 60 years of age, and the mortality rate is higher in this age group.
- Acute LGIB
  - In the United States, ranges from 20.5 to 27 per 100,000 persons per year
  - More common in men than women
  - Incidence increases with age
- OGIB
  - Exact numbers unknown
  - Accounts for about 5% of all cases of GIB
- EV
  - Approximately 10% of GIB cases are the result of EV.
  - 30% of patients with compensated and 60% to 70% with decompensated cirrhosis have EV at presentation.
  - Risk of bleeding is 30% in the first year after diagnosis.

Risk Factors

- Alcohol use
- Peptic ulcer disease
- NSAIDs
- Anticoagulation
- Cirrhosis
- Presence of EV
- Gastritis
- Esophagitis
- Advanced age
- Malignancy
- Colonic polyps
- Respiratory failure in the critically ill
- Coagulopathy in the critically ill
- Male gender
- Smoking

Prevention and Screening

- Treatment for *H. pylori* when identified
- Close monitoring of patients on anticoagulation therapy
- FOBT/FIT yearly for patients > 50 years of age to detect occult bleeding
- Colonoscopy every 10 years starting at age 50 or every 3 to 5 years starting at age 40 to 45 years for patients with history of colon cancer or polyps (or younger in select cases)
- Alternative to colonoscopy is a flexible sigmoidoscopy, CT colonography, or double-contrast enema every 5 years starting at age 50
- Daily monitoring of coagulation studies, CBC, and stool for occult blood in the hospitalized patient
- Alcohol and smoking cessation counseling
- Nonselective beta-blocker therapy for patients with EV

Assessment

History
- UGIB
  - Positive orthostatic vital signs
  - Pale skin
  - Altered mental status with severe blood loss
  - PUD
  - Use of NSAIDs
  - Anticoagulation
  - Nausea
  - Vomiting
- LGIB
  - Chronic
    - Positive orthostatic VS
    - Pale skin
    - Fatigue
  - Acute
    - Altered mental status
    - Hypotension
- OGIB
  - Pale skin
  - Positive FOBT/FIT
  - Smoking history
  - Fatigue
  - Shortness of breath
- EV
  - Nausea
  - Vomiting
  - Cirrhosis
  - Use of alcohol
  - Abdominal discomfort

Physical Examination

- UGIB
  - Hematemesis
  - Melena
  - In acute bleed with large-volume blood loss
    - Signs of hypovolemic shock
    - Positive orthostatic vital signs
    - Pale skin
  - Palmar erythema
  - Icterus
- LGIB
  - Hyperactive bowel sounds
  - Hematochezia
    - Bright-red or maroon
  - Melena
    - > 100 mL of blood for 1 melenic stool
    - Blood has been in GI tract for at least 14 hours
  - Chronic blood loss
    - Tachycardia
    - Positive orthostatic VS
    - Hypotension
  - Acute blood loss
    - Signs of hypovolemic shock
    - Gross rectal bleeding
- OGIB
  - Pale skin
  - May be no physical manifestations
- EV
  - Same as UGIB

Diagnostic Studies

- UGIB
  - CBC
  - Serum chemistry panel
  - Liver function studies
  - Type and crossmatch
  - Electrocardiogram
  - Endoscopy
  - Capsule endoscopy
- LGIB
  - CBC
  - Anemia workup to confirm iron deficiency anemia
    - Iron, total-iron binding capacity, ferritin, peripheral smear
  - Anoscopy
  - Sigmoidoscopy

- Colonoscopy
- Nuclear bleeding scans and angiography
- Push enteroscopy
  - Specially designed scope to examine the entire duodenum and part of the jejunum
- Capsule imaging

- OGIB
  - FOBT/FIT
  - CBC
  - Anemia workup as above
  - Endoscopy
  - Video capsule endoscopy
  - Push enteroscopy
- EV
  - CBC
  - Type and crossmatch
  - Serum chemistry panel
  - Coagulation studies
  - Arterial blood gases
  - Endoscopy after stabilization

Differential Diagnosis

- UGIB
  - Gastric ulcer
  - Duodenal ulcer
  - EV
  - Esophagitis
  - Malignancy
  - Angiodysplasia
- LGIB
  - Diverticulosis
  - Angiodysplasia
  - Ischemic colitis
  - Radiation-induced colitis
  - Neoplasm
  - Infectious colitis
- OGIB
  - Small intestinal erosion
  - Vascular anomalies
- EV
  - Budd-Chiari syndrome
  - Cirrhosis
  - Duodenal ulcers
  - Gastric cancer
  - Mallory Weiss tear
  - Portal vein obstruction

Management

Nonpharmacologic Treatment
- UGIB
  - Significant blood loss
    - 2 large-bore IV lines—16-gauge
      - Volume resuscitation
        - Crystalloid
          - Blood/blood products
            - Maintain hematocrit at 25% to 30%
            - Hematocrit should rise 4% for each unit transfused.
            - Fresh frozen plasma
    - Central line insertion
    - NG tube placement
  - Endoscopy
    - After stabilization
    - Perform within 6 to 24 hours of bleeding episode
    - Identifies the source of bleeding
    - Determines the risk of rebleeding and guides triage
    - Administer therapy
    - Cautery
    - Injection
    - Endoclips/bands
  - Discontinue NSAIDs, anticoagulation
  - Supplemental oxygen
  - Foley catheter for significant blood loss
  - Intra-arterial embolization
  - Transvenous intrahepatic portosystemic shunt (TIPS) for portal hypertension
- LGIB
  - Significant blood loss
    - Same as UGIB
    - NGT to rule out upper tract source
  - Discontinue NSAIDs, anticoagulation
  - Supplemental oxygen
  - Foley catheter for significant blood loss
  - Therapeutic colonoscopy
    - Epinephrine injection
    - Cautery
    - Endoclips/bands
  - Inta-arterial embolization
  - Surgical treatment
    - Required in < 5% of patients
    - Indicated for ongoing bleeding that requires more than 4 to 6 units of blood within 24 hours or more than 10 total units when attempts at endoscopic or angiographic therapy have failed
    - Localized resection or total colectomy with ileorectal anastomosis when accurate localization is not possible

- EV
  - Significant blood loss
    - Same as for UGIB
  - Supplemental oxygen
  - Foley catheter
  - Central line to monitor CVP
    - Maintain CVP at 10 mm Hg or less
    - If pulmonary catheter in place, keep wedge pressure at 8 mm Hg or less
    - Cautious hydration and blood product replacement
    - In the presence of active bleeding
      - Excessive volume resuscitation can increase portal pressure and increase risk of rebleeding.
      - Fresh frozen plasma 20 mg/kg loading dose, then 10 mg/kg every 6 hours for INR > 1.8 to 2.0
      - Platelet transfusion for levels < 50,000/mcL
  - Emergent endoscopy
    - Performed within 2 to 12 hours after stabilization
    - Excludes other causes
    - Therapy
      - Banding
      - Sclerotherapy
  - Balloon tube tamponade
  - Minnesota
  - Sengstaken-Blakemore
  - Provides initial control in 60% to 90% of patients
  - Used as temporizing measure only for bleeding that cannot be controlled with pharmacologic or endoscopic therapies
  - Complications
    - Gastric balloon rupture
      - Airway occlusion
    - Esophageal rupture
      - Severe back pain
      - Ulcerations of the gastric or esophageal mucosa
  - Portal decompressive procedures
    - TIPS
    - Emergency portosystemic shunt surgery
    - May be performed for rebleeding despite medical therapy
  - Candidacy for liver transplantation should be assessed in all patients with chronic liver disease and bleeding from portal hypertension.

Pharmacologic Treatment

- UGIB
  - Intravenous PPI
    - Esomeprazole or pantoprazole 80 mg bolus, then 8 mg/hr for 72 hours
  - Oral PPI
    - Esomeprazole 40 mg or lansoprazole 60 mg 2 times daily for 5 days
  - IV H_2 blockers
  - Octreotide
    - Continuous infusion
    - 100 mcg bolus followed by 50 to 100 mcg/hr
  - Vasopression 0.2 units/minutes
    - Do not stop abruptly or use in patients with coronary artery disease.
    - Recommended use < 12 hours
- EV
  - Antibiotic prophylaxis
    - Cirrhotic patients have > 50% chance of developing a bacterial infection during hospitalization.
      - Bacterial peritonitis
      - Pneumonia
      - Urinary tract infection
    - Fluoroquinolones
    - Third-generation cephalosporins
  - Octreotide
    - 50 mcg IV bolus followed by 50 mcg/hr
  - Vasopression
    - 0.2 to 0.4 unit/minute—maximum 0.8 unit/minute
    - May cause coronary artery spasm
  - Vitamin K
    - In cirrhotic patients with abnormal PT, administer 10 mg subcutaneously
  - Lactulose
    - Encephalopathy may complicate an episode of GI bleeding.
    - In patients with encephalopathy, lactulose should be administered in a dosage of 30 to 45 mL/hr p.o. until evacuation occurs, then 15 to 45 mL/hr every 8 to 12 hours as needed to promote 2 or 3 bowel movements daily
  - Prevention of rebleeding
    - Beta-blockers
      - Propanolol or labetalol 20 mg 2 times daily initially
      - Titrate for tolerance—slowly titrated upward for decrease in heart rate by 25% or if rate reaches 55 beats per minute

Special Considerations

- UGIB and LIGB are self-limiting in about 80% of patients.
- Patients hospitalized with LIGB are less likely to present with shock or orthostasis, or require transfusions.
- The color of stools may help to determine upper or lower GIB.
  - Brown stools mixed or streaked with blood—rectosigmoid or anus

- Large volume of bright-red blood indicates a colonic source
- Maroon stools suggest a lesion in the right colon or small intestine.
- Black stools (melena) indicate a source proximal to the ligament of Treitz.
- Bloody diarrhea with cramping, abdominal pain, urgency, or spasm of the anal sphincter is associated with inflammatory bowel disease, infectious colitis, or ischemic colitis.

When to Consult, Refer, or Hospitalize

- Patients with acute GI bleeding should be hospitalized, and those who are hemodynamically unstable should be placed in the medical intensive care unit; low- to moderate-risk patients may be admitted to a step-down unit or medical ward.
- Gastroenterology consult for management of cirrhotic patients, endoscopy, and liver transplant evaluation
- General surgery consult for surgical intervention

Follow-up

Expected Outcomes
- UGIB
  - After stabilization and endoscopy therapy, patient should be maintained on PPI therapy and treated for *H. pylori* if indicated.
  - Repeat endoscopy a few weeks after episode
  - Avoid NSAIDs
- LGIB
  - After acute bleeding episode, follow-up endoscopy with recurrent bleeding episodes
- OGIB
  - Monitoring of CBC and ongoing diagnostic studies to determine the cause of bleeding
- EV
  - Reduction of risk for rebleeding with beta-blockers, and definitive therapy as stated above
  - Nitroglycerin or long-acting nitrate may be added to help decrease portal hypertension.

Complications
- UGIB
  - Persistent bleeding
  - Upper endoscopy
    - Aspiration pneumonia
    - Perforation
    - In patients with CAD: dysrhythmias, ischemic ST changes
- LGIB
  - Abdominal surgery complications
    - Ileus
    - Sepsis
    - Poor wound healing
    - Myocardial infarction

- EV
  - Severe and persistent UGIB
    - Vascular collapse
    - Cardiomyopathy
    - Dysrhythmias
  - Sepsis
  - Encephalopathy
  - Complications associated with therapeutic procedures
    - Balloon tamponade
      - Aspiration pneumonia
      - Esophageal perforation
      - Lesion of gastric/esophageal mucosa
      - Pressure necrosis to lips, mouth, nasal passages
    - Sclerotherapy
      - Perforation of the esophagus
      - Esophageal ulceration and bleeding
      - Pleural effusion
      - Fever
      - Chest pain
      - Esophageal stricture
    - Variceal banding
      - Rebleeding
    - Surgical procedures
      - Hepatic encephalopathy
    - Liver transplant
      - Rejection
      - Sepsis

ACUTE HEPATIC FAILURE

Description

- Acute hepatic failure is the disruption of one or more of the five major liver functions.
  - Maintenance of acid–base balance through lactate metabolism
  - Detoxification
  - Glucose and lipid metabolism
  - Protein synthesis (clotting factors and albumin)
  - Phagocytic clearance of organisms and circulating debris
  - A three-tiered categorization of acute hepatic failure
  - Hyperacute
    - Developing in less than a week

- Acute
  - Evolving over 1 to 4 weeks
- Subacute
  - Occuring over 5 to 26 weeks
- May be fulminant or subfulminant
  - Fulminant
    - Development of hepatic encephalopathy within 8 weeks after the onset of liver disease
    - Coagulopathy with INR > 1.5
  - Subfulminant
    - Occurs when the above appears between 8 weeks and 6 months after the onset of acute liver disease

Etiology

- Acetaminophen toxicity
- Idiosyncratic drug reactions
- Viral hepatitis
  - Acute hepatitis A or B superimposed on chronic hepatitis C
- Poison mushrooms—*Amanita phalloides*
- Shock
- Hyper- or hypothermia
- Budd-Chiari syndrome
- Malignancy—most commonly lymphomas
- Reye's syndrome
- Fatty liver of pregnancy
- Disorders of fatty acid oxidation
- Autoimmune hepatitis
- Parovirus B19 infection

Incidence and Demographic

- About 1,600 cases of acute liver failure occur each year in the United States.
- Acetaminophen toxicity accounts for 45% of these cases.
  - Suicide attempts account for 44% of acetaminophen-induced hepatic failure.
  - Unintentional overdose because of decreased clearance from preexisting liver disease accounts for about 48%.
  - The risk is increased in the diabetic and obese population.
  - Viral hepatitis accounts for about 12% of all cases.
  - Patients with acute liver failure from acetaminophen toxicity have a better prognosis than those from another etiology.
  - Patients with stage 3 or 4 encephalopathy have a poor prognosis.

Risk Factors

- Acetaminophen use
- Critical illness
- Viral hepatitis
- Obesity
- Diabetes
- Use of hepatotoxic medications
- Congenital conditions

Prevention and Screening

- Patient education regarding the use of acetaminophen
  - 4 g/24 hours
  - 2 g/24 hours for those with liver disease
- Maintain normal weight.
- Control of diabetes
- Treatment of underlying causes
- Hepatitis B vaccination

Assessment

History
- Use of nephrotoxic agents
- Viral hepatitis
- Critical illness
- Fever
- Irritability
- Confusion
- Nausea and vomiting

Physical Assessment
- Jaundice
- RUQ tenderness
- Tremors
- Hyperventilation
- Asterixis
- Hypoxemia
- Ascites
- Peripheral edema
- Hepatomegaly
- Hepatic encephalopathy—see cirrhosis for grading

Diagnostic Studies

- Complete metabolic panel (includes liver function tests)
  - Transaminase levels are usually elevated.
    - With acetaminophen toxicity, levels may be > 10,000 μ/L.
  - Marked hyperbilirubinemia
  - Hypoglycemia
- Amylase
  - 10% of patients have elevated amylase levels.
- Lipase
- Complete blood count
  - Leukocytosis
- Coagulation studies
  - Prolonged prothrombin time
- Serum ammonia level
  - Usually elevated
- DIC (disseminated intravascular coagulation) panel
- Serum lactate
- Arterial blood gases
- Acetaminophen level
- Autoimmune markers
  - Antinuclear antibody
  - Anti–smooth-muscle antibody
- Drug screen
- Liver ultrasound (Doppler)
- Abdominal CT/MRI
- Liver biopsy
  - Contraindicated in coagulopathy
  - Helpful to diagnose autoimmune hepatitis, metastatic liver disease, lymphoma, or herpes simplex hepatitis

Differential Diagnosis

- Acute fatty liver of pregnancy
- Hemorrhagic viruses
- Idiopathic drug reaction
- Paramyxovirus
- Tyrosinemia
- Yellow phosphorus poisoning

Management

Nonpharmacologic Treatment
- Identify the cause.
- Intensive care unit for those with stage 2 encephalopathy
  - Airway protection
  - Encephalopathy/cerebral edema
    - CT scan of the head
    - Avoid sedation.
    - Head of bed at 30 degrees
    - Intracranial pressure monitoring
  - Cardiovascular monitoring
  - Manage coagulopathy
    - Correct abnormalities only in the presence of bleeding or when a procedure is planned.
      - Fresh frozen plasma
      - Recombinant factor VIIa
      - Platelet transfusions
  - Manage poisonings
  - Liver transplantation

Pharmacologic Treatment
- Acetaminophen toxicity
  - Acetylcysteine
    - Best when administered within 8 hours
    - Loading dose 140 mg/kg p.o.
      - 70 mg/kg p.o. every 4 hours x 17 doses
    - Do not wait for acetaminophen levels.
    - Give first maintenance dose after start dose.
    - Repeat dose if patient vomits within 1 hour.
- Phalloides mushroom
  - Penicillin G IV1 mg/kg/day
  - Silibinin 20 to 50 mg/kg/day p.o.
  - Oral charcoal 50 grams p.o. or through nasogastric tube

Special Considerations

- Acute hepatic failure has a wide variety of causes and must be diagnosed early.
- Ingestion of 6 grams of acetaminophen may be fatal.
- Because of the role of the liver in maintaining hemostasis, acute hepatic failure is often accompanied by gastrointestinal bleeding.
- Medications extensively metabolized by the liver should be avoided.
- Only hepatic failure from acetaminophen has an effective specific therapy; supportive care is the basis for treating most patients.

When to Consult, Refer, or Hospitalize

- All patients with acute hepatic failure require hospitalization.
- Multiple consults may be necessary.
  - Gastroenterology
  - Pulmonology
  - Critical care medicine
  - Neurology
  - Rheumatology
  - Infectious disease

Follow-up

Expected Outcomes
- Prognosis is dependent on the cause.
- Best prognosis is for patients ages 10 to 40.
- MELD score used as prognostic indicator
- Approximately 50% to 60% of patients with fulminant hepatic failure because of hepatitis A survive.
  - Survival from other causes of viral hepatitis is much less favorable.
- Acetaminophen toxicity
  - Consider liver transplant if King's College criteria are met.
- Non-acetaminophen toxicity
  - Consider liver transplant if King's College criteria are met.
- Wilson disease
  - Usually fatal without liver transplant

Complications
- Hepatic encephalopathy
- Cerebral edema
- Intracranial hemorrhage
- Seizures
- Hemorrhage
- Sepsis
- Electrolyte and acid–base imbalances

ACUTE VIRAL HEPATITIS

Description

- Acute viral hepatitis is a systemic infection primarily affecting the liver.
- Liver becomes inflamed by a specific hepatotropic virus, medications, or other toxic agents
- Acute hepatitis—infection < 6 months in duration

- Chronic hepatitis—infection lasting 6 months or longer
- Six types of hepatotropic viruses have been identified.
  - A (HAV)
    - Incubation period 15 to 45 days
    - Excreted in feces for up to 2 weeks before clinical illness
    - No chronic carrier state
    - Acute illness subsides over 2 to 3 weeks
      - Complete clinical recovery and laboratory recovery in 9 weeks
    - Low mortality rate
  - B (HBV)
    - Incubation period 6 weeks to 6 months (average 12 to 14 weeks)
    - Onset insidious
    - Fulminant hepatitis may be abrupt, with death in a few days.
  - C (HCV)
    - Incubation period 6 to 7 weeks
    - Clinical illness often mild
  - D (HDV)
    - Incubation period 45 to 60 days
  - E (HEV)
    - Incubation period 15 to 60 days
    - Illness generally self-limited
  - G (HGV)
    - HGV has not been shown to cause hepatitis.

Etiology

- HAV: RNA hepatovirus
  - Fecal-oral route
  - Crowding, poor sanitation
- HBV: 42-nm hepadnavirus with a partially double-stranded DNA genome
  - Inner core protein (hepatitis B core antigen, HBcAg)
  - Outer surface coat (hepatitis B surface antigen, HBsAg)
  - Eight different genotypes (A–H)
  - Present in saliva, semen, and vaginal secretions
  - Transmission
    - Sexual contact with multiple partners
      - Risk between monogamous partners: 4% to 5% over 20 years
    - IV drug use
    - Needlestick
      - 0% to 7%
    - Contaminated blood and blood products
    - Body piercing and tattoos
    - Perinatal
    - Chronic carrier state responsible for most liver cirrhosis

- HCV: single-stranded RNA virus
  - Blood-borne
  - 50% related to IV drug use
  - Source of infection may be uncertain
  - Only 4% of cases related to blood transfusion
  - Risk of sexual and perinatal transmission low
- HDV: defective RNA virus
  - Causes hepatitis only in the presence of hepatitis B infection, specifically with HBsAG
  - Blood-borne
  - This virus is cleared when HBV is resolved.
  - Combined infection with HBV has a worse prognosis
- HEV: 29 to 32-nm RNA hepevirus—seen mainly in Central and Southeast Asia, the Middle East, and North Africa
  - Transmission via fecal-oral route
- HGV: flavivirus percutaneously transmitted and associated with chronic viremia lasting at least 10 years
  - Has been detected in 1.5% of blood donors, 50% of IV drug users, 30% of hemodialysis patients, 20% of hemophiliacs, and 15% of patients with chronic hepatitis B or C
  - Does not appear to cause significant liver disease

Incidence and Demographics

- HAV: In 2008, the number of cases reported was 2,585; estimated number of acute clinical cases was 11,000; estimated number of new infections was 22,000.
  - Percent of persons ever infected: 29.1% to 33.5%
- HBV: In 2008, the number of cases reported was 4,033; estimated number of acute clinical cases was 12,000; estimated number of new infections was 38,000.
  - Percent of persons ever infected: 4.3% to 5.6%
  - Number of individuals living with chronic infection: 800,000 to 1.4 million persons
  - Annual number of chronic liver disease deaths associated with viral disease: 3,000
  - Men at greater risk than women
  - Patients with chronic hepatitis B at higher risk for cirrhosis and hepatocellular carcinoma
- HCV: In 2008, the number of cases reported was 878; estimated number of acute clinical cases was 2,900; estimated number of new infections was 18,000.
  - Percent of persons ever infected: 1.3% to 1.9%
  - Number of persons living with chronic infection: 2.7 to 3.9 million individuals
- HDV: In the early 1970s and 1980s, HDV was endemic in Mediterranean countries and Central and Eastern Europe—up to 80% of patients with HBV were infected.
  - Annual number of chronic liver disease deaths associated with viral disease: 12,000
  - In the United States, HDV occurred in IV drug users—new cases are infrequent because of control of HBV infection.
  - Cases seen today are mostly from individuals infected many years previously who survived the initial insult of HDV and now have inactive cirrhosis.
- HEV: see above description—rare in the United States; consider in patients who have traveled in endemic areas
  - Mortality rate is 20% in pregnant women.
- HGV: see above description

Risk Factors

- HAV
  - Exposure to contaminated food and water
  - Overcrowded conditions
  - Poor sanitation
  - Poor handwashing
- HBV
  - Blood transfusion recipient
  - Needle-sharing between IV drug users
  - Exposure to infected body fluids
  - Sexual activity with multiple partners
  - Healthcare workers
- HCV
  - Same as HBV
  - Cocaine use
  - Body piercing, tattoos
  - Hemodialysis
- HDV
  - Infection with HBV
  - Travel to endemic countries
- HEV
  - Travel to endemic countries
- HEG
  - IV drug users
  - Hemodialysis
  - History of chronic hepatitis B or C
  - Hemophilia

Prevention and Screening

- Avoid high-risk behavior.
- Proper handwashing
- Improve overcrowded conditions.
- Safe sex practices
- Screening of blood products
- Screen women who are pregnant for HBV.
- Hepatitis B vaccine for healthcare workers
- Hepatitis vaccines
  - HAV
- Target populations
  - International travelers
  - Chronic liver disease
  - High-risk sexual behaviors
  - IV drug users
    - HAV
      - Havrix

- 1,440 elisa units (1 mL) IM
- Booster at 6 to 18 months
- Vaqta
  - 50 units (1 mL) IM
  - Booster at 6 to 18 months
- Twinrix (A & B)
  - 0.5 mL IM
  - Repeat at 1 and 6 months
- Immunoglobulin
  - 0.02 to 0.06 mL/kg IM for exposed contacts or individuals traveling to areas for up to 6 months; use higher dose if individual will be in the area for up to 6 months where hepatitis A is common
  - 0.06 mL/kg IM every 4 to 6 months for travelers staying > 3 months
- HBV
  - Target population
    - Healthcare workers
    - Individuals with high-risk behavior
      - Recombivax HB
      - Engerix-B
        - 10 to 20 mcg initially, depending on preparation
        - Repeated at 1 and 6 months
        - Alternative schedules
          - 0, 1, 2, and 12 months
          - 0, 7, 21 days plus 12 months
- None available for hepatitis C, D, E, G

Assessment

- Symptoms of acute viral hepatitis are similar.
- Severity of symptoms varies among the various types, ranging from asymptomatic infection without jaundice to fulminant hepatitis.
- Pre-icteric phase
  - Fatigue
  - Malaise
  - Anorexia
  - Nausea
  - Vomiting
  - Headache
  - Aversion to smoking or drinking alcohol
- Icteric phase
  - Weight loss
  - Pruritus
  - RUQ pain
  - Clay-colored stool
  - Jaundice
  - May appear mildly to acutely ill

History
- HAV
  - History of travel
  - Occupational risk
  - Upper respiratory symptoms
  - Diarrhea
  - Constipation
  - 1 to 2 weeks of
    - Anorexia
    - Nausea
    - Malaise
    - Fever
- HBV
  - May have asymptomatic seroconversion
  - Anorexia
  - Nausea
  - Malaise
  - Arthralgias
  - Arthritis
- HCV
  - May be mild
  - Similar symptoms as hepatitis A and B
- HDV
  - Similar to hepatitis B
- HEG/HEG
  - Similar to hepatitis B
  - Abdominal pain

Physical Examination
- HAV
  - Jaundice
  - Hepatomegaly
- HBV
  - Jaundice
  - Macular skin rash
  - Hepatomegaly
  - Splenomegaly
- HCV
  - Jaundice in approximately 25% of patients
- HDV
  - Same as for hepatitis B
- HEV/HGV
  - Jaundice

Diagnostic Studies
- The following are positive lab values for the various hepatitis viruses.
- HAV
  - CBC
    - WBC normal to low
    - Occasionally large, atypical lymphocytes
    - Low-grade hemolysis
  - Urinary studies
    - Mild proteinuria
    - Bilirubinuria
  - Liver function studies
    - Elevated AST or ALT
      - Occurs early
    - Elevated bilirubin and alkaline phosphatase follow elevated liver enzymes.
    - May see modest drop in serum albumin
  - Acute
    - Anti-HAV IgM
      - Peak during the first week
      - Disappear within 3 to 6 months
  - Later in disease
    - Anti-HAV IgG—stays for life
      - Rise after 1 month in the disease
      - Indicates previous exposure, noninfectivity, immunity
- Imaging studies usually not indicated
- HBV
  - Liver function studies
  - CBC
  - Acute
    - HBsAg
      - First evidence of infection
      - Persists throughout clinical illness
      - Persistence longer than 6 months: indicates chronic hepatitis B
    - HBcAb IgM: serum levels rise following HBsAG appearance
    - Anti-HBc IgM
    - HBeAg is positive, may appear only briefly
    - HBV DNA
      - Parallels the presence of HBeAg
      - May persist in very low levels long after recovery
  - Recovery
    - HBsAg
      - Typically disappears with recovery, but can remain positive with chronic HBV infection
    - Anti-HBs
      - Signals that recovery has occurred
      - Noninfectivity
      - Protection from recurrent infection
      - Immunity with vaccination
        - Anti-HBc IgG
          - Marker of past or current infection
        - Anti-HBc

- Marker of acute, chronic, or resolved HBV
- Not a marker of vaccine-induced immunity
- Chronic
  - HBsAG
    - With active and low viral replication
    - With heterotypic anti-HBs (in about 10% of cases)
    - With anti-HBc IgG, if present without anti-HBc IgM
  - HBV-DNA: used to monitor patients with chronic hepatitis B infection
- Abdominal US, CT to exclude biliary obstruction
  - Nonspecific finding—echogenicity of the liver parenchyma

- HCV
  - CBC
  - Liver function tests
    - Waxing, waning ALT
    - ALT may be used to guide efficacy of treatment.
  - Thyrotropin level
  - Screen for coinfection with HIV or HBV.
  - Screen for alcohol or drug abuse.
  - Screen for depression.
  - Acute
    - Anti-HCV
      - First-line test
      - Highly sensitive
        - If negative, infection unlikely
        - If positive, hepatitis C infection is present until proved otherwise
    - EIA
      - Enzyme immunoassay
      - Can yield results an average of 8 weeks after the onset of infection
      - May have false positive results
    - RIBA
      - Recombinant immunoblot assay
      - Use to confirm infection; however, not needed in presence of positive anti-HCV
    - OraQuick HCV Rapid Antibody Test
      - Test strip can be used with saliva, whole blood, serum, or plasma
    - HCV RNA assay
      - Blood sample
  - Ultrasound of the liver
  - Liver biopsy
    - Used for assessing the severity and activity of HCV-related liver disease
- HDV
  - Acute
    - Anti-HDV IgM positive initially, then positive for anti-HDV immunoglobulin G
    - The finding of antigen A antibody to HDV is nearly always associated with chronic HDV infection.
    - HDV RNA
- HEV & HGV
  - Diagnosis made by exclusion of other hepatitis viruses.
  - Anti-HEV IgM
  - HEV RNA

Differential Diagnosis

- HAV
  - HBV
  - HCV
  - Infectious mononucleosis
  - CMV
  - Spirochetal diseases
  - Rickettsial diseases
  - Drug-induced liver disease
  - Autoimmune hepatitis
- HBV
  - Alcoholic hepatitis
  - Cholangitis
  - Hemochromatosis
  - Hepatic carcinoma
  - HAV
  - Autoimmune hepatitis
- HCV
  - Autoimmune hepatitis
  - Cholangitis
- HDV
  - Bile duct strictures
  - Budd-Chiari syndrome
  - Cholangitis
- HEV
  - CMV
  - Epstein-Barr virus
  - Mononucleosis

Management

Nonpharmacological Treatment
- HAV/HBV
  - Bedrest for severe symptoms
  - IV hydration if unable to take oral fluids
  - Avoid overfeeding
    - High-carbohydrate diet
    - Low-protein diet
    - No fatty foods
  - Avoid physical exertion, alcohol, and hepatotoxic agents
  - Avoid morphine sulfate
- Transjugular intrahepatic portosystemic shunt (TIPS) procedure for massive ascites, advanced liver disease with portal hypertension not responsive to therapy
- Liver transplant

Pharmacologic Treatment

- HAV
  - Oxazepam—not metabolized by the liver
  - Anti-emetics
- HBV
  - No medical therapy of acute HBV—supportive medical management
  - Chronic HBV
    - Interferon-alpha
    - Lamivudine
    - Adefovir dipivoxil
    - Tenofovir
- HCV
  - Peginterferon alfa-2a
    - 6 to 24 weeks
    - Treatment is reserved for patients whose serum HCV RNA levels fail to clear after 3 months.
- HDV
  - If present, resolves with the resolution of HBV

Special Considerations

- HAV
  - Isolation is not necessary, must wash hands after bowel movements
  - Vaccination after prescreening for prior immunity is recommended for patients with chronic hepatitis B or C and other chronic liver disease.
- HBV
  - In many cases, jaundice never develops.
  - With onset of jaundice, prodomal symptoms may worsen, followed by progressive clinical improvement—stools may be clay-colored.
  - The acute illness subsides over 2 to 3 weeks with complete clinical recovery by 16 weeks.
  - In 5% to 10% of cases, there is a more protracted course.
  - < 1% of cases will have a fulminant course.
- HCV
  - Fulminant hepatitis is rare.
  - Increased risk of hepatocellular carcinoma at a rate of 3% to 5% per year

When to Consult, Refer, or Hospitalize

- Consult with specialist for all cases of hepatitis.
- Refer to a gastroenterologist, infectious disease specialist, or both for uncertain diagnosis, fulminant hepatitis, or chronic hepatitis.
- Admit
  - For encephalopathy
  - INR > 1.6
  - Patient cannot maintain hydration
  - Liver biopsy

Follow-up

Expected Course
- HAV
  - Clinical recovery usually complete in 3 months
  - Does not cause chronic liver disease
- HBV
  - Clinical recovery complete in 3 to 6 months
  - Mortality rate is 0.1% to 1%, higher with superimposed hepatitis D
  - Chronic hepatitis develops in 1% to 2% of immunocompetent adults.
  - Cirrhosis develops in up to 40% of those with chronic hepatitis B.
- HCV
  - Mortality rate is < 1%; higher in older adults
  - Chronic hepatitis develops in about 85% of cases of acute HCV infection.
  - Cirrhosis develops in 30% of cases of chronic hepatitis C.

Complications
- Hepatic necrosis
- Chronic hepatitis
- Cirrhosis
- Hepatic failure
- Hepatocellular carcinoma
- Insulin resistance
- Hepatic steatosis
- With HCV: 20% to 30% risk of non-Hodgkin's lymphoma

LARGE BOWEL OBSTRUCTION

Description

- Large bowel obstruction (LBO) is a mechanical or functional obstruction of the large intestine that disrupts normal function.
- Acute colonic pseudo-obstruction (ACPO) is thought to be the result of an autonomic imbalance because of decreased parasympathetic tone or excessive sympathetic stimulation.

Etiology

- Approximately 60% of LBOs are the result of malignancies.
- Diverticular disease
- Colonic volvulus
- Endometriosis

Incidence and Demographics

- It is 3 to 4 times less frequent than small bowel obstruction.

Risk Factors

- Presence of rectal or colon cancer
- Diverticular disease
- Advanced age
  - Individuals > 60 years of age are at increased risk for ACPO.

Prevention and Screening

- Screening colonoscopies per guidelines
- High-fiber diet
- Low-fat diet
- Management of endometriosis

Assessment

History
- Nausea
- Vomiting
- Crampy abdominal pain
- Chronic constipation with laxative use
- ACPO
  - Similar to mechanical LBO and usually develops over 3 to 7 days

Physical Examination
- Abdominal distention
- Tenderness
  - Abdominal rigidity, fever, and severe tenderness point to peritonitis from perforation
- Guaic-positive stool
- Palpable rectal or lower sigmoid mass on rectal examination

Diagnostic Studies
- CBC
- Serum chemistry panel
- Lactate level
- Coagulation panel
- Type and crossmatch
- Upright chest radiograph
  - Detect free air in perforation

- Abdominal flat and upright plain films
  - Identifies sigmoid or cecal volvulus
- Abdominal CT with IV, oral, and/or rectal contrast
  - "Bird's beak" pattern suggests colonic volvulus

Differential Diagnosis

- Constipation
- Diverticular disease
- Small bowel obstruction
- Colorectal carcinoma

Management

Nonpharmacologic Treatment
- NG tube for vomiting
- NPO
- Surgical intervention
  - Frequently indicated

Pharmacologic Treatment
- Fluid and electrolyte replacement
- Broad-spectrum antibiotics
  - Clindamycin 400 to 900 mg IV every 8 hours
  - Metronidazole 1 gm IV loading dose then 0.5 gm IV every 6 hours or 1 gm IV every 12 hours
  - Aztreonam 2 gm IV every 8 hours
  - Cefoxitin 2 gm IV every 8 hours

Special Considerations

- Suspect bowel perforation in patients with sustained tachycardia, fever, and abdominal pain.
- Malignancy should be suspected in all patients with LBO.

When to Consult, Refer, or Hospitalize

- Early surgical consult

Follow-up

Expected Outcomes
- If treated early, outcome good
- If underlying cause is cancer, then prognosis depends on the cancer prognosis

Complications
- Perforation
- Sepsis
- Intraabdominal abscess
- Death

MESENTERIC ISCHEMIA

Description

- Mesenteric ischemia is an uncommon vascular disorder with a high mortality rate.
- Occurs when there is inadequate perfusion to intestinal tissue
- Characterized by the etiology
  - Arteriocclusive mesenteric ischemia (AOMI)
  - Nonocclusive mesenteric ischemia (NOMI)
  - Mesenteric venous thrombosis (MVT)
- Chronic intestinal ischemia as a result of progressive narrowing of the arterial circulation to the intestine from atherosclerotic disease

Etiology

- Occlusive ischemia is the result of an embolus or progressive thrombosis in a major artery or vein supplying the intestine.
  - Emboli originate from the heart in > 75% of cases.
  - Patients taking oral contraceptives
  - Protein S or C deficiency
  - Malignancy
  - Antithrombin III deficiency
  - Systemic disease
    - Systemic lupus erythemtosus
    - Disseminated intravascular coagulopathy
    - Polyarteritis nodosa
    - Thrombotic thrombocytopenic purpura
  - Visceral infection
  - Portal hypertension
  - Abdominal surgery
  - Abdominal trauma
- Nonocclusive occurs from arteriolar vasospasm in response to low flow states such as shock, congestive heart failure, vasoconstrictive medications, aortic stenosis, or cardiac dysrhythmias
  - If left untreated, early mucosal ulceration will progress to full-thickness injury.
- Chronic ischemia
  - Atherosclerosis

Incidence and Demographics

- Mesenteric ischemia accounts for 0.1% of hospital admissions.
- Mortality rates range from 60% to 100%, depending on the source of the obstruction.
  - Mortality rates decrease when this condition is treated early and prior to the development of peritonitis.
- Occurs equally in both genders
- Typically occurs in the older population, usually in those > 60 years of age; however, with predisposing factors, it may occur in younger patients

Risk Factors

- Advanced age
- Abdominal surgery
- Congestive heart failure
- Aortic stenosis
- Smoking
- Use of oral contraceptives
- Genetics
  - Prothrombin gene 20210G/A mutation has been linked to thrombosis of digestive vessels
- Cocaine use
- Atherosclerosis
- Abdominal trauma
- Cardiac dysrhythmias
- Hypotension

Prevention and Screening

- Avoidance of hypotensive, low-flow states
- When vasopressors are used, use lowest dose that is therapeutic and for the shortest duration.
- Lipid-lowering agents
- Smoking cessation
- Diagnosis and treatment of hypercoagulable disorders
- Identify patients at high risk for early diagnosis

Assessment

History
- Occlusive ischemia
  - Abdominal pain
    - Severe, acute, nonremitting
    - Generalized or periumbilical
    - Out of proportion to physical findings
  - Nausea
  - Vomiting

- Transient diarrhea
- Bloody stools
- Nonocclusive ischemia
  - Anorexia
  - Generalized abdominal pain
- Chronic ischemia
  - Weight loss
  - Self-limited food intake
  - Abdominal pain/cramping after a meal, lasting 1 to 3 hours
  - Chronic diarrhea

Physical Examination
- Occlusive ischemia
  - Early in the course, the abdominal examination may be unremarkable.
    - Hypoactive bowel sounds
    - Mild abdominal distention
  - Later findings
    - Signs of peritonitis
    - Cardiovascular collapse
- Nonocclusive ischemia
  - Generalized abdominal pain
  - Bloody stools
  - Abdominal distention

Diagnostic Studies
- CBC
  - Leukocytosis
- Serum chemistry panel with liver function studies
- Coagulation panel
- Arterial blood gas analysis
  - Metabolic acidosis
- Amylase
  - Elevated
- Lipase
- Lactic acid
  - Elevated
- Type and crossmatch
- Cardiac enzymes
- Electrocardiogram
- D-dimer
- Platelet activating factor
- Plain abdominal films
  - May show free air and indicate perforation
  - Bowel wall edema
  - Air in the bowel wall
- CT abdomen
  - With and without contrast

- Mesenteric angiography
  - Best performed intraoperatively
  - Gold standard for chronic mesenteric ischemia
- Ultrasound may be used as a screening tool for chronic ischemia.

Differential Diagnosis

- Abdominal aneurysm
- Acute appendicitis
- Cholangitis
- Cholelithiasis
- Lactic acidosis
- Myocardial infarction
- Large bowel obstruction
- Small bowel obstruction
- Pancreatitis
- Renal calculi
- Hypovolemic shock

Management

Nonpharmacologic Treatment
- Gold standard for diagnosis and treatment of occlusive disease is laparotomy
  - Surgical exploration should not be delayed if suspicion for occlusive mesenteric
  - Ischemia is high
  - Goal is to resect compromised bowel and restore blood supply
  - Embolectomy or bypass of occluded vessel
- Total parenteral nutrition may be needed for recovery.
- For nonocclusive disease, correct the underlying problems.
- NG tube for decompression
- Chronic disease
  - Angioplasty with endovascular stenting
    - 80% long-term success rate

Pharmacological Treatment
- Broad spectrum antibiotics if peritonitis is suspected
  - Clindamycin 400 to 900 mg every 8 hours
  - Metronidazole 1 gram IV loading dose followed by 0.5 g every 6 hours or 1 g every 12 hours
  - Aztreonam 2 g IV every 8 hours
  - Ticarcillin 4 g IV every 6 hours
  - Cefoxitin 2 g IV every 8 hours

Special Considerations

- With the exception of small bowel obstruction, ischemic colitis is the most common form of acute ischemia.
- High index of suspicion is the key element in diagnosing mesenteric ischemia early

When to Consult, Refer, or Hospitalize

- Patients with acute mesenteric ischemic colitis should be hospitalized in the intensive care unit (ICU).
- Mesenteric ischemia may occur while patient hospitalized for another condition—early recognition will warrant transfer to the ICU
- Chronic mesenteric ischemia may require hospitalization for workup and intervention.
- Consult general surgery, interventional radiology, and other consultants as underlying conditions warrant.

Follow-up

Expected Outcomes
- Restoration of blood flow to the intestine
- Mortality rate is high and dependent on when the condition is diagnosed and the underlying cause.

Complications
- Sepsis/shock
- Multi-organ system failure
- Bowel necrosis
- Death

ACUTE PANCREATITIS

General Description

- Acute pancreatitis is inflammation of the pancreas causing release of pancreatic enzymes into surrounding tissue.
- There is usually complete recovery of pancreatic function; if there is not, then patient develops chronic pancreatitis.

Etiology

- Majority of cases are from biliary tract disease resulting from a large gallstone blocking the pancreatic duct or from excessive alcohol abuse
  - Pancreatic enzymes are leaked and cause local and systemic symptoms.
- Other causes include hypercalcemia, hyperlipidemia, viral infections, renal failure, abdominal trauma, vasculitis, and some medications.
  - Didanosine (DDI)
  - Pentamidine
  - Furosemide
  - Hydrochlorothiazide
  - Divalproex sodium
  - Valproic acid
  - NSAIDs
  - Tetracyclines

Incidence and Demographics

- Approximately 40 cases per year per 100,000 adults
- Equal distribution between genders
- The annual incidence in Native Americans is 4 per 100,000; in Whites, it is 5.7 per 100,000; and in Blacks, it is 20.7 per 100,000.
- Average age 35 to 45 years

Risk Factors

- Alcohol abuse
- Gallstones
- Hyperlipidemia
- Hyperparathyroidism
- Hypercalcemia
- Abdominal trauma
- Viral infections
  - Mumps
  - Coxsackie virus
  - Cytomegalovirus
  - Hepatitis
  - Epstein-Barr
  - Rubella
- Medications—see Etiology
- Carcinoma of the pancreas
- Peptic ulcer disease

Prevention and Screening

- Alcohol cessation counseling/treatment
- Low-fat, low-cholesterol diet
- Early recognition of viral infections
- Treatment for hyperparathyroidism, hypercalcemia, peptic ulcer disease
- Identification and monitoring of gallstones
- Identify and avoid or minimal use of inciting medications

Assessment

History
- Abrupt onset of epigastric or left upper quadrant pain, often with radiation to the back
  - Described as steady and severe
- Pain is increased with movement or lying supine, improves with sitting or leaning forward
- Nausea
- Vomiting
- History of alcohol intake or a heavy meal prior to the onset of symptoms
- Fever
- Recent surgery or invasive procedure
- Family history of hypertriglyceridemia
- History of previous biliary colic

Physical Examination
- Epigastric or left upper abdominal tenderness, distention, guarding, and rigidity
- Occasionally, a left upper quadrant mass can be palpated because of inflammation or pseudocyst
- Mild jaundice
- Diminished or absent bowel sounds
- Tachycardia
- Tachypnea
- Hypotension
- Bibasilar crackles, greater on the left because of the contiguous spread of inflammation
- Pallor
- Diaphoresis
- Severe necrotizing pancreatitis
  - Cullen sign
  - Grey-Turner sign
  - Erythematous skin nodules

Diagnostic Studies
- CBC
  - Leukocytosis: > 12,000 mcL
- Serum chemistry: complete metabolic panel, which includes liver function studies
  - May see elevated serum glucose (β-cell injury)
  - Electrolyte imbalance from third spacing of fluids

- Alkaline phoshatase, ALT, AST may be mildly elevated
- Serum calcium may be decreased in severe acute disease.
- In chronic disease, labs may be normal.
- Serum amylase
  - Preferably amylase P
  - Levels three times higher than normal strongly suggest acute pancreatitis.
- Serum lipase
  - Are also elevated and remain high for 12 days
  - Chronic pancreatitis: levels may be elevated when amylase is normal
- C-reactive protein
- Arterial blood gases if patient is dyspneic
- Kidney, ureters, bladder (KUB) plain film with the patient in the upright position
- Abdominal ultrasound as a screening test
- Abdominal CT is the most reliable imaging tool.
- In the case of biliary pancreatitis, when a dilated obstructed common bile is diagnosed and an elevated plasma bilirubin of > 5 mg/dL, an ERCP with a sphincterotomy is indicated in the first 72 hours
- Ranson's criteria—assesses severity of acute pancreatitis at the first 48 hours
  - Three or more of these criteria predict a severe course complicated by pancreatic necrosis with a sensitivity of 60% to 80%.
    - Age > 55 years
    - WBC > 16,000/mcL
    - Serum glucose > 200 mg/Dl
    - Serum lactic dehydrogenase > 350 units/L
    - Aspartate aminotransferase > 250 units/L
  - If the following develop in the first 48 hours, it indicates a worsening prognosis.
    - Hematocrit drop of more than 10 percent
    - BUN increase of > 5 mg/dL
    - Arterial PO2 of < 60 mm Hg
    - Serum calcium < 8 mg/dL
    - Base deficit > 4 mEq/L
    - Estimated fluid sequestration of > 6 L
- Mortality rates correlate with the number of criteria present (Table 9–2).

Table 9–2. Ranson's Criteria

Number of criteria	Mortality rate
0–2	1%
3–4	16%
5–6	40%
7–8	100%

Adapted from *Current Medical Diagnosis and Treatment, 2011*, by S. McPhee & M. Papadakis (Eds.), 2011, New York: McGraw-Hill, p. 667.

Differential Diagnosis

- Acute cholecystitis
- Acute intestinal obstruction
- Perforated duodenal ulcer
- Leaking aortic aneurysm
- Kidney stone
- Acute mesenteric ischemia
- Gastroenteritis
- Pancreatic cancer
- Hepatitis

Management

Nonpharmacologic Treatment
- Mild disease
  - Bowel rest
  - Bedrest
  - May or may not require NG tube
  - Resume p.o. feedings when pain resolved—begin with clear liquids, advance as tolerated
- Severe disease
  - Nasogastric tube for intractable vomiting
  - Accurate intake and output
  - Hemodynamic monitoring, central line with severe fluid loss and hypotension
  - Close monitoring of vital signs and hemodynamic status
  - Pulse oximetry
  - CT-guided aspiration of necrotic areas as needed
  - ERCP for common duct stone removal
  - Stent across pancreatic duct or orifice to reduce risk of post-ERCP pancreatitis

Pharmacologic Treatment
- Fluids—may require aggressive fluid management
- Analgesics for pain
- Antibiotics in severe cases associated with septic shock or if a phlegmon is identified on CT
- Vaspressors for refractory shock after fluid resuscitation
- Nutritional support with TPN or enteral feedings (as tolerated)
- Biliary pancreatitis associated with cholangitis
  - Ampicillin
  - Third-generation cephalosporins

Special Considerations

- Idiopathic acute pancreatitis is commonly caused by occult biliary microlithiasis and may be the result of sphincter of Oddi dysfunction that involves the pancreatic duct.
- Between 15% and 25% of cases are idiopathic.
- Smoking may increase the risk of alcoholic and idiopathic pancreatitis.

When to Consult, Refer, or Hospitalize

- Surgical consult for severe, acute pancreatitis
- Gastroenterology
- Nearly all cases of acute pancreatitis should be admitted.

Follow-up

Expected Outcomes
- Mortality rates have declined from approximately 10% to 5% since the 1980s.
- Mortality for severe pancreatitis is at least 10% to 20% for those with sterile necrosis and up to 25% for patients with infected necrosis.
- Half of deaths occur in the first 2 weeks.
- Recurrences are common in alcoholics.
- Risk of chronic pancreatitis after an episode of acute alcoholic pancreatitis is 13% in 10 years and 16% in 20 years

Complications
- Acute fluid collection—ascites
- Pseudocyst
- Intraabdominal infections
- Pancreatic necrosis
- Acute respiratory distress syndrome
- Pancreatic hemorrhage

PEPTIC ULCER DISEASE

Description

- Peptic ulcer disease (PUD) is a painful ulceration in the gastric or duodenal mucosa that occurs as a result of irritation and penetration of the protective lining of the stomach and/or intestine by acid secretion.
- Ulceration extends through the muscularis mucosa and is usually 5 mm or greater in diameter.

Etiology

- Nonsteroidal anti-inflammatory drugs (NSAIDS)
- *H. pylori* infection associated with 95% of duodenal ulcers
- Acid hypersecretory states (Zollinger-Ellison syndrome)—caused by a gastrin-secreting tumor
- Uncommon causes include cytomegalovirus (CMV), systemic mastocytosis, Crohn's disease, lymphoma, and some medications such as alendronate.
- Up to 10% are idiopathic.

Incidence and Demographics

- In the United States, approximately 500,000 new cases occur each year and 4 million relapses occur each year.
- Duodenal ulcers occur five times more frequently than gastric ulcers and are found in the duodenal bulb or pyloric channel 95% of the time.
- In the stomach, benign ulcers are located most commonly in the antrum (about 60% of the time).
- Ulcers occur slightly more commonly in men.
- May occur in any age group—however, duodenal ulcers are most common in patients age 35 to 50, and gastric ulcers are more common in the 55- to 70-year-old age group
- Duodenal ulcer disease has been declining for the past 30 years.
- Gastric ulcers are increasing because of the widespread use of NSAIDs and low-dose aspirin.

Risk Factors

- Smoking
- Long-term use of NSAIDs
- Alcohol, dietary factors, and stress do not appear linked to peptic ulcer disease.
- Aging—because of decreased gastric mucosal mechanisms
- Concurrent use of anti-platelet therapy (low-dose aspirin, clopidogrel), anticoagulation medication (warfarin), or corticosteroids

Prevention and Screening

- Weigh the benefits of NSAID therapy against the risks of cardiovascular and GI complications.
  - Use the lowest possible dose for the shortest duration possible.
- Test for and treat *H. pylori* infections.
- For patients on NSAID therapy, proton pump inhibitors (PPIs) once daily are effective for the prevention of NSAID-induced gastric and duodenal ulcers
- The prostaglandin analog misoprostol decreases the incidence of NSAID-induced gastric and duodenal ulcers by 50% to 75% when given at doses of 100 to 200 mcg 4 times daily—it is used less commonly than PPIs.
- Smoking cessation
- Take NSAIDs with food

Assessment

History
- Classic symptom is epigastric pain (dyspepsia)—present in 80% to 90% of patients
- Clinical history cannot distinguish between gastric and duodenal ulcers.
- Pain is well-localized to the epigastrum and is not severe.
- Gnawing, dull, aching, or hungerlike pain/pangs

- About 50% of patients have relief of pain with food or antacids with a recurrence of pain 2 to 4 hours later—especially with duodenal ulcers.
- Many patients report no association with food.
- Two-thirds of duodenal ulcers and one-third of gastric ulcers cause nocturnal pain that awakens the patient.
- A change from typical waxing and waning discomfort to constant or radiating pain may indicate ulcer penetration or perforation.
- Many patients have symptomatic periods that may last several weeks with asymptomatic intervals lasting months to years (called periodicity).
- Nausea and anorexia may occur with gastric ulcers.
- Severe vomiting and weight loss are not usually seen with uncomplicated PUD and may suggest gastric outlet obstruction or malignancy.

Physical Examination
- May be normal in uncomplicated disease
- Mild, localized epigastric tenderness with deep palpation
- Stool for occult blood is positive in about one-third of patients

Diagnostic Studies
- CBC
  - Anemia from acute or chronic blood loss
  - Leukocytosis may suggest ulcer penetration or perforation.
- Liver function studies
  - Elevated serum amylase may indicate perforation into the pancreas.
- Fasting (12 hours) serum gastrin level to screen for Zollinger-Ellison syndrome
  - Hold histamine receptor antagonists for 24 hours and PPIs for 1 week because they may interfere with testing and falsely elevate gastrin levels.
- Test for *H. pylori.*
  - When diagnosed by endoscopy: gastric mucosal biopsies for rapid urease test and histological examination
  - When ulcer diagnosed by upper gastrointestinal series or patient has a history of PUD, use fecal antigen assay or urea breath testing (*H. pylori* generates urease).
  - Serum testing should only be done if fecal antigen assay or urea breath testing is not available, because of its lower sensitivity/specificity.
- Upper endoscopy-esophagogastroduodenoscopy (EGD)
  - Procedure of choice for diagnosis of gastric and duodenal ulcers
  - Duodenal ulcers are rarely malignant—for that reason, biopsies of the ulcer margin are taken.
  - If no evidence of cancer, dysplasia, or atypical cells, the patient may be monitored without further biopsy.
  - If any of the above is present, a follow-up endoscopy is performed at 12 weeks after the start of therapy to document complete recovery.
  - Nonhealing ulcers are a suspicious sign of malignancy.
- Barium upper gastrointestinal series
  - Less-sensitive for the detection of ulcers and less accurate for differentiating benign from malignant tumors
  - Mostly replaced by upper endoscopy

Differential Diagnosis

- Atypical gastroesophageal reflux
- Cholecystitis
- Pancreatitis
- Diverticulitis
- Biliary tract disease
- Gastric carcinoma
- Cardiovascular disease
- Esophageal rupture
- Ruptured aortic aneurysm

Management

Nonpharmacologic Treatment
- Stop or limit NSAIDs if possible.
- Maintain optimal nutrition—balance diet at regular intervals.
- Smoking cessation
- Surgery for refractory ulcers is rarely performed—NSAID use and *H. pylori* must be ruled out.

Pharmacologic Treatment
- Treatment of *H. pylori*–associated ulcers
  - Goals of treatment are to relieve symptoms, promote ulcer healing, and eliminate *H. pylori* infection.
  - Uncomplicated ulcers should be treated for 10 to 14 days with one of the PPI-based eradication regimens.
  - Active *H. pylori*–associated ulcer
    - Regimen 1
      - Treat for 10 to 14 days
      - PPI orally 2 times daily
      - Clarithromycin 500 mg orally 2 times daily (if patient has been previously treated with a macrolide, choose another regimen)
    - Regimen 2
      - PPI orally 2 times daily
      - Bismuth subsalicylate two tablets orally 4 times daily
      - Tetracycline 500 mg orally 4 times daily
      - Metronidazole 250 mg orally 4 times daily *or*
      - Bismuth subcitrate potassium 140 mg/metronidazole
      - Tetracycline 125 mg (Pylera) 3 capsules orally 4 times daily
      - Avoid use of metronidazole in areas of high resistance or in patients who have failed therapy with a metronidazole regimen.
      - Pylera is an approved combination of bismuth subcitrate, metronidazole, and tetracycline in one capsule.
      - Preferred regimen for patients previously treated with a macrolide or with a penicillin allergy

- Regimen 3
  - PPI orally 2 times daily
  - Days 1 to 5: amoxicillin 1 gram orally 2 times daily
  - Days 6 to 10: clarithromycin 500 mg and metronidazole 500 mg, both orally twice daily
  - After completion of the eradication therapy, continue PPI once daily for 4 to 6 weeks if ulcer is > 1 cm or complicated.
  - Confirm successful treatment with urea breath test, fecal antigen test, or endoscopy at least 4 weeks after completion of antibiotic treatment and 1 to 2 weeks after PPI treatment.

- Treatment of ulcer not related to *H. pylori*
  - Look for other causes.
    - NSAIDs
    - Zollinger-Ellison syndrome
    - Gastric cancer
      - Regimen #1
        - PPI
        - Uncomplicated duodenal ulcer: treat for 4 weeks
        - Uncomplicated gastric ulcer: treat for 8 weeks
      - Regimen #2
        - H2 receptor antagonists
        - Uncomplicated duodenal ulcer: cimetidine 800 mg, ranitidine or nizatidine 300 mg, famotidine 40 mg orally once daily at bedtime for 6 weeks
        - Uncomplicated gastric ulcer: cimetidine 400 mg, ranitidine or nizatidine 150 mg, famotidine 20 mg for 8 weeks
- Complicated ulcers: PPIs are preferred choice of therapy
- All patients should be tested for *H. pylori* and treated if it is present.
- Prevention of reoccurrence
  - NSAID-induced ulcer: prophylactic therapy for high-risk patients (prior ulcer disease or ulcer complications, corticosteroid or anticoagulant use, age > 60 years, serious comorbid disease)
    - PPI once daily
    - COX-2 selective NSAID (celecoxib contraindicated in patients with increased risk of cardiovascular disease)
    - Misoprostol 200 mcg orally 4 times daily
    - Long-term maintenance therapy for patients with recurrent ulcers who are either *H. pylori* negative or have failed eradication therapy
      - PPI orally once daily
      - H2 receptor antagonist orally at bedtime: cimetidine 400 to 800 mg, nizatidine or ranitidine 150 to 300 mg, famotidine 20 to 40 mg

Table 9–3. Oral Proton Pump Inhibitors	
Omeprazole 20–40 mg	Rabeprazole 20 mg
Lansoprazole 15–30 mg	Pantoprazole 40 mg
Esomeprazole 40 mg	PPIs are administered 30 minutes before meals daily.

Special Considerations

- Pregnancy—misoprostol may induce uterine contractions leading to spontaneous abortion

When to Consult, Refer, or Hospitalize

- Refer to gastroenterologist for symptoms of GI bleeding, persistent vomiting, weight loss, severe epigastric pain, patients over age 50 with new onset dyspepsia, all gastric ulcers, persistent symptoms after therapy, or symptom recurrence.

Follow-up

Expected Outcomes
- Evaluate at 2 weeks of therapy and again after completion.
- All gastric ulcers should be reevaluated by endoscopy with cytology after treatment to document their eradication and to exclude malignancy.

Complications
- Ulcer perforation
- Penetration
- Hemorrhage
- Gastric outlet obstruction

PERITONITIS

Description

- Peritonitis is inflammation of the serosal membrane that lines the abdominal cavity and organs within it.
- The peritoneum reacts to pathologic stimuli with a predictable inflammatory response.
- Peritonitis may be infectious or sterile, depending on the underlying pathology.
- Primary, secondary, peritoneal abscess, tertiary

Etiology

- Primary (hematogenous dissemination)
  - Spontaneous bacterial peritonitis (SBP)
  - Infection of ascites fluid
  - Complication of cirrhosis
  - *Escherichia coli* most common organism
  - Also common: *Klebsiella, Pneumococcus, Entercoccus*
- Secondary (related to a pathological process)
  - Most common form encountered in clinical practice
  - Perforation or necrosis of a hollow visceral organ
  - Continuous ambulatory peritoneal dialysis (CAPD)
  - Boerhaave syndrome
  - Malignancy
  - Trauma—blunt/penetrating
  - Iatrogenic
    - Endoscopic procedures
    - Wound dehiscence
    - Inadvertent bowel injury (e.g., surgery)
  - Peptic ulcer perforation
  - Cholecystitis
  - Stone perforation from gallbladder
  - Choledochal cyst (rare)
  - Pancreatitis
  - Ischemic bowel
  - Incarcerated hernia—internal/external
  - Closed-loop obstruction
  - Crohn's disease
  - Meckel diverticulum
  - Diverticulitis
  - Ulcerative colitis
  - Crohn's disease
  - Appendicitis
  - Colonic vulvulus
  - Pelvic inflammatory disease (PID)
- Most common cause of postoperative peritonitis is anastomotic leak—5 to 7 days after surgery
- Offending organisms
  - Gram-positive organisms predominate in the upper GI tract unless patient on gastric acid suppression, then gram-negative organisms predominate
  - Contamination from a distal small bowel or colon source contains a mixture of aerobic and anaerobic bacteria—predominantly gram-negative organisms.
  - Gram-negative
    - *E. coli*
    - *Enterobacter* species
    - *Klebsiella* species
    - *Proteus* species

- Gram-positive
  - *Streptococcus* species
  - *Enterococcus* species
- Anaerobic
  - *Bacteroides fragilis*
  - *Eubacterium* species
  - *Clostridium* species
  - Anaerobic *Streptococcus* species
- Peritoneal abscess
  - Infected fluid collection contained by fibrinous exudates, omentum, adjacent visceral organs, or a combination of these
  - Occurs most frequently in the subhepatic area, pelvis, paracolic gutters, and perisplenic areas
- Tertiary peritonitis (persistent and recurrent)
  - Persistent or recurrent peritonitis following adequate therapy
  - Occurs more frequently in immunocompromised patients and those with extensive comorbidities
- Chemical peritonitis
  - Sterile
  - Irritants such as bile, blood, barium, inflammation without bacterial involvement

Incidence and Demographics

- Overall incidence varies with etiology
- Up to 30% of patients with cirrhosis will develop SBP.

Risk Factors

- Peptic ulcer disease
- Diverticulitis
- Malignancy
- Trauma
- Cirrhosis
- Pancreatitis
- Appendicitis
- Biliary disease
- PID
- Ischemic bowel
- Irritable bowel disease
- Advanced age
- See Etiology

Prevention and Screening

- Proper training when initiating CAPD
- Abstinence from alcohol with cirrhosis
- Control of peptic ulcer disease and diverticulosis
- Close monitoring of the postoperative patient

Assessment

History
- Acute abdominal pain
  - Exacerbated by motion
  - Localized, generalized; referral to shoulder, thorax
- Fever
- Nausea
- Anorexia
- Vomiting
- Constipation
- Shortness of breath

Physical Examination
- Tachycardia
- Dyspnea
- Hypotenison
- Intravascular volume depletion, vasodilation (sepsis)
- Abdominal distention
- Rebound tenderness or tenderness to palpation
- Generalized rigidity
- Decreased or absent bowel sounds
- May have hyperresonance to percussion
- Rectal exam often elicits increased abdominal pain.
- In females, vaginal and bimanual examination may indicate PID.
- Ascites

Diagnostic Studies
- CBC
  - Leukocytosis: > 11,000 cells/μL
  - With left shift
  - May see leucopenia in the immunocompromised patient
  - Hemoconcentration
- Serum chemistry
  - Elevated BUN/creatinine—prerenal because of dehydration
- Coagulation studies
  - May be prolonged if underlying liver disease or in sepsis

- Arterial blood gases
  - Metabolic and respiratory acidosis
- Liver function studies
- Amylase and lipase
  - Elevated amylase levels
- Urinalysis
  - To rule out UTI, pyelonephritis, renal stone disease
  - WBCs: Microhematuria may be present with abdominal infections.
- Stool sample
  - To identify infectious enterocolitis
- Blood cultures: aerobic and anaerobic
- β-HCG
- Peritoneal fluid
  - Leukocyte count > 10,000/mm^3
  - Lactate dehydrogenase (LDH) > 225 mu/mL
  - Protein levels greater than 1 g/dL
  - Presence of polyorganisms with gram stain or culture
- Plain films of the abdomen
  - Free air
    - Present in most cases of gastric and duodenal perforation
    - Less frequent with perforations of the small bowel or colon
    - Unusual with perforation associated with appendicitis
- Ultrasound
  - Identify ascites
  - Intraabdominal mass
  - Used for guided aspiration and placement of drains
  - Identify abscesses
- Abdominal CT scan
  - Peritoneal abscesses
  - Used when diagnosis cannot be made on clinical grounds or with plain film x-ray
- MRI
  - Limited used for identifying abscesses
- SBP peritoneal fluid
  - Protein < 1 g/dL
  - Polymorphonuclear (PMN) cell count > 250/mm^3
  - Bacteria with gram stain
  - Lactic acid level > 32 mg/dL
  - Glucose > 50 mg/dL
  - LDH < 225 mu/mL

Differential Diagnosis

- Cholecystitis
- Pancreatitis
- Divertculitis
- Colitis
- Ileitis
- PID
- Peptic ulcer disease
- Incarcerated hernia
- Intussusception
- Ulcerative colitis
- Crohn's disease

Management

Nonpharmacologic Treatment
- NPO
- Nutrition and metabolic support
- Hemodynamic monitoring
  - Vital signs
  - Pulmonary artery catheter
  - Arterial line
- Diagnostic paracentesis
- Measurement of intraabdominal pressures
- Percutaneous drainage of abscesses
  - Placement of drains
- Surgical intervention
  - Definitive source control and elimination of bacteria from the abdominal cavity
  - Open surgery
  - Laparoscopy

Pharmacologic Treatment
- SBP
  - Third-generation cephalosporin
  - Avoid aminoglycosides in patients with liver disease
  - Usually a 10-day course
- Secondary and tertiary peritonitis
  - Initially, empiric coverage
  - In community-acquired infections
    - Second- or third-generation cephalosporin
    - Quinolone with or without metronidazole
    - Broad-spectrum penicillins
- Peritoneal dialysis
  - Intraperitoneal vancomycin
  - Intraperitoneal cefazolin

Special Consideration

- Infections in the peritoneum are divided into generalized (peritonitis) and localized (intraabdominal abscess).
- If untreated, acute peritonitis may be fatal.
- Approach to treatment targets correction of the underlying process, administration of antibiotics, and supportive therapy to prevent or minimize complications from multi-organ system failure.

When to Consult, Refer, or Hospitalize

- All patients should be hospitalized.
- Surgical consult
- Infectious disease consult

Follow-up

Expected Outcomes
- Mortality rate of about 30% if diagnosis and treatment delayed
- Up to 70% of patients who survive have recurrent episodes in 1 year with mortality about 50%.
- Recurrence rate may be decreased with long-term antibiotic therapy.
- Uncomplicated, simple abscesses have a mortality rate < 5%.
- Mortality rate for intraabdominal abscesses is 10% to 20%.
  - Worse outcomes for advanced age, malnutrition, or malignancy
- Mortality may rise to 90% with quadruple organ failure.
- Patients > 65 years old have a threefold risk of developing generalized peritonitis and sepsis from gangrenous or a perforated appendicitis and perforated diverticulitis.
- Follow-up care is directed by underlying etiology.
- Patients with perforated PUD, Crohn's disease, or pancreatitis often require lifelong medical therapy.

Complications
- Surgical site infection/dehiscence
- Impaired wound healing
- Complications related to surgical intervention
  - Bleeding
  - Erosion
  - Fistula formation
    - Enterocutaneous
    - High output
  - Bowel obstruction
- Abdominal compartment syndrome
- SBP

SMALL BOWEL OBSTRUCTION

Description

- Small bowel obstruction (SBO) is blockage of the lumen of the small intestine that disrupts normal bowel function.
- Leads to proximal distention of the intestine because of accumulation of GI secretions and swallowed air
- The bowel dilatation causes increased secretion of intestinal cells, which causes fluid accumulation with increased peristalsis above and below the obstruction that manifests as frequent loose stools and flatus early in the course.
- May be a mechanical cause or because of an ileus in which there is no structural problem

Etiology

- Postsurgical adhesions are the most common cause.
- Malignant tumor
- Hernia
- Inflammatory bowel disease
- Volvulus
- Trauma
- Feces
- Foreign bodies
- Intussusception

Incidence and Demographics

- Accounts for approximately 20% of hospital admissions
- Mortality for adhesive SBO is 1% to 2%.
- The presence of strangulation increases the mortality to about 20%.
- The incidence of readmission for SBO following surgery in the first few postoperative weeks is 5% to 25%.

Risk Factors

- Previous abdominal surgery
- Hernia
- Malignancy
- Presence of inflammatory bowel disease
- Ingestion of foreign body
- Constipation

Prevention and Screening

- Identify patients at high risk.
- Treatment of tumors, hernia
- Avoid ingestion of foreign bodies.
- Avoid constipation, impaction
- Close monitoring of inflammatory bowel disease

Assessment

History
- History of abdominal surgery
- Presence of inflammatory bowel disease
- Cramping mid-abdominal pain
  - Pain becomes less severe as distention progresses.
- With strangulation, pain is more localized, without the colicky component.
- Obstipation, failure to pass flatus
- Partial obstruction—watery, mucuoid diarrhea
- Symptoms of dehydration

Physical Examination
- Episodic vomiting
  - Proximal obstruction
  - Distal obstruction
- High-pitched, tinkling bowel sounds
- Abdominal distention—hallmark finding
- Tenderness, rigidity, fever, and signs of shock indicate the presence of a contaminated peritoneum.
- Visible peristalisis

Diagnostic Studies
- CBC
  - Leukocytosis with left shift
  - Normal WBC does not exclude strangulation
- Serum amylase
  - May be elevated
- Plain film supine and upright abdominal radiography
  - Distended fluid- and gas-filled loops of small intestine in a "stepladder" pattern
  - Complete obstruction when gas is absent in distal intestine
- Abdominal ultrasound
  - Highly specific for SBO
  - Abdominal CT
  - Used to differentiate adynamic ileus, partial obstruction, and complete obstruction
  - Small bowel feces sign
    · Presence of fecal matter mingled with gas bubbles in the lumen of dilated loops of small intestine
    · Seen in a small percentage of patients

Differential Diagnosis

- Alcoholic ketoacidosis
- Acute appendicitis
- Cholangitis
- Cholecystitis
- Constipation
- Endometriosis
- Gastroenteritis
- Large bowel obstruction
- Ovarian torsion
- Pancreatitis
- Urinary tract infection
- Adynamic ileus
- Intestinal pseudo-obstruction

Management

Nonpharmacologic Treatment
- NG tube
- NPO
- 20% to 30% of patients can be managed medically without surgical intervention.
- Foley catheter
- Surgical intervention
  - Always indicated for strangulating SBO
  - Laparoscopic
  - Open exploratory laparatomy

Pharmacologic Treatment
- Restoration of fluid and electrolytes
- Broad-spectrum antibiotics for strangulating SBO
  - Cefoxitin
  - Cefotetan

Special Considerations

- Key considerations for management
  - Recognize the obstruction.
  - Identify partial from complete obstruction.
  - Differentiate simple from strangulating SBO.
  - Determine underlying cause.
- The abdominal pain becomes constant and diffuse as distention develops.
- Intestinal pseudo-obstruction is a chronic motility disorder that mimics SBO and is exacerbated with narcotic use.
- Adynamic ileus is mediated through the sympathoadrenal system and may occur after any peritoneal insult.
  - Occurs to some degree after any abdominal surgery

When to Consult, Refer, or Hospitalize

- Surgical consult when SBO diagnosed
- Consult gastroenterology
- All patients with suspected SBO should be hospitalized for evaluation.

Follow-up

Expected Outcomes
- About one-third of patients with SBO will recover without surgical intervention.
- Resolution is marked by decreasing abdominal distention, passing of flatus or bowel contents, decreasing NG outputs, and ability to tolerate oral intake.

Complications
- Sepsis
- Intraabdominal abscess
- Wound dehiscence
- Aspiration
- Short bowel syndrome—following multiple surgeries
- Death

ULCERATIVE COLITIS

Description

- Ulcerative colitis (UC) is a chronic, relapsing inflammatory disease of the colon and rectal mucosa, resulting in diffuse friability and erosions with bleeding.
- May be limited to the rectum or involve the entire colon
- Characterized by acute exacerbations and remissions

Etiology

- Cause unknown, but genetic and environmental factors are implicated
  - Genetic
    - Occurs in families
    - Genetic markers linked to UC
  - Environmental
    - Diet
      - High sugar content
      - Low-fiber
    - Accutane use
  - Autoimmune phenomena

Incidence and Demographics

- Typically occurs between the ages of 15 and 35, with a second smaller peak in the 70-year-old age group
- May occur as early as 5 years of age
- Occurrence is 30% higher in women
- In the United States, new diagnoses are 10–12 per 100,000 persons annually
- Incidence lower in Hispanic, Asian, and Native American populations
- Rates are higher among people living in an urban environment than those living in a rural setting.
- Higher incidence in those with a higher socioeconomic status

Risk Factors

- Tenfold increased risk when first-degree relatives are affected
- Jewish descent
- Urban dwellers
- High-sugar, low-fiber diet

Prevention and Screening

- High-fiber, low-refined-sugar diet
- Familial predisposition

Assessment

History
- Bloody diarrhea
- Crampy lower abdominal pain
  - Typically, left lower quadrant
  - Relieved by defecation
- Fecal urgency
- Tenesmus
- Noturnal diarrhea
- Severe cases
  - Fever
  - Anemia
  - Anorexia
  - Weight loss
- Extra-intestinal symptoms occur in approximately 25% of cases.
  - Oligoarticular arthritis
  - Ankylosing spondylitis
  - Uveitis
  - Oral aphthous ulcers
  - Pyoderma gangrenosum

- Erythema nodosum
- Uric acid renal stones
- Digital examination may reveal bright-red blood and mucus.

- Extra-intestinal manifestations
  - Skin rashes
  - Iritis

Diagnostic Studies
- CBC
  - Anemia
  - Leukocytosis
- Erythrocyte sedimentation rate
  - Elevated
- C-reactive protein
  - Elevated
- Serum chemistry with liver function studies
  - Albumin may be low.
- Stool studies
  - Used to exclude infection
- Culture
- Ova and parasites
  - C. *dificile* toxin
- Colonoscopy
  - Should not be done in severe active disease because of the risk of perforation
  - Performed when symptoms improve
- Sigmoidoscopy
  - Diagnostic
  - Friable and inflamed mucosa
  - Purulent exudates and ulcers
  - Biopsy to differentiate from infectious colitis
- Plain abdominal radiographs
  - To exclude toxic megacolon
  - Atonic and dilated colon > 6 cm is associated with symptoms of toxicity.

Differential Diagnosis

- Crohn's disease
- Trauma
- Enterocolitis
- Infectious colitis
- Irritable bowel syndrome
- Ischemic colitis
- Appendicitis
- Hemolytic uremic syndrome
- Radiation-induced proctitis
- Henoch-Schönlein purpura
- Rectal cancer
- Colon cancer

Management

Nonpharmacologic Treatment
- Well-balanced, high-fiber diet
- Avoid caffeine and gas-producing foods
- Surgical intervention
  - Curative with proctocolectomy
    - Ileal pouch–anal anastomosis—high rate of fecal continence
  - Indications
    - Severe colitis that does not respond to treatment
    - Toxic megacolon that fails to improve in 48 to 72 hours
    - High-grade dysplasia
    - Severe hemorrhage
    - Obstruction or stricture with suspicion of malignancy

Pharmacologic Treatment
- Fiber supplements or bulk forming agents if not achieved with diet
  - Bran powder
  - Psyllium
  - Methylcellulose
- Anti-inflammatory agents in mild disease to induce remission
  - 5-aminosalicylic acid (5-ASA)
    - Sulfasalazine 1 to 2 g p.o. 2 times daily
      - Hypersensitivy and intolerance limits its use.
    - Mesalamine 800 to 1,600 mg p.o. 3 times daily
  - Corticosteroids
    - Prednisone 40 to 60 mg p.o. daily as starting dose
    - Hospitalized patients
      - Hydrocortisone 100 mg IV 3 times daily *or*
      - Methylprednisolone 25 mg IV 2 times daily
  - Cyclosporine
    - 2 to 4 mg/kg/day IV as a bridge to 6-MP/AZA in patients with severe disease who have failed steroid therapy
    - Monitor levels to reduce the risk of nephrotoxicity.
    - Patients with low serum cholesterol may be at risk for seizures.
    - All patients at risk for infection
  - 6-Mercaptopurine (6-MP) and Azathioprine (AZA)
    - 6-MP
      - 1 to 1.5 mg/kg/day p.o.
    - AZA
      - 2 to 3 mg/kg/day p.o.
    - Used for maintaining remission
    - Slow onset
    - Patients at risk for life-threatening leucopenia
    - WBC should be checked within 2 weeks of starting or stopping these medications.
  - Infliximab
    - 5 to 10 mg/kg infusion at 0, 2, and 6 weeks as induction therapy, then 5 mg/kg IV infusion as maintenance
- Treatment length is dictated by symptoms

Special Considerations

- Pregnancy
  - Flares typically occur in the first trimester.
  - Should postpone pregnancy until 1 year after remission
  - May use sulfasalazine with folic acid during pregnancy to maintain remission
- Prednisone is safe in pregnancy; immunosuppressants are not.

When to Consult, Refer, or Hospitalize

- Consult gastroenterology for initial diagnosis and management.
- Consult general surgery for intervention when severe disease does not respond to treatment.
- Hospitalize for fulminant colitis with symptoms of high fever, sepsis, profuse bloody diarrhea, abdominal pain, and dehydration.

Follow-up

Expected Outcomes
- Acute exacerbations are usually controlled with medication, with lifelong exacerbations.
- Hospitalization is not usually required.
- Severe disease resistant to therapy may be cured with surgery in about 20% of cases.
- Colon cancer screening and biopsy every 1 to 2 years, beginning 7 to 8 years after disease onset
  - Colon cancer incidence triples in patients with UC for > 10 years.

Complications
- Toxic megacolon
- Perforation
- Strictures
- Anemia
- Colorectal cancer

REFERENCES

Barkley, T., & Myers, C. (2008). *Practice guidelines for acute care nurse practitioners.* St. Louis, MO: Saunders.

Bartlett, J., Auwaerter, P., & Pham, P. (2010). *Antibiotic guide, diagnosis, and treatment of infectious diseases.* Sudbury, MA: Jones & Bartlett Learning.

Beers, M., Porter, R., Jones, T., Kaplan, J., & Berkwits, M. (Eds.). (2006). *The Merck manual of diagnosis and therapy.* Whitehouse Station, NJ: Merck Research Laboratories.

Cappell, M. S., & Batke, M. (2008). Mechanical obstruction of the small bowel and colon. *Medical Clinics of North America, 92*(3), 575–97, viii.

Chait, M. (2007). Lower gastrointestinal bleeding in the elderly. *Annals of Long-Term Care, 15*(4), 147–154.

Chang, Y. W. (2006). Indication of treatment for esophageal varices: Who and when. *Digestive Endoscopy, 18*(1), 10–15.

Cooper, D., Kraink, A., Lubner, S., & Reno, H. (Eds.) (2007). *The Washington manual of medical therapeutics* (32nd ed.). Philadelphia: Wolters Kluwer/Lippincott Williams & Wilkins.

Diaz, J. J., Bockari, F., Mowery, N. T., Ocosta, J. A., Block, E. F., Bromberg, W. J ., et al. (2008). Guidelines for management of small bowel obstruction. *Journal of Trauma, 64*(6), 1651–1664.

Fauci, A., Braunwald, E., Kasper, D., Hauser, S., Longo, D., Jameson, J., & Loscalzo, J. (Eds.). (2008) *Harrison's principles of internal medicine* (17th ed.) New York: McGraw Hill.

Garcia-Tsao, G., Sanyal, A.J., Grace, N.D., & Carey, W. D. (2007). Prevention and management of gastroesophageal varices and variceal hemorrhage in cirrhosis. *American Journal of Gastroenterology, 102*(9), 2086–2102.

Habermann, T., & Ghosh, A. (2008). *Mayo Clinic internal medicine concise textbook.* Rochester, MN: Mayo Clinic Scientific Press.

Marini, J., & Wheeler, A. (2010). *Critical care medicine, the essentials.* Philadelphia: Wolters Kluwer/Lippincott Williams & Wilkins.

McKean, S., Bennett, A., & Halasyamani, L. (Eds.). (2008). *Hospital medicine.* Philadelphia: Wolters Kluwer/Lippincott Williams & Wilkins.

McPhee, S., & Papadakis, M. (2011). (Eds.). *Current medical diagnosis and treatment.* New York: McGraw Hill.

Multignani, M., Iacopini, F., & Perri V. (2009). Endoscopic gallbladder drainage for acute cholecystitis—technical and clinical results. *Endoscopy, 41*(6), 539–546.

Society of American Gastrointestinal and Endoscopic Surgeons. (2007). *Guidelines for diagnostic laparoscopy.* Retrieved from http://www.sages.org/publication/id/12

Wells, B., DiPiro, J., Schwinghammer, T., & DiPiro, C. (Eds.). (2009). *Pharmacotherapy handbook.* New York: McGraw Hill.

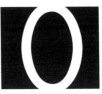

Hematologic Disorders

Pamela Smith, MSN, RN, ACNP-BC, CCRN
Elizabeth Petit de Mange, PhD, MSN, BSN, NP-BC, RN; and
Tiffany Boysen, MSN, APRN-BC, CCRN

GENERAL APPROACH

- Most common anemia in all age groups is iron deficiency anemia.
- Do not assume that anemia in a patient with chronic inflammatory disease is "anemia of chronic disease."
- Do not begin treatment for B_{12} deficiency without assessing and treating folate deficiency.
- Hematopoiesis is slowed in older adults when the presence and number of progenitor cells decline; 60% of all anemias are seen in people over age 65.

Definitions

- *Anemia:* Hematocrit (Hct) < 37% for females, < 42% for males; or Hgb < 12 for females, < 14 for males, or a red blood cell (RBC) count < 4.0 x 10^6/mcL for females and < 4.5 x 10^6/mcL for men
- *Mean corpuscular (cell) volume* (MCV): represents the size of the RBC and is calculated from the hemoglobin, hematocrit, or RBC count. Used in differentiation of types of anemia.
- *Ferritin:* represents iron storage in the serum. May be elevated during infection or chronic inflammation and decreased in iron deficiency.
- *Hypochromic:* erythrocytes containing decreased level of Hgb, causing the cells to appear "paler" on smear

- *Hyperchromic:* erythrocytes containing increased level of Hgb, causing cells to appear "darker" on smear
- *Macrocytic anemia:* decreased Hct/Hgb/RBC with associated MCV > 100
- *Megaloblastic anemia:* anemia characterized by a large, nucleated, embryonic type of cell that is a precursor of erythrocytes in an abnormal erythropoietic process seen almost exclusively in pernicious anemia
- *Microcytic anemia:* decreased Hct/Hgb/RBC with associated MCV < 80
- *Normocytic anemia:* decreased Hct/Hgb/RBC with associated MCV 80–100
- *RDW:* red blood cell distribution width, a statistical index of the variation in red cell widths
- *Total iron binding capacity (TIBC):* Amount of iron in serum plus amount of transferrin available in serum (transferrin is a transport protein that regulates iron absorption); decreased in anemia of chronic disease

RED FLAGS

- Blood values helpful in identifying anemias can be found in Table 10–2
- Anemia in the presence of splenomegaly requires further diagnostic evaluation
- *Deficiency of coagulant factor VIII (Hemophilia A) or factor IX (Hemophilia B)* is rare and presents in males during first few years of life as excessive bruising, bleeding after circumcision, bleeding hours or days after injury, hematuria, or hemorrhage or hematoma after minor injury. Laboratory results include normal platelet count, partial thromboplastin time (PTT) greatly prolonged, factor VIII low in hemophilia A, factor IX low in hemophilia-B. Refer to hematologist for management

Table 10–1. Normal Ranges for RBC Studies

Test	Females	Males
Hematocrit	36%–48%	40%–53%
Hemoglobin	12–16 g/dL	13.5–17.7 g/dL
RBC (10^6/μl)	4.0–5.4	4.5–6.0
MCV	80–100 fL	80–100 fL
MCH	26–34 pg	26–34 pg
MCHC	31%–37% g/dL	31%–37% g/dL
Reticulocyte count	0.5%–1.5% of RBC	0.5%–1.5% of RBC
Serum iron	50–170 mcg/dL	65–175 mcg/dL
TIBC	250–450 mcg/dL	250–450 mcg/dL
Ferritin	10–120 ng/mL (avg. 55)	20–250 ng/mL (avg. 125)

Note. MCH = mean corpuscular hemoglobin; MCHC = mean corpuscular hemoglobin concentration; RBC = red blood cells; TIBC = total iron binding capacity; fl = femtoliter (10^{-15} liter); pg = pictogram (10^{-12} g); ng = nanogram (10^{-9} g); μl= microliter (10^{-6})

Reprinted from *Family Nurse Practitioner: Nursing Review and Resource Manual* by E. Blunt (Ed.), 2009, Silver Spring, MD: American Nurses Credentialing Center, p. 797.

Table 10–2. Blood Values Helpful in Differentiating Anemias

Anemia	MCV	Appearance of red cell
Iron deficiency	< 80 fL	Normocytic or microcytic, hypochromic
Folate deficiency	> 100 fL	Macrocytic, hyperchromic
Vitamin B$_{12}$	> 100 fL	Macrocytic, hyperchromic
Chronic disease	Normal	Normochromic, normocytic or microcytic
Sideroblastic	< 80 fL	Hypochromic
Sickle cell	< 80 fL	Sickle cells, normochromic
G6PD	Normal	Heinz bodies, bite cells, blister cells
Thalassemia	< 80 fL	Microcytic
Drug-induced	Normal	Normocytic, normochromic
Aplastic	Normal	Normocytic, normochromic
Post-hemorrhagic	Normal	Normocytic, normochromic

Reprinted from *Family Nurse Practitioner: Nursing Review and Resource Manual*, by E. Blunt (Ed.), 2009, Silver Spring, MD: American Nurses Credentialing Center, p. 797.

NORMOCYTIC ANEMIAS

ANEMIA OF CHRONIC DISEASE

Description

- A mild hypoproliferative anemia associated with chronic disease, infections, and malignancies that has persisted for > 1 to 2 months; probably a consequence of long-term disease with inflammatory process
- Diagnosis of exclusion from active blood loss or production abnormalities associated with iron or folate intake

Etiology

- The pathophysiology of anemia of chronic disease is not well understood, but may be the result of decreased RBC life span, erythropoietin reduction, and problems of iron transfer.
- Occurs as a result of renal disease, liver disease, endocrine disorders, rheumatoid arthritis, infections, and some forms of cancer

Incidence and Demographics

- The second most common anemia in the world; incidence parallels the rate of chronic inflammatory disease
- The most common anemia in older adults

Risk Factors

- Chronic diseases: renal, liver, endocrine disease; rheumatoid arthritis; infection; and some cancers

Prevention and Screening

- Attention to good nutrition
- CBC screening for those with chronic disease

Assessment

History
- Chronic disease
- Fatigue, dyspnea on exertion, irritability, listlessness, easy fatigability

Physical Examination
- Perform a complete physical exam for signs of the underlying disease
- Signs of anemia, depending on severity: pallor, tachycardia, tachypnea on exertion

Diagnostic Studies
- CBC, reticulocyte count, iron studies (serum iron, TIBC, ferritin); studies pertinent to underlying disorder; repeat iron studies important for diagnosis and management
- Characteristic labs: Hgb usually 8 to 12 g/dL, Hct 25% to 35%, MCV 75 to 85 as Hgb falls < 10, often low serum iron and TIBC, and normal or increased ferritin (TIBC is increased and ferritin decreased in iron deficiency), serum erythropoietin normal, but not generally assessed

Differential Diagnosis

- Iron deficiency anemia
- Multifactorial anemia
- Chronic renal insufficiency
- Liver disease (usually alcohol-related)
- Post-hemorrhagic anemia
- Endocrine disorders: hypothyroidism
- AIDS
- Aplastic anemia

Management

Nonpharmacologic Treatment
- Treat underlying disease
- Ensure appropriate nutrition
- Transfusion only in severe, symptomatic cases

Pharmacologic Treatment
- Recombinant erythropoietin (Epogen, Procrit) in selected patients

How Long to Treat
- Treatment required as long as underlying disease and anemia persist

Special Considerations

- A similar profile to iron deficiency may eventually develop, with patient becoming mildly microcytic and hypochromic as Hgb falls to < 10 g/dL.
- Patients with AIDS often have anemia of chronic disease. As disease progresses, pancytopenia may occur because of marrow damage. At that point, checking serum erythropoietin level may help determine if patient will benefit from recombinant erythropoietin injections.
- Anemia of renal disease relates to severity of renal failure, because of decreased erythropoietin production; may benefit from erythropoietin
- In patients with diabetes mellitus, anemia is frequently severe early in the disease process.

When to Consult, Refer, or Hospitalize

- Refer if diagnosis is questionable.
- Refer to confirm underlying cause (e.g., rheumatologist for collagen or vascular problem, oncologist for cancer, nephrologist for renal disease, infectious disease specialist for infections)

Follow-up

- Frequent monitoring of blood pressure, CBC, iron studies with recombinant erythropoietin therapy

Expected Outcomes
- Anemia will improve or worsen as the underlying disease improves or progress
- Patient can often tolerate fairly low Hct and Hgb, as low as 30/10, if they develop gradually

Complications
- Possible exacerbation of cardiopulmonary disease, particularly in the elderly (anemia results in less oxygen delivered to tissues, heart rate and cardiac output increase to compensate, heart may begin to fail)

APLASTIC ANEMIA

Description

- Aplastic anemia is characterized by intrinsic bone marrow dysfunction or failure; pluripotent stem cell expression is impaired, so pancytopenia with hypercellularity of the bone marrow is seen.
- Intrinsic marrow dysfunction produces defective RBC synthesis; it produces anemia, neutropenia, thrombocytopenia, and pancytopenia.

Etiology

- Autoimmune suppression of hematopoiesis is most common cause, but it may be precipitated by viral illness, autoimmune suppression, drug or chemical exposure, tumor, radiation, or an inherited disorder.
- Inherited: Fanconi's anemia, Schwachman-Diamond syndrome

Incidence and Demographics

- Not common in the United States
- 50% idiopathic; 20% drug or chemical exposure (chloramphenicol—rare); 10% viral

Risk Factors

- Family history, some medications (anticonvulsants, antibiotics, gold), radiation, exposure to some toxic chemicals such as insecticides, herbicides, organic solvents, paint removers, and others

Prevention and Screening

- Most cases cannot be prevented.
- There are no general screening methods recommended.
- Individuals should avoid contact exposure to certain chemicals such as insecticides, herbicides, organic solvents, paint removers, and other toxic chemicals. This is especially important for those who have already had aplastic anemia caused by toxic chemicals. Recurrent exposure may increase the risk of a reoccurrence of the disease.
- Individuals who have had exposure to toxic chemicals or have had aplastic anemia in the past should have regular physical examinations.
- Individuals should report the following signs and symptoms early: fever, fatigue, weight loss, weakness, sore throat, dyspnea, palpitations, and bleeding.

Assessment

History
- Insidious onset of fever, fatigue, weight loss, weakness, sore throat, dyspnea, palpitations
- Bleeding problems such as menorrhagia, rectal bleed, epistaxis
- History of potential sources of exposure to toxic agents: medications, chemical exposure at work, hobbies, and so forth
- History of associated anomalies: kidney, hypospadias, short stature

Physical Examination
- General: pallor, petechiae, bruises
- Thorough physical for tumors, signs of infection, signs of bleeding
  - Cardiac exam: systolic ejection murmur may be present
  - Eyes: retinal flame hemorrhage
  - Rectal: occult or rectal bleeding

Diagnostic Studies
- Pancytopenia is pathognomonic
- Severe anemia, decreased reticulocytes
- CBC with differential, peripheral smear, bleeding studies, TIBC, urinalysis, bone marrow, liver function, CT of thymus as indicated
- Lab results: normochromic, normocytic anemia; TIBC normal; hematuria
- Bone marrow shows hypoplasia, fatty infiltration

Differential Diagnosis

- Leukemia
- Hypersplenism
- Systemic lupus erythematosus (SLE)
- Myelodysplasia
- Sepsis

Management

Nonpharmacologic Treatment
- Education and supportive care
- A well-balanced diet decreases risk of infection
- Manage underlying cause
- Perform human leukocyte antigen (HLA) testing on patients and immediate families for inherited conditions

Pharmacologic Treatment
- Immunosuppression therapy, oxygen
- Severe cases: bone marrow transplant is considered (may be age-dependent)
- May consider stem cell transplant
- RBC transfusions should only be used when absolutely necessary.
- Platelet infusions if platelet count drops below 10,000/mm^3

How Long to Treat
- Lifelong treatment may be required unless effective bone marrow transplant is curative

Special Considerations

- Must avoid further exposure to etiologic agents

When to Consult, Refer, or Hospitalize

- Refer immediately to hematologist when diagnosis is suspected; work with hematologist throughout therapy

Follow-up

Expected Outcomes
- Often favorable outcome depending on age and treatment response
- Untreated cases are fatal; successful bone marrow transplant is curative.

Complications
- Infection, leukemia, heart failure, hemorrhage

HYPOCHROMIC ANEMIAS

IRON DEFICIENCY ANEMIA

Description

- Microcytic, hypochromic anemia because of decreased iron stores, poor iron utilization, or poor iron reutilization

Etiology

- Hemorrhage, occult malignancy, increased need (pregnancy and growth spurts), impaired absorption, inadequate dietary intake

Incidence and Demographics

- Prevalent in all ages and populations in the United States
- Seen in 7% to 10% of adult population; 10% to 20% of infants and toddlers; 15% to 45% of women who are pregnant; 20% women overall
- More common in women than men because of menstruation and pregnancy

Risk Factors

- Insufficient intake of iron from low dietary intake, poor bioavailability of the dietary iron, or malabsorption. Low intake is the most common etiologic factor seen in infants, toddlers, teens, older adults, and those who are institutionalized
- Increased loss of iron because of disease process, including Meckel's diverticulum, peptic ulcer disease, polyps, hemangiomas, parasitic infections, or cow's milk enteropathy. Losses may also occur from menorrhagia, chronic use of NSAIDS, uncommonly recurrent epistaxis, and possibly strenuous exercise
- Conditions such as achlorhydria, gastric surgery, celiac disease, or pica, which cause impaired absorption
- Conditions such as neoplasm, duodenal or gastric ulcers, diverticulosis, or ulcerative colitis
- Repeated blood donations

Prevention and Screening

- Dietary supplements if patient has risk factors
- Selective screening for at-risk populations such as some older adults and women who are menstruating

Assessment

History
- Initially asymptomatic; insidious onset of gradually progressing fatigue, dyspnea on exertion, irritability, listlessness, easy fatigability, dysphagia, postural hypotension
- Possible palpitations, shortness of breath, impaired muscular performance
- Diet history: low in iron, pica, drug or chemical exposure
- Family history of iron deficiency anemia
- Review of systems (ROS) for blood loss, symptoms of gastrointestinal problems, neoplasms

Physical Examination
- Observe for pallor or chlorosis (peculiar greenish pallor)
- Angular stomatitis, ulcerations or fissure of the mouth
- Ozena—chronic atrophy of the nasal mucosa
- Dry skin and mucous membranes
- Koilonychia—thinning and flattening of the nails and then spooning
- Auscultate heart for systolic flow murmurs
- Splenomegaly
- Brittle hair, tachycardia, tachypnea

Diagnostic Studies
- CBC with differential and smear, TIBC, serum iron, ferritin, special tests to determine underlying bleed
- Laboratory findings (see the following table): Hgb < 12 g/dL in adults; serum ferritin level < 10 nanograms/mL in women and < 20 nanograms/mL in men; low Hct; "pencil cells" on smear, MCV and MCH decrease, RDW > 15, increased TIBC > 400 mcg/dL, low serum iron < 30 mcg/dL; transferrin saturation < 15%; MCV < 80 mcg/dL; reticulocyte count elevated in cases of blood loss, decreased in iron deficiency; increased platelet count > 400,000; bone marrow absent for iron staining
- Bone marrow aspiration if severe, questionable diagnosis, or resistant to treatment

Table 10-3. Comparison of Differential Laboratory Findings in Microcytic Anemias

Laboratory Finding	Thalassemia Trait	Lead Poisoning	Iron Deficiency	Anemia of Chronic Disease
Hgb	Decreased	Decreased	Decreased	Decreased
MCV	Decreased	Decreased	Decreased	Normal
Ferritin	Normal	Normal	Decreased	Increased
FEP (free erythrocyte porphyrins)	Normal	Very High	High	Mild Increase

Reprinted from *Family Nurse Practitioner: Nursing Review and Resource Manual*, by E. Blunt (Ed.), 2009, Silver Spring, MD: American Nurses Credentialing Center, p. 804.

Differential Diagnosis

- Thalassemia
- G6PD deficiency
- Infection
- Cancer
- Chronic diseases
- Lead poisoning
- Hypothyroidism
- Renal failure

Management

Nonpharmacologic Treatment
- Diagnose and treat underlying cause
- Normal dietary intake meets only daily losses, not therapeutic; RDA iron = 10 mg/day for men and up to 15 mg/day for women and children; must increase iron intake
- No dairy product or antacid within 2 hours of oral iron
- Symptomatic care of treatment side effects (constipation, nausea, cramps, diarrhea)

Pharmacologic Treatment
- Oral iron supplements: up to 300 mg of elemental iron divided 3 to 4 times a day for adolescents and adults
  - 325 mg of ferrous sulfate contains 65 mg of elemental iron
  - Oral iron therapy is safer and less costly than IM or IV iron
  - Reduce dose to decrease GI side effects; no real benefit to more expensive preparations
  - Vitamin C will help increase absorption; meals will decrease absorption by up to 50%
  - Concurrent use of stool softener will help with GI side effects
- Parenteral iron if poor absorption or inability to tolerate oral iron
  - IV iron dextran—side effect of anaphylaxis
  - Test dose of 25 mg in 50 mL of normal saline should be infused over 5 to 10 minutes
  - Have methylprednisolone, diphenhydramine, and 1:1,000 epinephrine 1 mg ampule immediately available during and after infusion
- Blood transfusion is not recommended for iron supplementation

How Long to Treat
- Treat until deficiency corrected; expect to see improvement within 4 weeks; return to baseline blood levels in 8 weeks; continue therapy 3 to 6 months to replace iron stores

Special Considerations

- If unresponsive to therapy, reevaluate underlying cause and compliance

When to Consult, Refer, or Hospitalize

- Refer to hematologist if patient is not responsive to treatment or underlying cause cannot be determined

Follow-up

- Follow-up recommended after 1 month and every 6 months if resolved, until stable

Expected Outcomes
- Cure expected; increase in Hgb of 1 g/week expected
- Prolonged course of treatment may be required because of noncompliance

Complications
- May have unidentified underlying source of bleeding
- Heart failure (late, untreated)

MEGALOBLASTIC ANEMIAS

VITAMIN B$_{12}$ DEFICIENCY

Description

- A megaloblastic, macrocytic anemia in which MCV is > 100 resulting from a deficiency of intrinsic factor, which leads to inadequate vitamin B$_{12}$ absorption (< 170 picograms/mL) and impaired red blood cell synthesis

Etiology

- Pernicious anemia: Caused by congenital enzyme deficiency so B$_{12}$ cannot be absorbed; overgrowth of intestinal organisms, autoimmune reaction involving gastric parietal cells, gastrectomy
- Malabsorption: GI parasites, GI surgery, Crohn's disease, chronic alcoholism, strict vegetarians (rare)
- In older adults the stomach is less acidic; B$_{12}$ needs acid to be absorbed

Incidence and Demographics

- Onset at age 50–60; median age at diagnosis = 60
- Women slightly > men

Risk Factors

- Age (commonly presents around age 60), family history of pernicious anemia
- Chronic alcoholism
- GI surgery, Crohn's disease, immunologic diseases

Prevention and Screening

- Adequate dietary intake—meat and dairy products
- Routine screening for B_{12} level in dementia and malnutrition

Assessment

History
- Insidious onset of peripheral numbness, personality changes, memory loss, anorexia, diarrhea, glossitis, distal paresthesias, ataxia
- Assess for risk factors, underlying causes
- Should be considered in differential diagnosis of dementia

Physical Examination
- Characteristic beefy red, shiny tongue
- Abdominal tenderness, organomegaly, tachycardia, tachypnea, pallor, hepatosplenomegaly
- Neurologic signs: numbness, sensory ataxia, limb weakness, spasticity, changes in deep tendon reflexes, decreased vibratory sense, impaired proprioception, impaired fine motor movement, positive Romberg test, progressive mental status impairment

Diagnostic Studies
- CBC with differential
- Peripheral smear
- LDH
- Serum B_{12} levels
- Consider Schilling test with and without intrinsic factor to test B12 absorption
- Consider bone marrow aspiration
- Laboratory results: serum B_{12} levels < 170 picograms/mL; Hct decreased; MCV markedly elevated; decreased reticulocyte count; WBC and platelet count reduced, elevated LDH
- On smear: A large, nucleated, embryonic type of cell that is a precursor of erythrocytes in an abnormal erythropoietic process
- Schilling's test documents decreased oral B_{12} absorption

Differential Diagnosis

- Folic acid deficiency
- Myelodysplasia
- Liver dysfunction
- Side effects of medications
- Alcoholism
- Bleeding or hemorrhage
- Hypothyroidism

Management

Nonpharmacologic Treatment
- Education and supportive therapy; maintain balanced diet, good health and hygiene

Pharmacologic Treatment
- Initial: 800 to 1000 mcg of vitamin B_{12} IM daily for 4 to 8 weeks
- Maintenance: 100 to 1000 mcg monthly
- Oral cobalamin 1000 mcg daily is alternative replacement.
- May require iron supplementation for the first month of therapy during rapid regeneration of RBCs

How Long to Treat
- Lifelong

Special Considerations

- If patient presents with abnormal neurologic signs, the symptoms might be irreversible.
- Might have hypokalemia in first week of treatment
- Do not begin treatment for B_{12} deficiency without assessing for and treating folate deficiency also.
- Check serum B_{12} levels in patients with distal polyneuropathies (even if no anemia or macrocytosis seen).
- Oral B-complex vitamin only valuable when B_{12} deficiency is nutritional

When to Consult, Refer, or Hospitalize

- Refer as needed for underlying cause; refer for follow-up endoscopy every 5 years to rule out malignancy

Follow-up

Expected Outcomes
- Response rapid; good prognosis if treatment within 6 months of neurological signs

Complications
- Stomach cancer
- Permanent central nervous system (CNS) signs or symptoms

FOLIC ACID DEFICIENCY

Description

- Anemia as a result of inadequate folic acid present for DNA synthesis and RBC maturation
- Lack of folic acid (folate) causes macrocytic, normochromic, and megaloblastic anemia
- Also associated with increased incidence of embryonic neural tube defects

Etiology

- Folic acid–deficient diet, malabsorption syndromes, or increased demand for folic acid (pregnancy)

Incidence and Demographics

- All races and age groups
- Most common at ages 60 to 70 years

Risk Factors

- Pregnancy, elderly, alcoholism
- Malnourished or malabsorption syndromes; hemodialysis patients
- Medications that interfere with folic acid absorption (e.g., trimethoprim, phenytoin, oral birth control pills, phenobarbital, sulfamethoxazole/trimethoprim, sulfasalazine)

Prevention and Screening

- Adequate intake of folic acid: 400 mcg for women who are pregnant, 200 mcg for all others

Assessment

History
- Indigestion, constipation, diarrhea, anorexia, lethargy
- Fatigue, weakness, headache, dizziness, dyspnea on exertion, depression, apathy

Physical Examination
- Pallor, atrophic glossitis (red, shiny tongue), stomatitis
- Change in mental status, confusion but no focal neurologic deficits
- Tachycardia, wide pulse pressure, heart murmur
- Peripheral neuropathy

Diagnostic Studies
- CBC
- RBC folate more reliable for diagnosis than serum folate
- Serum B12
- TIBC
- LDH
- RDW
- Laboratory results: Serum folate < 3 nanograms/mL, RBC folate < 150 nanograms/mL, Hct decreased, Hgb normal, RDW elevated, TIBC normal, LDH and MCV elevated > 100 mcg/mL; MCHC normal, Schilling test normal, serum B12 normal

Differential Diagnosis

- Vitamin B_{12} efficiency
- Myelodysplastic syndromes
- Pernicious anemia
- Hypothyroidism

Management

Nonpharmacologic Treatment
- Education and supportive therapy; good oral hygiene
- Folate-rich diet: green leafy vegetables, red beans, wheat bran, fish, bananas, asparagus
- Need for frequent rest

Pharmacologic Treatment
- Folic acid replacement 400 mcg for pregnant women, 200 mcg for all others
  - Prescription supplements usually contain 1 mg folic acid, but be aware that supplementation of greater than 400 mcg may mask B12 deficiency

How Long to Treat
- Treat until anemia corrected, usually about 2 months until folic acid stores replenished
- Duration of treatment depends on elimination of underlying cause

Special Considerations

- Folate body stores can be depleted in about 4 months.
- Women not on birth control who are potentially child-bearing should routinely take folic acid preparations to decrease incidence of embryonic neural tube defects.

When to Consult, Refer, or Hospitalize

- Not usually needed; refer patients who do not improve with therapy

Follow-up

- In 2 months and periodically thereafter

Expected Outcomes
- Good prognosis

Complications
- Failure to thrive
- Neural tube defects of infants born to deficient women

HEMOLYTIC ANEMIAS

Hemolytic conditions produce anemias in which accelerated RBC destruction occurs as a result of an intrinsic genetic RBC defect as seen in hemoglobinopathies (sickle cell and thalassemia), in metabolic enzyme deficiencies (G6PD), or in cytoskeleton disorders (spherocytosis or elliptocytosis). The intrinsic destruction could also be acquired as seen in paroxysmal nocturnal hemoglobinuria or alcoholic cirrhosis. Extrinsic causes of hemolysis include antibody-mediated processes such as autoimmune reactions, drug-related reactions, transfusion reactions, and reactions to infections.

Important Features

- Peripheral blood smear shows spherocytosis, and may be hyperchromic
- Coombs test will be positive in immune hemolysis.
- An elevated reticulocyte count in the patient with anemia is the most useful indicator of hemolysis.

- Other laboratory findings include increased unconjugated bilirubin (indirect), decreased heptoglobin, possible increase in LDH, increased urine hemoglobin, increased urine bilirubin. Hemosiderin is a delayed sign and may represent chronic hemolysis.
- Bone marrow shows normoblastic erythroid hyperplasia.
- The most common and clinically observed hemolytic anemias are discussed here.

SICKLE CELL ANEMIA

Description

- Sickle cell disease (SSD) is a group of hemoglobin disorders characterized by production of hemoglobin S (HbS), the most common of which is sickle cell anemia (HbSS). Other common genotypes are sickle cell C (HbSC) and sickle beta-thalassemia (HbS beta-thalassemia). Severe hemolytic anemia may be produced in which abnormal hemoglobin (the result of a DNA point mutation in the B-globin chain) leads to chronic hemolytic anemia, with recurrent painful crises in individuals who are homozygous for hemoglobin S.
- Sickle cell disorders are characterized by chronic hemolytic anemia.

Etiology

- Hemoglobin S readily deforms the RBC into a sickle shape; the sickle cells hemolyze, and clusters of sickle cells occlude small blood vessels.
- Autosomal recessive gene (hemoglobin S gene from each parent)
- Sickle cell trait (Hgb AS) is seen when one normal Hgb gene and one sickle hemoglobin–producing gene are inherited from the parents; this will not cause sickle cell disease.

Incidence and Demographics

- Sickle cell anemia present in about 1 in 400 to 500 Blacks; 8% to 10% of Blacks carry hemoglobin S gene.
- No gender predominance; onset in first year of life

Risk Factors

- Factors that precipitate sickle cell crisis
  - Deoxygenation of Hgb molecule, as in high altitude
  - Infection
  - Dehydration
  - Overexertion or stress
  - Hypoxia
  - Exposure to extreme temperatures, hot or cold

Prevention and Screening

- Screening for sickle cell trait and genetic counseling for couples at risk; prenatal diagnosis via chorionic villus sampling or amniocentesis
- Universal newborn screening
- Good health maintenance with anticipatory guidance for potential complications
- All regular immunizations as well as pneumococcal and influenza (yearly) vaccinations
- Recognition and avoidance of known pain-precipitating factors

Assessment

History
- Hemolytic anemia starting in first year of life
- Family history of sickle cell anemia or trait
- Sickle cell trait may be asymptomatic unless provoked by exertion at high altitudes
- Sickle cell anemia: acute, sudden, excruciating episodes with pain in long bones, back, chest, abdomen; priapism; chronic leg ulcers; delayed puberty

Physical Examination
- May include chronically ill appearance, jaundice
- Splenomegaly (primarily in children)
- Hot, tender, swollen joints
- Retinopathy
- Cardiomegaly (laterally displaced point of maximum impulse (PMI), systolic murmur
- Chronic lower leg ulcers, blood loss

Diagnostic Studies
- Hgb electrophoresis: definitive diagnostic test
- CBC: classic findings (by age 1 year) include Hct in the 20s, reticulocyte count in the 20s, normal MCV, slightly elevated WBC count, and elevated platelet count
- Peripheral blood smear: fragmented cells, long crescent-shaped irreversible sickled cells, target cells, Howell-Jolly bodies, and occasional nucleated red blood cells
- Elevated LDH and indirect bilirubin during increased hemolysis
- Laboratory results: Hgb decreased, MCV might be elevated slightly, chronic neutrophilia, increased platelet count, erythrocytes with classic sickle shape on peripheral smear, Hgb S predominates

Differential Diagnosis

- Other hemoglobinopathies (e.g., hemoglobin C, D, E)
- Compound hemoglobinopathies (e.g., hemoglobin SC disease, hemoglobin S beta-thalassemia)

Management

Nonpharmacologic Treatment
• Hydration, nonpharmacologic pain modalities, patient and family education and supportive care, genetic counseling

Pharmacologic Treatment
• Oxygen for hypoxia
• Hydration
• Manage pain (morphine or hydromorphone)
• Do not give iron (increases Hgb S production)
• Folic acid 1 to 2 mg p.o. daily
• Consider transfusion

How Long to Treat
• Lifelong

Special Considerations

• In some patients, hydroxyurea 500 to 750 mg daily may decrease number of painful crises (long-term safety unknown).
• Individuals have different patterns of crisis.
• Crises might increase during pregnancy.

When to Consult, Refer, or Hospitalize

• Refer all suspected cases to a hematologist; hospitalize for acute episodes of sickling.
• Consult with physician for specialized care in the primary care setting.
• Any temperature of >38.5° C (101.3° F) must be considered a medical emergency and the patient should be hospitalized immediately.
• Hospitalize for unrelieved pain lasting more than 8 hours, sepsis, pregnancy-related complications

Follow-up

Expected Outcomes
• Number of crises decrease in young adulthood, but complications increase
• Life expectancy is 40 to 50 years

Complications
• Anemia, bone infarct, cerebrovascular accident (CVA), cardiac enlargement, priapism, retinopathy, acute chest syndrome, infections, gallstones, hemosiderosis (secondary to multiple transfusions), increased fetal loss during pregnancy, and sepsis

THALASSEMIA

Description

- A group of hereditary disorders with hypochromic microcytic anemia because of gene deletion or point mutation; causes abnormal synthesis of alpha and beta-globin chains, resulting in abnormal hemoglobin synthesis and displacement of hemoglobin A1 with abnormal types—microcytosis is out of proportion to the degree of anemia

Etiology

- Autosomal recessive genetic disorder producing defective hemoglobinization of red blood cells. Normal adult hemoglobin, Hgb A, has four chains or globins, two alpha and two beta. Delta and gamma chains are similar to beta and are found in hemoglobin A2 (two gamma, two delta chains), and hemoglobin F (fetal Hgb, two delta and two gamma chains). Hemoglobin cannot be formed without the α chains; unaffected individuals have four copies of gene for α-globin.
- *Alpha-thalassemia* is a result of a gene deletion such that not enough alpha chains can be synthesized.
- *Beta-thalassemia* results when point mutation causes decreased or no synthesis of beta chains.
- *Thalassemia major* (beta) occurs when unbalanced hemoglobin chain synthesis results in severe anemia (usually presents in infants or young children).
- *Thalassemia intermedia* is a more minor form of beta-thalassemia; may or may not need transfusions
- *Thalassemia trait* (alpha or beta) is a milder form of anemia, not requiring aggressive therapy.

Incidence and Demographics

- Alpha-thalassemia: people originating from Southeast Asia, China, occasionally Africa
- Beta-thalassemia: people originating from the Mediterranean, also, less commonly, Asia and Africa; there are about 1,000 patients with severe thalassemia in the United States.
- Trait present in 3% to 5% of at-risk populations

Risk Factors

- One or both parents with any combination of alpha- and/or beta-thalassemia syndromes

Prevention and Screening

- Screening of prospective parents at risk (ideally prior to pregnancy), genetic counseling
- Prenatal diagnosis (fetal blood sampling or chorionic villus sampling) if desired

Assessment

History
- Alpha trait (one of four alpha genes affected) usually asymptomatic; alpha-thalassemia minor (two of four alpha genes affected) and beta-thalassemia (heterozygous form) are mild forms, usually asymptomatic; beta-thalassemia major (Cooley's anemia—both genes affected)—easy fatigueability, palpitations, shortness of breath with exertion, headaches
- Family or personal history of lifelong anemia
- Infants and children with thalassemia major will have symptoms of severe and chronic anemia: pallor, shortness of breath, lethargy
- Children and adults with thalassemia trait may present with history of unresponsive anemia or signs of iron toxicity.

Physical Examination
- Normal exam in thalassemia minor syndromes
- Pallor and enlarged spleen in alpha thalassemia with 1 alpha-globin gene (also called hemoglobin H disease)
- Multiple abnormalities in thalassemia major (homozygous beta thalassemia) starting in infancy: bony deformities, jaundice, enlarged spleen, and enlarged liver

Diagnostic Studies (see Table 10–4)
- CBC with attention to RBC morphology and hemoglobin electrophoresis, iron studies
- Laboratory results: microcytic, hypochromic, acanthocytes, target cells, serum iron, and TIBC normal to increased, serum ferritin > 100

Differential Diagnosis

- Iron deficiency anemia
- Combined hemoglobinopathies

Table 10–4. Diagnostic Studies Used in Thalassemia

Diagnostic Studies	Findings
Alpha-Thalassemia Trait	Hematocrit 28%–40% Very low MCV (60–75 mcg/mL) Reticulocyte count normal Iron parameters normal Mild anemia; significant microcytosis
Alpha-Thalassemia Minor and Beta-Thalassemia Minor	Hematocrit 28%–40% MCV 55–75 mcg/mL Reticulocyte count normal or slightly elevated Iron parameters normal Hemoglobin electrophoresis shows elevation HgB A2 to 4%–8% and occasional Hgb F to 1%–5%
Beta-Thalassemia Major	Hematocrit 10% MCV < 75 mcg/mL Peripheral blood smear: severe poikilocytoses, hypochromia, basophilic stippling, and nucleated red blood cells; virtually no Hgb A present; major hemoglobin present in Hgb F
Hemoglobin H Disease	Hematocrit 22%–32% MCV < 7 mcg/mL Peripheral blood smear markedly abnormal: hypochromia, microcytosis, poikilocytosis Reticulocyte count elevated Hemoglobin electrophoresis shows HgbH as 10%–40% of Hgb

Reprinted from *Family Nurse Practitioner: Nursing Review and Resource Manual*, by E. Blunt (Ed.), 2009, Silver Spring, MD: American Nurses Credentialing Center, p. 813.

Management

- No treatment needed for beta-thalassemia minor or alpha-thalassemia trait

Nonpharmacologic Treatment
- Severe thalassemia major: regular transfusions; bone marrow transplants in children; splenectomy if needed; patient and family education and supportive care

Pharmacologic Treatment
- Folic acid supplementation
- Iron chelation therapy with deferoxamine (Desferal)
- Appropriate immunizations (especially if splenectomy contemplated)
- Avoid iron supplements and iron-fortified foods; avoid oxidative drugs (e.g., sulfonamides)

How Long to Treat
- Lifelong

Special Considerations

- Support for family as coping with guilt is a major problem for parents

When to Consult, Refer, or Hospitalize

- Consult or refer when diagnosis is in question; refer all patients with thalassemia major or intermedia to hematologist, hospitalize for complications. Refer all patients with severe disease to specialty clinic experienced in iron chelation and transfusions

Follow-up

- Follow-up depends on severity of disease.

Expected Outcomes
- Thalassemia minor: benign
- Thalassemia intermedia: Patients have chronic hemolytic anemia but generally will only need transfusions when under stress; live into adulthood
- Children with thalassemia major die in their teens or even younger unless they receive regular transfusions and iron chelation therapy; with compliance, live well into adulthood

Complications
- Limited growth and bony deformities; iron overload (because of frequent transfusions), which can cause cirrhosis, diabetes, cardiac dysfunction (including arrhythmia); failure of sexual maturation; decreased life expectancy

COAGULATION DISORDERS

IDIOPATHIC THROMBOCYTOPENIA PURPURA (ITP)

Description

- An autoimmune disorder characterized by accelerated, spleen-mediated platelet destruction, resulting in a decreased platelet count (< 100,000/mL) that predisposes the patient to a decreased ability for primary clotting. May be acute (with spontaneous resolution within 2 months after an acute infection—usually children) or chronic (persists ≥ 6 months without identifiable cause—usually adults). IgG autoantibody binds to platelets; splenic macrophages bind to antibody-tagged platelets and destroy them.

Etiology

- Unknown, perhaps autoimmune response after viral illness

Incidence and Demographics

- Predominantly occurs in pediatric population; uncommon in geriatric population
- Slight seasonal peaks in winter and spring
- Adult female-to-male ratio = 2:1 for age range 20 to 40
- 13,000 new cases in the United States annually

Risk Factors

- No genetic predispositions described
- Acute infection (usually viral, e.g., varicella, EBV, CMV), HIV, cardiopulmonary bypass, hypersplenism, preeclampsia
- Medications such as heparin, sulfonamides, thiazides, quinine, cimetidine, gold
- History of autoimmune diseases (rheumatoid or collagen vascular symptoms, thyroid disease, hemolytic anemia) or chronic lymphocytic leukemia (CLL)

Prevention and Screening

- None

Assessment

History
- Insidious onset in otherwise well person
- Prolonged purpura, bruising tendency, gingival bleeding, menorrhagia, epistaxis, petechiae
- History of acute viral illness

Physical Examination
- Nonpalpable spleen is essential criterion
- Signs of GI bleeding, dysmorphic features

Diagnostic Studies
- Often diagnosed on routine CBC with differential and platelets; also get peripheral smear; consider HIV, liver function, CT abdomen, stool guaiac as needed
- Laboratory results: Platelets decreased, normal RBC and WBC morphology
- ANA testing if autoimmune disorder is suspected
- Bone marrow biopsy to evaluate for myelodysplasia

Differential Diagnosis

- Viral infection
- SLE
- Bone marrow disorders
- AIDS
- Drug-induced
- Hemolytic-uremic syndrome
- Liver disease
- Congenital thrombocytopenia (e.g., Fanconi syndrome)
- Sepsis

Management

Nonpharmacologic Treatment
- Education and supportive care
- Avoid medications that increase bleeding risk
- Decrease activities that might cause bruising, injury
- Monitor patient for platelet count, associated symptoms

Pharmacologic Treatment
- Initiate treatment if platelet count less than 20,000/mcL or patient is symptomatic
- Acute: prednisone 1 to 2 mg/kg q.d. for 4 weeks, then taper
- Chronic: 60 mg/day for 4 to 6 weeks, then taper
- Severe or emergency: IV gamma-globulin (IVGG) 1 gm/kg for 1 to 2 days (very expensive)
- HIV patients: 2 mg/kg/day in divided doses; preferred over steroids

- Platelet transfusion ONLY during life-threatening hemorrhage
- Splenectomy if platelets < 30,000 after 6 weeks of pharmacologic treatment (splenectomy response not good if IVGG response poor); pneumococcal vaccine several weeks prior to procedure
- If poor response after prednisone and splenectomy, may consider chemotherapy

How Long to Treat
- Until remission

Special Considerations

- Focus: bleeding, exclusion of other diagnoses

When to Consult, Refer, or Hospitalize

- Refer all suspected cases to hematologist; refer to surgeon for splenectomy

Follow-up

Expected Outcomes
- Acute = 80% to 85% remission, 15% become chronic; chronic = 20% spontaneous remission
- Response usually seen in 3 to 5 days after initiation of treatment

Complications
- Cerebral hemorrhage (1% mortality); other blood loss, pneumococcal infection

HEPARIN-INDUCED THROMBOCYTOPENIA

Description

- Hypercoagulable state caused by antibodies targeting heparin and platelet factor 4.

Etiology

- Heparin and platelet factor 4 binding causes immune response, resulting in production of antiplatelet factor 4/heparin antibodies. This is considered a normal occurrence, but a portion of patients will develop thrombocytopenia as a result. The antibodies cause platelet activation, which eventually leads to generation of thrombin and causes the patient to be in a hypercoagulable state.

Incidence

- Rarely associated with fondaparinux
- Low incidence with low-molecular-weight heparin
- Unfractionated heparin after total hip or knee replacement: > 1% to 5%
- Medical and obstetric patients: 0.1% to 1%

Risk Factors

- Patient has received unfractionated heparin, low-molecular-weight heparin, or fondaparinux

Prevention and Screening

- None

Assessment

History
- Patient has received unfractionated heparin, low-molecular-weight heparin, or fondaparinux
- Usual onset is 5 to 14 days of start of heparin
- Onset time may vary from within 24 hours to after heparin is discontinued.

Physical Examination
- Thrombosis; venous > arterial
- Necrosis at injection sites
- May have systemic allergic reactions following IV bolus of heparin, which include fever, hypotension, dyspnea, and cardiac arrest

Diagnostic Studies
- 50% decrease in baseline platelet count
- Rapid HIT-antibody assays
- Platelet factor 4 antibodies identification through serologic enzyme immunoassays
- Functional assays

Differential Diagnosis

- HIV
- Aplastic anemia
- Lymphoma
- Leukemia
- Effects of chemotherapy
- ITP
- DIC

Management

Nonpharmacologic Treatment
- Evaluate for lower extremity DVT.

Pharmacologic Treatment
- Discontinue all heparin-containing medications.
- Initiate alternative anticoagulation with direct thrombin inhibitors (lepirudin, argatroban, or heparinoid danaparoid)
- Once the platelet count has normalized, start warfarin to prevent thrombosis.
- Alternative anticoagulation may be discontinued after 5 days of overlapping warfarin.

How Long to Treat
- Warfarin should be continued for 2 to 3 months in patients without evidence of thrombosis and at least 6 months in those with thromboembolism.

When to Consult, Refer, or Hospitalize

- Possible surgical consult for amputation related to gangrene
- Consider hematology consult

Follow-up

Expected Outcomes
- Patient specific
- Increased risk in patients with surgical intervention on vascular system and history of renal impairment
- Inverse relationship between platelet count and risk of complications

Complications
- Arterial and venous thromboses
- Skin necrosis at injection sites
- Acute systemic reactions after IV bolus administration
- Gangrene

DISSEMINATED INTRAVASCULAR COAGULATION (DIC)

Description

- Increased, abnormal production of thrombin and fibrin
- Increased coagulation factor consumption and platelet aggregation

Etiology

- Sepsis
- Infection
- Malignancy
- Shock
- Complication of obstetrics
- Less common causes are head injury, burns, frostbite, and gunshot wounds

Incidence

- Affects up to 1% of hospitalized patients
- Equal in both sexes
- Septic patients with DIC have a 24.2% higher mortality rate than trauma patients with DIC

Risk Factors

- See Etiology

Assessment

History
- Presence of risk factor
- Signs of macrovessel thrombosis such as DVT or microvessel thrombosis such as renal failure
- Bleeding from three unrelated sites

Physical Examination
- Hypotension
- Tachycardia
- Fever
- Bruising or petechiae
- Possible hematuria
- Necrotic changes of lower extermities
- Localized infarction and gangrene

Diagnostic Studies
- Platelet count
- PT/PTT
- Plasma fibrinogen level
- Plasma D-dimer
- Rapidly evolving DIC—thrombocytopenia, more prolonged PT/PTT, declining plasma fibrinogen level, increased D-dimer
- Slowly evolving DIC—mild thrombocytopenia, normal to minimally prolonged PT/PTT, normal or moderately decreased plasma fibrinogen level, increased D-dimer

Differential Diagnosis

- ITP
- HIT
- Thrombocytopenia
- Medication side effects
- Viral infection
- Liver disease
- Anticoagulation
- Bone marrow suppression
- Hematologic malignancies

Management

Nonpharmacologic Treatment
- Supportive care
- Identify and treat underlying cause

Pharmacologic Treatment
- Broad-spectrum antibiotics if infection is underlying cause
- Platelet transfusion to correct thrombocytopenia
- Cryoprecipitate for correction of fibrinogen and factor VIII
- Fresh frozen plasma to increase other clotting factors
- Heparin is not recommended.

How Long to Treat
- Treat until DIC is resolved.

Special Considerations
- Heparin is a consideration in obstetric patients with a dead fetus and evolving DIC.

When to Consult, Refer, or Hospitalize

- DIC patients should be hospitalized
- Consider hematology consult if DIC does not improve.

Follow-up

Expected Outcomes
- Mortality rates differ depending on underlying cause.

Complications
- Multi-organ system failure
- Renal failure
- DVT
- Severe bleeding

ONCOLOGY

General Considerations

- Cancer is the second most common cause of death in the United States; however, the incidence is decreasing in both men and women as evidenced by data over the past 10 years.
- The incidence for all cancers of both genders decreased 0.8% per year from 1999 to 2005.
- Death from cancer has decreased over the past two decades, with 10 of the top 15 cancer sites showing a decrease in mortality events.
  - Decline in mortality has been seen in all ethnic and racial groups except for American Indians and Alaskan Natives.
- Esophageal cancer in men, pancreatic cancer in women, and hepatocellular cancer in both genders are the exception and have increased in mortality numbers.
- Modifiable risk factors
  - Tobacco use
    - Linked to 30% of all cancer deaths
    - At least 15 cancers are related to smoking, with lung cancer being the most notable—90% of lung cancer cases occur in smokers.
  - Poor nutrition
    - Fruit-and-vegetable-rich diets lower the risk of gastrointestinal malignancies
  - Physical inactivity
  - Excessive alcohol consumption
    - Linked to head and neck, esophageal, and liver cancers
  - Obesity
    - Associated with breast and uterine cancer in women, and colorectal, esophageal, and renal carcinoma in both genders
- Tumor staging
  - TNM (tumor, nodes, metastasis) system
  - Rules for staging set by the American Joint Committee on Cancer
  - Elements of staging
    - T: Tumor size and level of tumor invasion
      - T0: no evidence of tumor
      - Tis: Carcinoma in situ (limited to surface cells)
      - T1–4 :Increasing tumor size and involvement

- N: Absence or presence, extent of nodal metastasis
  - N0: No lymph node involvement
  - N1–4: Increasing degrees of lymph node involvement
  - Nx: Lymph node involvement cannot be assessed
- M: Presence or absence of systemic metastasis
  - M0: No evidence of metastasis
  - M1: Evidence of distant metastasis

- Once the TNM is identified, then an overall stage is assigned
  - Stage 0
    - Cancer in situ (limited to surface cells)
  - Stage I
    - Limited to the tissue of origin, evidence of tumor growth
  - Stage II
    - Limited local spread of cancer cells
  - Stage III
    - Extensive local and regional spread
  - Stage IV
    - Distant metastasis
- Tumor grading
  - Tumor cells that have been obtained during a biopsy are examined.
  - The abnormality of the cells determines the grade given, which increases from 1 to 4.
  - Grade 1
    - Cells are slightly abnormal and well-differentiated.
  - Grade 2
    - Cells are more abnormal and moderately differentiated.
  - Grade 3
    - Cells are very abnormal and poorly differentiated.
  - Grade 4
    - Cells are immature and undifferentiated.
- Ten most common cancers in the United States—in order of most to least prevalent
  - Males
    - Prostate
    - Lung and bronchus
    - Colon and rectum
    - Urinary
    - Lymphoma
    - Melanoma
    - Kidney and pelvis
    - Leukemia
    - Oral cavity
    - Pancreas
  - Females
    - Breast

- Lung and bronchus
- Colon and rectum
- Uterine corpus
- Lymphoma
- Thyroid
- Kidney and renal pelvis
- Ovary
- Pancreas

RED FLAGS

- Paraneoplastic syndromes
  - Effects initiated by a tumor product
  - Effects of destruction of normal tissues by the tumor
  - Effects from an unknown mechanism
  - Clinically important
    - Paraneoplastic syndromes may accompany limited neoplastic growth and provide early information in some types of cancer
    - The metabolic or toxic effects of the syndrome may be more dangerous than the underlying cancer itself.
    - Effective treatment of the tumor should also include the paraneoplastic syndrome associated with it.
- Anorexia
- Weight loss
- Malaise
- Fever

LUNG CANCER

Description
- Lung cancers are divided into small cell lung cancer (SCLC) and non–small cell lung cancer (NSCLC)
- Non–small cell is further divided into adenocarcinoma, squamous cell carcinoma, and large cell carcinoma
  - Adenocarcinoma
    - Arises from the bronchial mucosal glands
    - Is the most frequent NSCLC in the United States
    - Usually occurs in a peripheral location in the lung
    - May manifest as "scar carcinoma"
    - This subtype is seen most often in nonsmokers.
      - Bronchoalveolar carcinoma

- This is a distinct subtype of adenocarcinoma.
- Appears as interstitial lung disease on CXR
- Grows along alveolar septa
- May be a solitary peripheral nodule, multifocal disease, or rapidly progressing
- Squamous cell
  - Is seen as a cavitary lesion in a proximal bronchus
  - Presence of keratin pearls are detected with cytologic studies.
  - Associated with hypercalcemia
- Large cell
  - Is seen as a large peripheral mass on CXR
  - Has sheets of highly atypical cells with focal necrosis
  - No evidence of keratinization or gland formation
- Non–small cell carcinoma accounts for about 85% of all lung cancers.

Etiology

- The cause of lung cancer is tobacco smoking in as many as 90% of patients (78% of men and 90% of women).
  - Tobacco smoke contains more than 300 harmful substances with at least 40 known carcinogens.
  - The number of cigarettes smoked and the length of the smoking history is directly related to the development of lung cancer.
  - Risk is highest among those currently smoking and the lowest in nonsmokers.
    - In one large trial, smokers had a 16-fold increase in lung cancer risk.
  - The risk of lung cancer declines after the person stops smoking.
    - Relative risk remains high in the first 10 years then declines to twofold 30 years after quitting.
  - Passive smoking
    - Secondhand smoke may be implicated in about 25% of lung cancers.
- Asbestos exposure
- Radon
  - Correlation seen in uranium miners
  - Household exposure has not been clearly shown to cause lung cancer.
- Genetic susceptibility

Incidence and Demographics

- In the United States, there were over 200,000 cancers of the lung and bronchus in 2009.
- Lung cancer is the most common malignancy in the world—in 2007 there were approximately 1.5 million new cases diagnosed globally.
- Global lung cancer trends have followed trends with smoking but lag behind by several decades.
- The incidence peaks between the ages of 55 and 65 years.
- Lung cancer accounts for 29% of all cancer deaths (31% in men and 26% in women).

Risk Factors

- Cigarette, cigar, or pipe use
- Secondhand smoke
- Asbestos exposure
- Radon exposure
- HIV infection
- Exposure to beryllium, nickel, copper, chromium, or cadmium
- Higher mortality in women who have NSCLC when taking estrogen-progestin for more than 5 years
- Inherited predisposition
- Ionizing radiation
- Air pollution
- Vitamin A and E deficiencies

Prevention and Screening

- Smoking cessation
- Limit exposure to second hand smoke.
- Limit exposure to known carcinogens as listed in risk factors.
- HIV screening
- Diet rich in fiber and vegetables
- Use of aspirin reduced deaths in adenocarcinoma of the lung
- Screening for high-risk patients (current or former smokers > 50 years of age) is controversial.
  - Screening chest x-ray not recommended
  - Low-dose, noncontrast, thin-slice, helical or spiral CT is emerging as tool for lung cancer screening
    - More sensitive than chest x-ray for detecting lung nodules
    - Risks and benefits of screening must be presented to patients
    - Will detect lung cancer in 1% to 4% of patients screened over a 5-year period but will also detect false-positive lung lesions in 25% to 75% of cases

Assessment

- 5% to 15% may be asymptomatic.
- Symptomatic lung cancer is generally seen in advanced disease.

History
- Nonspecific symptoms
  - Weight loss
  - Chest pain
  - Loss of appetite
- Lung symptoms
  - Shortness of breath
  - Central or endobronchial growth
    - Cough

- Hemoptysis
- Fever
- Peripheral growth of the primary tumor
  - Dyspnea
  - Pleural or chest wall pain, or both
- Regional spread of the tumor in the thorax
  - Esophageal compression with dysphagia
  - Recurrent laryngeal nerve paralysis with diaphragmatic elevation
    - Hoarseness
    - Phrenic nerve paralysis
      - Dyspnea
  - Pancoast's syndrome
    - Tumor growth into lung apex
      - Shoulder pain with radiation to ulnar distribution of the arm
- Metastasis
  - Bone pain (bone metastasis)
  - Abdominal or right upper quadrant pain (liver metastasis)
  - Central nervous system involvement
    - Headache
    - Altered mental status
    - Seizure
    - Meningismus
    - Ataxia
    - Nausea, vomiting, or both

Physical Examination
- Central or endobrochial growth
  - Wheezing
  - Stridor
  - Post obstructive pneumonitis
- Peripheral growth of the primary tumor
  - Lung abscess from tumor cavitation
- Lower airway obstruction
  - Asymmetric breath sounds
  - Pleural effusion
  - Pneumothorax
- Regional spread of the tumor in the thorax
  - Tracheal obstruction
  - Sympathetic nerve paralysis with Horner's syndrome
    - Results from neurological damage to the cervical nerve
  - Acute spinal cord compression
    - Paraplegia
    - Sensory deficits
  - Malignant pleural effusions
  - Pancoast's syndrome or tumor
    - Radiologic destruction of the first and second ribs

- Atrophy of the muscles of the arm and hand caused by brachial plexus and sympathetic ganglia tumor
  - Superior vena cava syndrome
- Paraneoplastic syndrome
  - Cushing's syndrome
  - Lambert-Eaton myasthenic syndrome
    - Gradual onset of proximal lower extremity weakness
    - Proximal upper extremity weakness less noticeable
    - Syndrome may be worse in the morning and then improve during the day.
    - Ptosis is common.
  - Hypercalcemia
  - Syndrome of inappropriate antidiuretice hormone
  - Enlargement of extremities, painful swollen joints
- Metastasis
  - Bone pain
  - Neurological dysfunction
    - Brain metastasis
    - Spinal cord compression
- Pericardial tamponade

Diagnostic Studies
- Tissue diagnosis—biopsy
  - Bronchial or transbronchial
  - Node biopsy via mediastinoscopy
  - Biopsy at the time of definitive surgical resection—thoracotomy
  - Percutaneous biopsy of enlarged lymph nodes, soft tissue mass, lytic bone lesion, bone marrow or pleural lesion
  - Fine needle aspiration via CT guidance
  - Adequate cell recovery from a pleural effusion
  - Video-assisted thoracoscopy (VATS)
  - Ultrasound-guided thoracentesis
- Chest x-ray
  - Compare to previous films
  - Central lesions
    - Squamous cell carcinoma
    - Small cell carcinoma
- Peripheral lesions
  - Adenocarcinoma
  - Large cell carcinoma
  - Bronchoalveolar cell carcinoma
  - Cavitation
    - Squamous cell carcinoma
    - Large cell carcinoma
  - Early mediastinal-hilar involvement
    - Small cell cancer
- Full staging workup
  - NSCLC
    - Use the TNM International Staging System.
      - Particularly useful for curative attempts with surgery or radiotherapy

- The TNM factors are combined to form staging groups.
  - At presentation, one-third of patients have localized disease
    - Stage I or II, IIIa disease
    - Localized for curative attempt with surgery or radiotherapy
  - One-third have distant metastatic disease.
    - Stage IV
  - One-third have local or regional disease.
    - May or may not be amenable to curative therapy
    - Stage IIIA, IIIB disease
  - Staging system provides useful prognostic information
  - **T – Primary tumor**
    - T0
      - No primary tumor
    - T1
      - Tumor ≤ 3 cm, surrounded by lung or visceral pleura, not more proximal that the lobar bronchus
    - T1a
      - Tumor ≤ 2 cm
    - T1b
      - Tumor > 2 cm but ≤ 3 cm
    - T2
      - Tumor > 3 but ≤ 7 cm or tumor with any of the following:
        - Invades visceral pleura, involves main bronchus ≥ 2 cm distal to the carina, atelectasis/obstructive pneumonia extending to hilum but not involving the entire lung
    - T2a
      - Tumor > 3 cm but ≤ 5 cm
    - T2b
      - Tumor > 5 cm but ≤ 7 cm
    - T3
      - Tumor > 7 cm
        - Or directly invading chest wall, diaphragm, phrenic nerve, mediastinal pleura, or parietal pericardium
        - Or tumor in the main bronchus < 2 cm distal to the carina
        - Or atelectasis/obstructive pneumonitis of entire lung
        - Or separate tumor nodules in the same lobe
    - T4
      - Tumor of any size with invasion of the heart, great vessels, trachea, recurrent laryngeal nerve, esophagus, vertebral body, or carina
      - Or separate tumor nodules in a different ipsilateral lobe
  - **N – Regional lymph nodes**
    - N0
      - No regional metastasis
    - N1
      - Metastasis in ipsilateral peribronchial, peprihilar lymph nodes and intrapulmonary nodes, or both, including involvement by direct extension

- · N2
    - Metastasis in ipsilateral mediastinal lymph nodes, subcarinal lymph nodes, or both
  - · N3
    - Metastasis in contralateral mediastinal, contralateral hilar, ipsilateral or contralateral scalene, or supraventricular lymph nodes
  - **M – Distant metastasis**
    - · M0
      - No distant metastasis
    - · M1a
      - Separate tumor nodules in a contralateral lobe
      - Or tumor with pleural nodules or malignant pleural dissemination
    - · M1b
      - Distant metastasis
- Small-cell cancer
  - · Two-stage system
  - · Limited-stage disease
    - Seen in about 30% of patients
    - Confined to one hemithorax and regional lymph nodes (includes mediastinal, contralateral hilar, and ipsilateral supraclavicular nodes)
    - Usually confined to area that is small enough to be treated with radiation
  - · Extensive-stage disease
    - Seen in about 70% of patients
    - Extends beyond the boundaries of limited stage disease—both lungs
  - · Clinical studies—physical examination, x-rays, CT and bone scans, and bone marrow examinations are used to stage
  - · Contralateral supraclavicular nodes, recurrent laryngeal nerve involvement, and superior vena caval obstruction can be limited stage.
  - · Cardiac tamponade, malignant pleural effusion, and bilateral pulmonary parenchymal involvement usually qualify as extensive stage because the organs within a curative radiation port cannot safely tolerate curative radiation doses.
- Complete blood count
- Serum chemistries
- Liver function studies
- CT scan of chest and upper abdomen
  - CT of the head for altered mental status
- MRI
  - Not part of routine staging
  - Useful when spinal cord compression is suspected
- Radionuclide imaging
  - Bone scans
- Positron emission tomography (PET)
  - Excellent for solitary pulmonary nodules
  - Most useful for non–small cell carcinoma
- Sputum cytology
  - Greatest yield with large, central tumors
  - If positive, allows for more invasive diagnostic testing

- Bronchoscopy
  - Allows direct visualization of the tumor
- Transthoracic percutaneous fine-needle aspiration
  - Less invasive than bronchoscopy
  - Performed with CT guidance
- Spirometry
  - Evaluate peak expiratory flow for airflow obstruction

Differential Diagnosis

- Bronchitis
- Pleural effusion
- Pneumonia
  - Bacterial
  - Empyema
  - Abscess
  - Immununocompromised
  - Mycoplasma
  - Viral
- Pneumothorax
  - Iatrogenic
  - Spontaneous
  - Pneumomediastinum
  - Tension
  - Traumatic
- Superior vena cava syndrome
- Tuberculosis

Management

- Smoking cessation

Nonpharmacologic and Pharmacologic Treatment
- Treatment decisions are based on the whether the tumor is classified as small cell lung carcinoma or non–small cell carcinoma
- Small cell
  - Surgery plays a limited role
    - With limited-stage disease
      - Surgical resection such as lobectomy, wedge resection, pneumonectomy with mediastinal lymph node removal and biopsy
      - Chemotherapy combination every 3 weeks for 4 to 6 cycles
        - Cisplatin
        - Carboplatin
        - Etoposide
      - May also have concurrent radiotherapy based on the clinical stage
      - Response rate with limited disease is 60% to 80% and a 10% to 30% complete response rate

- Extensive disease
  - Combination chemotherapy
    - Cisplatin
    - Carboplatin
    - Etoposide
    - Irinotecan
  - May include radiation therapy to symptomatic sites
    - Superior vena cava
    - Bone metastasis
    - Spinal cord compression
    - Response rates lower with extensive disease, about 50% and almost always partial
  - Tumor regression is usually rapid, within the first two cycles
  - The overall survival rate for both stages is about 6%.
  - For extensive small cell cancer without treatment, average life expectancy is 2 to 4 months, with treatment about 6 to 12.
- Non–small cell carcinoma
  - Stage-based management
    - Stage 0: limited to lining of air passages
      - Surgical resection with least extensive technique
        - Segmentectomy
        - Wedge resection
      - Endoscopic photodynamic therapy
      - Electrocautery
      - Cryotherapy
      - Nd-YAG laser therapy
      - High incidence of second primary cancers developing
    - Stage I
      - Surgery is the treatment of choice
        - Lobectomy or segmental, wedge, or sleeve resection
        - Radiation therapy with curative intent for potentially resectable tumors in patients with medical contraindications to surgery
        - Clinical trials of adjuvant chemoprevention
        - In highly selective patients: endoscopic photodynamic therapy and other endobronchial therapies—clinical trials
      - 5-year survival is 60% to 80%
    - Stage II
      - Surgical options
        - Lobectomy, pneumonectomy, or segmental, wedge or sleeve resection
        - Radiation therapy with curative intent for potentially operative tumors in those with contraindications for surgery
        - Adjuvant chemotherapy after curative surgery
        - Clinical trials—radiation after curative surgery
      - 5-year survival is 40% to 50%
    - Stage IIIa
      - Resected/resectable disease
        - Surgery followed by adjuvant chemotherapy
        - Clinical trials—combined modalities—chemotherapy, radiation therapy, surgery

- Unresectable disease
  - Chemoradiation therapy
  - Radiation therapy alone for those unable to tolerate combined therapy
- Superior sulcus tumors
  - Radiation therapy and surgery
  - Radiation therapy alone
  - Surgery alone in selected cases
  - Chemotherapy with radiation therapy and surgery
  - Clinical trials—combined modalities
  - Chest wall tumor
    - Surgery
    - Surgery and radiation therapy
    - Radiation therapy alone
    - Chemotherapy combined with radiation therapy, surgery, or both
  - The overall survival rate for stage IIIa lung cancer is 23%, but varies among the different cancers in this classification
- Stage IIIb
  - Chemotherapy combined with radiation therapy
  - Radiation therapy alone
  - The 5-year survival rate is about 10%. The mean survival time with treatment is 13 months.
- Stage IV
  - Doublet of chemotherapy with cisplatin or carboplatin and paclitaxel, gemcitabine, docetaxel, vinorelbine, irinotecan, and pemetrexed
  - Paclitaxel, carboplatin, and bevacizumab for patients with nonsquamous histology, no brain metastases or no hemoptysis
  - Epidermal growth factor (EGFR) tyrosine kinase inhibitors in patients with EGFR mutations
  - Cisplatin, vinorelbine, and cetuximab for those with NSCLC expressing EGFR
  - Maintenance pemetrexed in patients with stable or responding disease after four cycles of nonpemetrexed-platinum combination therapy
  - Endobronchial laser therapy, brachytherapy, or both for obstructing lesions
  - External beam radiation therapy (EBRT)

Special Considerations

- Patients with central nervous system(CNS) metastasis, immunosuppression, superior vena cava syndrome, Pancoast tumor, or Ogilvie intestinal psedueo-obstruction may require a specific work-up.
  - CNS metastasis
    - Head CT, with and without contrast
    - Headache and cerebral edema may respond to dexamethasone 10 mg IV
    - Neurosurgical consult

- Whole-brain irradiation or resection
- Seizures are treated with anticonvulsants
  - Brain metastases and no history of seizures do not generally need anticonvulsant therapy
- Immunosuppression with cancer and infection
  - CBC
  - Electrolytes
  - If diarrhea is present:
    - Urinalysis and culture
    - Blood cultures from peripheral sites
    - Cultures from any indwelling catheters
    - Stool cultures for *Clostridium difficile*
    - Broad-spectrum antibiotics
    - Granulocyte colony-stimulating factor
- Pancoast tumor
  - MRI is best diagnostic study to identify superior sulcus tumors
  - Admit for transthoracic needle aspiration
  - Bronchoscopy for endobronchial involvement
- Superior vena cava syndrome
  - Lung cancer is the cause in 60% to 80% of cases.
  - Elevate the head, cautious fluid administration, supplemental oxygen
  - Definitive treatment: radiotherapy, chemotherapy, or vena caval stenting
  - Diuretics and glucocorticoids (methylprednisolone) may help with symptoms.
- Ogilvie intestinal pseudo-obstruction
  - Abdominal x-ray reveals massive dilation of the colon and small intestine, with or without air-fluid levels
  - Electrolytes
  - Nasogastric tube, rectal tube
  - Admit for possible colonic decompression and treatment of underlying cause—lung cancer producing autoantibodies to the myenteric neural plexus

When to Consult, Refer, or Hospitalize

- Oncology to manage treatment strategies, thoracic surgery for resection when applicable, and other subspecialties as needed
- Hospitalize for surgery, chemotherapy, and to manage complications of treatment and/or disease

Follow-up

Expected Outcomes
- See survival rates

Complications
- Spinal cord compression
- Superior vena cava syndrome
- Metabolic complications

- Hypercalcemia
- Hyponatremia
- SIADH

- Complications of therapy
  - Febrile netropenia from bone marrow suppression
  - Bleeding from bone marrow suppression
  - Renal failure
  - Ototoxicity
  - Peripheral neuropathy

COLORECTAL CANCER

Description

- A complex disease with progression from premalignant lesions (adenomas, polyps) to invasive adenocarcinoma
  - Adenomatous polyps that are at least 1 cm in size, with villous features or high-grade dysplasia, are associated with a higher risk of cancer.
- Adenocarcinomas are the majority of colorectal cancers (98%).
- Other rare colorectal cancers are carcinoid (0.4%), lymphoma (1.3%), and sarcoma (0.3%).
- About 20% of colon cancers develop in the cecum, 20% in the rectum, 10% in the rectosigmoid junction, and 25% in the sigmoid colon.
- The National Comprehensive Cancer Network (NCCN) defines rectal cancer as a malignancy located within 12 cm of the anal verge by rigid proctoscopy

Etiology

- The etiology for most cases appears to be related to environmental factors
- Diet high in animal fat and processed meat
- Insulin resistance leads to increased levels of insulin, which results in higher circulating levels of insulin-like growth factor type I (IGF-I); this growth factor may stimulate proliferation of the intestinal mucosa.
- Inflammatory bowel disease
- Alcohol intake of more than 30 g per day is associated with an increased of developing colorectal cancer (ingestion of beer a greater risk than wine), with rectal cancer being a greater risk than colon cancer.

Incidence and Demographics

- Cancer of the large bowel is second only to lung cancer as a cause of cancer death in the United States.
- 153,760 new cases occurred in 2007 and 52,180 deaths were the result of colorectal cancer.

- Incidence rate has remained relatively unchanged during the past 30 years, but the mortality rate has decreased, especially in women.
- The lifetime risk of developing colorectal cancer is approximately 6%.
- Incidence is higher in Western nations than in Asian and African countries.
- Males have a higher incidence than females; left colon carcinomas are more likely in males and right colon cancers in females.

Risk Factors

- Age
  - The risk increases after age 45 years, and 90% occur in patients over 50 years of age.
- Family history
  - Familial adenomatous polyposis (FAP)
  - Hereditary nonpolyposis colorectal cancer (HNPCC)
    - Amsterdam criteria
      - Three or more relatives diagnosed with HNPCC-associated cancer (colorectal, endometrium, small bowel, ureter, renal pelvis)
      - One affected person is a first-degree relative of the other two.
      - One or more cases of cancer are diagnosed before age 50.
      - FAP has been excluded.
      - Tumors have undergone a pathology review.
- Personal history
  - Adenomatous polyps
  - Inflammatory bowel disease (IBD)
  - Peutz-Jeghers syndrome
  - Breast cancer
  - Ovarian cancer
  - Endometrial cancer
  - Prostate cancer
- Dietary factors
  - Ingestion of animal fat found in red meat
  - Processed meat
- Elevated serum cholesterol
- Tobacco use

Prevention and Screening

- Primary prevention
  - Chemoprotective compounds
    - Aspirin
    - NSAIDS
    - Estrogen replacement therapy
- Screening
  - The early detection of localized, superficial cancers in asymptomatic persons increases the surgical cure rate.

- Most screening programs focus on digital rectal examination and fecal occult blood testing.
  - Digital rectal examination should be part of any routine physical examination in adults over 40.
  - About 50% of patients with documented colorectal cancer have a negative fecal occult blood test.
  - Individuals with a positive occult blood test should undergo further medical evaluation—sigmoidoscopy, barium enema, colonoscopy, or a combination of these.
  - Starting at age 50, asymptomatic individuals having no colorectal cancer risk factors should have an annual hemoccult test and flexible sigmoidoscopy every 5 years.
- Total colon examination (colonoscopy or double-contrast barium enema) every 10 years as an alternative to hemoccult testing with periodic flexible sigmoidoscopy.
- Other screening tests
  - Virtual colonoscopy
  - Stool DNA testing (SDNA)
    - Evaluates for genetic alterations that lead to cancer formation

Assessment

History
- Symptoms vary with the anatomic location of the tumor
- Ascending colon due to chronic blood loss
  - Fatigue
  - Malaise
  - Palpatations
  - Angina
- Transverse/descending colon
  - Abdominal cramping
  - Obstruction
- Rectosigmoid
- Hematochezia
- Tenesmus
- Narrowing of the caliber of stool
- Altered bowel habits

Physical Examination
- May not have any overt signs
- Abdominal tenderness
- Palpation of discrete mass
- Positive hemoccult
- Digital rectal examination
  - Rectal tumors can be assessed for size, ulceration, and presence of an pararectal lymph nodes.
  - Fixation of tumor to surrounding structures can be assessed.
  - Evaluation of sphincter function—used to determine if patient is a candidate for rectal-sparing procedure

Diagnostic Studies
- Staging
  - The prognosis is related to the depth of tumor penetration in the bowel wall and the presence of both regional lymph node involvement and distant metastases.
  - The TNM or Duke staging system is used.
  - Cuthbert E. Dukes introduced the ABC staging system in 1932 for rectal cancer
  - Stage I (Duke Staging A)
    - T1
      - No deeper than submucosa
      - 5-year survival > 95%
      - 23% of this stage at presentation are in the colon.
      - 34% of this stage at presentation are in the rectum.
    - T2
      - Not through muscularis
      - 5-year survival > 90%
  - Stage II (Duke Staging B)
    - T3
      - Through muscularis
      - 5-year survival 70% to 80%
      - 31% of this stage at presentation are in the colon.
      - 25% of this stage at presentation are in the rectum.
  - Stage III (Duke Staging C)
    - N1
      - 1–3 lymph node metastases
      - 5-year survival 50% to 70%
      - 26% of this stage at presentation are in the colon and the rectum.
    - N2
      - ≥ 4 lymph node metastases
      - 5-year survival 25% to 60%
  - Stage IV
    - M
      - Distant metastasis
      - 5-year survival < 5%
      - 20% of this stage at presentation are in the colon.
      - 15% of this stage at presentation are in the rectum.
- Digital rectal examination
- Fecal occult blood test
- Colonoscopy with biopsy
- CBC
- Serum chemistry
- Liver function studies
- Carcinoembryonic antigen (CEA)
  - Useful for monitoring therapy
- CT of the abdomen and pelvis
- Chest x-ray

Differential Diagnosis

- Arteriovenous malformation (AVM)
- Carcinoid/neuroendocrine tumors and rare tumors of the GI tract
- Crohn's disease
- Diverticulosis, small intestine
- Gastrointestinal lymphoma
- Ileus
- Ischemic bowel
- Small intestinal carcinomas
- Ulcerative colitis

Management

Nonpharmacologic Treatment

- Rectal cancer
  - Surgical—recurrence rate for surgery alone is 30% to 50%
    - Transanal excision
    - Endocavitary radiation
    - Transanal endoscopic microsurgery
    - Sphincter-sparing procedures
      - Low anterior resection
      - Colo-anal anastomosis
      - Abdominal perineal resection
  - Stage I rectal cancer patients do not require adjuvant therapy because of their high cure rate with surgical intervention.
  - Surgical resection for stage II rectal cancer should be done 4–10 weeks after completion of chemotherapy and radiotherapy.
  - Adjuvant radiation therapy
  - Intraoperative radiation therapy
  - High-risk patients (poorly differentiated tumor histology, lymphovascular invasion) should be considered for adjuvant chemotherapy and radiotherapy.
- Colon cancer
  - Radiation
    - Role is limited in colon cancer but remains a standard modality
    - No role in adjuvant therapy
    - In metastatic settings, it is limited to palliative therapy for selected metastatic sites such as bone or brain metastases.
    - Selective radiation therapy—stereotactic radiotherapy (CyberKnife) and tomotherapy
  - Surgical
    - Surgery is the only curative modality for localized colon cancer (stage I–III)
    - Potentially the only curative option with limited metastatic disease in liver and/or lung (stage IV)
    - General principles for all operations
      - Removal of the primary tumor with adequate margins, including areas of lymphatic drainage
      - Laparoscopy is an option

- Cecum and right colon
  · Right hemicolectomy
- Proximal or middle transverse colon
  · Extended right hemicolectomy
- Splenic flexure and left colon
  · Left hemicolectomy
- Sigmoid colon
  · Sigmoid colectomy
- Hereditary nonpolyposis colon cancer (HNPCC)
  · Total abdominal colectomy with ileorectal anastamosis
- Colonic stents to relieve obstruction
- Diet
  · High intake of fruits, vegetables, poultry, and fish
- Physical activity reduces the risk of reoccurrence and mortality of colon cancer

Pharmacologic Treatment
- Rectal cancer
  - Metastatic disease is treated with chemotherapy.
  - Adjuvant chemotherapy
    · 5-fluorouracil (5-FU)
    · Pro-drug 2-deoxy-5-floxuridine (5-FUDR) is rapidly converted to 5-FU and is used for metastatic liver disease via continuous intrahepatic infusion.
  - Patients with locally advanced rectal cancer should be treated with primary chemotherapy and radiotherapy.
    · The combination with fluorouracil improves local control, distant spread, and survival.
  - NCCN guidelines for patients with high-risk or intermediate-risk stage II disease recommend combination therapy with infusional fluorouracil, folinic acid, and oxaliplatin (FOLFOX)
  - FOLFOX is not indicated for good- or average-risk state II rectal cancer.
  - For stage III or IV rectal cancer, a combination of folinic acid, fluorouracil, and irinotecan (FOLFIR) is recommended.
  - Cetuximab should not be used in patients with *KRAS* mutation.
  - In recent studies, panitumumab combined with FOLFOX4 (fluorouracil, leucovorin, and oxaliplatin) or FOLFIRI (fluorouracil, leucovorin, and irinotecan) significantly improved progression-free survival.
- Colon cancer
  - Metastatic disease is treated with systemic chemotherapy.
  - Systemic chemotherapy
    · 5-Fluorouracil is the mainstay for colon cancers—for both adjuvant and metastatic treatment.
    · In the past 10 years, combination therapies have provided increased efficacy and prolonged progression-free survival.
      - In addition to 5-fluorouracil, oral fluoropyrimidines (cepecitabine) and tegafur are being used for monotherapy or in combination with oxaliplatin and irinotecan.
      - Some standard combination therapies include a continuous infusion of fluorouracil (FOLFIRI, FOLFOX) or capecitabine (CAPOX, XELOX, XELIRI).
    · Adjuvant (postoperative) chemotherapy
      - Standard therapy for stage III and some patients with stage II colon cancer has

been fluorouracil in combination with levamisoe and leucovorin.
- This has been tested in several large trials and has been shown to reduce individual 5-year risk of cancer recurrence and death by about 30%.
- The addition of oxaliplatin to fluorouracil (FOLFOX4 and FLOX) showed a significant improvement in 3-year disease-free survival for patients with stage III colon cancer in large randomized trials (MOSAIC and NASBP-C06).
- Biologic agents
  · Bevacizumab was the first anti-angiogenesis medication to be approved in clinical practice.
  · Two other approved biological agents are epidermal growth factor receptor (EGFR)–targeted monoclonal antibodies.
    - Cefuximab is approved as monotherapy or in combination with irinotecan in patients with metastatic colorectal cancer refractory to fluoropyrimidine and oxaliplatin therapy.
    - Panitumumab is indicated as monotherapy for patients with colorectal cancer in whom combination therapy failed or was not tolerated.

Special Considerations

- Advancing age is a well-known risk factor.
- Timeline for progression from early premalignant lesion to malignant cancer ranges from 10 to 20 years.
- Right-sided lesions are more likely to bleed and cause diarrhea.
- Left-sided tumors are usually detected later and can present with bowel obstruction.

When to Consult, Refer, or Hospitalize

- Refer to gastroenterology for colonoscopy in symptomatic patients
  - Change in bowel habits
  - Hematochezia
  - Mass on abdominal examination
  - Mass on digital rectal examination
  - Iron deficiency anemia
  - Suspected cancer or adenomatous polyps
- All patients with proven rectal cancer should be referred to a surgeon for resection.
- Patients with stage III or IV disease should be referred to an oncologist.
- Admit to treat complications of the cancer or chemotherapy
  - Bowel obstruction
  - Acute bleeding
  - Refractory nausea and vomiting
  - Renal failure
- Admit for palliative care in advanced metastatic disease

Follow-up

Expected Outcomes
- See preceding survival rates
- Approximately 85% of colon cancer recurrences occur within 3 years after resection of the primary tumor.
- Patients with stage II and III resected colon cancer should undergo regular surveillance for at least 5 years after resection.
- Serum CEA should be checked every 3 months with stage II or III disease for at least 3 years and every 6 months in years 4 and 5.
- CT of the chest and abdomen should be performed annually for at least 3 years.
- All patients with colon cancer should have preoperative or postoperative colonoscopy.
- If no high risk pathology or increased susceptibility is identified on the first colonoscopy, follow-up colonosocopy should be performed at 3 years after surgery, then if normal, once every 5 years

Complications
- Bowel obstruction
- Recurrence of the cancer
- Metastasis
  - Liver
  - Lung
- GI bleeding
- Ureteral obstruction
- Peritonitis
- Toxic megacolon

BREAST CANCER (FEMALE)

Description

- Invasive cancers develop through a series of molecular alterations at the cellular level that results in outgrowth and spread of breast epithelial cells with uncontrolled growth.
- There are four subclasses of discrete breast tumor subtypes
  - Luminal A
    - Most common subtype
    - Less aggressive
    - Lower histological grade
    - Good prognosis
    - Hormone-responsive
    - Associated with increasing age
  - Luminal B
    - Similar to luminal A
    - Worse outcome than luminal A

- Basal
  - Aggressive subtype
  - High grade histology and high mitotic rate
  - Risk at younger age (< 40 years)
  - More likely premenopausal Black women
- HER2+
  - Less common, highly aggressive subtype
  - High-grade histology
  - Risk at young age (< 40 years) greater than luminal subtypes
  - African-American race may be a risk factor.

Etiology

- See Description

Incidence and Demographics

- Breast cancer will develop in one of eight American women.
- The mean age and the median age of women with breast cancer is 61 years.
- In 2009, there were about 192,370 new cases of breast cancer and 40,170 deaths in the United States.
- Approximately 75% of women who are diagnosed with breast cancer do not have an obvious risk factor.
- Current lifetime risk for breast cancer in the United States is 12.7% for all women, 13.3% for non-Hispanic White women, and 9.98% for Black women.
- Death rates have steadily declined since 1990, and this is thought to be the result of early detection and improved treatment strategies.

Risk Factors

- Advanced age
- Family history
  - Two or more relatives
  - One first-degree relative
  - Family history of ovarian cancer in women < 50 years of age
- Personal history
  - Positive BRCA1/BRCA2 mutation
  - Breast biopsy with atypical hyperplasia
  - Breast biopsy with lobular carcinoma in situ (LCIS) or ductal carcinoma in situ (DCIS)
  - Endometrial cancer
- Reproductive history
  - Early age at menarche (< 12 years of age)
  - Late age of menopause
  - Late age of first term pregnancy (> 30 years) or nulliparity

- Use of combined estrogen/progesterone hormone replacement therapy (HRT)
- Adult weight gain
- Sedentary lifestyle
- Alcohol consumption
- Risk assessment models
  - National Surgical Adjuvant Breast and Bowel Project (NSABP)
    - Modified Gail Model
      - Basis for prophylactic use of tamoxifin
      - Tamoxifin approved for women aged 35 years or older who have a 5-year Gail risk of breast cancer of 1.67% or more
    - U.S. National Cancer Institute's Breast Cancer Risk Assessment Tool
      - Gail Model 2
      - Most accurate for non-Hispanic White women who receive annual mammograms
      - May overestimate risk in younger women who do not receive annual mammograms
    - CARE model
      - Demonstrated high correlation between the number of breast cancers predicted and the number of breast cancers observed in Black women

Prevention and Screening

- Annual screening mammography
  - U.S. Preventive Services Task Force (USPSTF) guidelines
    - Aged 40–49 years—individualized screening
    - Routine screening for women aged 50–74 biennially
    - Recommends screening stop for women aged 75 and older
  - American College of Obstetricians and Gynecologists (ACOG)
    - Screening mammography every 1–2 years for women aged 40–49 years and annually for women 50 years of age or older.
  - Breast self-examination (BSE)
    - Perform monthly
    - Has not been found to reduce breast cancer mortality; however, with improved treatment strategies for early, localized disease, BSE and clinical breast examination are still recommended, especially in women under 40 years of age.
  - Clinical breast examination (CBE)
    - Annually
    - When combined with mammography, screening sensitivity is improved, especially in younger women and those who have a mammography biennially
  - Alternative screening methods
    - Digital mammography
    - Ultrasound
    - MRI
      - Not recommended by the American Cancer Society for use in women that have a < 15% lifetime risk
- Prevention
  - National Surgical Adjuvant Breast Project (NSABP)
    - Breast Cancer Prevention Trial (BCPT) P-1
      - Trial evaluated tamoxifen as a preventative agent

- Those who received tamoxifen for 5 years had a 50% reduction in noninvasive cancers compared with those taking a placebo.
- Selective estrogen receptor modulator (SERM)—raloxifene
  - Used for osteoporosis but is also effective in preventing breast cancer
  - Multiple Outcomes of Raloxifene Evaluations (MORE) trial
    - After taking the medication for 8 years, an overall reduction in breast cancer of 66% was seen
  - The Study of Tamoxifen and Raloxifene (STAR) P-2 trial
    - Conducted by the NSABP
    - Demonstrated that tamoxifen and raloxifene are equivalent in preventing invasive breast cancer in high-risk populations.
    - DCIS occurred more often in women treated with raloxifene.
- Aromatase inhibitors (AI)
  - Have shown success in treating breast cancer with fewer side effects
  - Trials are underway to determine if AI has a role in prevention.
    - International Breast Cancer Intervention Study II (IBIS-II)
    - National Cancer Institute of Canada Clinical Trials Group (NCIC CTG)
- Diet
  - Decreasing dietary fat intake
- Exercise

Assessment

- TNM staging system is used—American Joint Committee on Cancer
  - Primary tumor (T)
    - TX: primary tumor cannot be assessed
    - T0: no evidence of primary tumor
    - Tis: (DCIS) carcinoma in situ
    - Tis: (LCIS) carcinoma is situ
    - Tis: Paget's disease of the nipple with no tumor
    - T1: tumor 2 cm or smaller in greatest diameter
    - T2: tumor > 2 cm but not > 5 cm in greatest diameter
    - T3: tumor > 5 cm in greatest diameter
    - T4: tumor of any size with direct extension to (a) the chest wall or (b) skin only
  - Regional lymph nodes
    - Nx: regional lymph nodes cannot be assessed (previously removed)
    - N0: no regional lymph node metastasis
    - N1: metastasis in movable ipsilateral axillary lymph nodes
    - N2: metastasis in ipsilateral axillary lymph node(s) fixed or matted, or clinically assessed in the ipsilateral internal mammary nodes with evidence of axillary lymph noded metastasis
    - N3: metastasis in ipsilateral infraclavicular or supraclavicular lymph node(s) with or without axillary lymph node involvement or clinically assessed ipsilateral internal mammary lymph node(s) in the presence of axillary lymph node involvement
  - Distant metastasis
    - Mx: distant metastasis cannot be assessed
    - M0: no distant metastasis
    - M1: distant metastasis

- Staging
  - Stage 0
    - Tis, N0, M0
  - Stage I
    - T1, N0, M0
  - Stage IIA
    - T0, N1, M0
    - T1, N1, M0
    - T2, N0, M0
  - Stage IIB
    - T2, N1, M0
    - T3, N0, M0
  - Stage IIIA
    - T0, N2, M0
    - T1, N2, M0
    - T2, N2, M0
    - T3, N1–2, M0
  - Stage IIIB
    - T4, N0, M0
    - T4, N1, M0
    - T4, N2, M0
  - Stage IIIC
    - Any T, N3, M0
  - Stage IV
    - Any T, Any N, M1

History
- Breast pain (5%)
- Skin changes of the breast
  - Thickening
  - Swelling
  - Redness
- Nipple abnormalities
  - Ulceration
  - Retraction
  - Spontaneous bloody drainage

Physical Examination
- Painless lump in the breast (70% of patients' initial complaint)
  - Nontender
  - Firm mass
  - Poorly delineated margins because of local infiltration
  - Lesions < 1 cm may be difficult for the examiner to feel, but may be felt by the patient.
- Often detected on mammogram before identified by patient or healthcare provider
- Inspection
  - Abnormal variations in breast size and contour
  - Minimal nipple retraction
  - Slight edema, redness
  - Asymmetry of the breasts

- Dimpling of the skin
- Enlarged lymph nodes
  - Axillary
  - Supraclavicular
  - Metastases tend to involve regional lymph nodes
  - Firm or hard axillary nodes larger than 1 cm are typically the result of metastases.
  - Axillary nodes matted or fixed to skin or deep structures indicate advanced disease (stage III).
  - Firm or hard nodes in the supraclavicular nodes are suggestive of metastatic disease and should be biopsied.
  - Ipsilateral supraclavicular or infraclavicular nodes containing cancer indicate that the tumor is in an advanced stage (III or IV).
- Edema of the ipsilateral arm is also a sign of advanced cancer resulting from the infiltration of regional lymphatics.

Diagnostic Studies

- Biopsy
  - Fine needle aspiration cytology (FNA cytology)
    - Easily performed with extremely low morbidity
    - Subject to sampling problems
      - Deep lesions may be missed
      - Noninvasive cancers usually cannot be distinguished from invasive ones
      - Low false positive (1% to 2%)
      - False negative: about 10%
  - Large-needle (core needle) biopsy
    - May be done in the clinic setting with local anesthesia
    - Sampling problems due to improper positioning of the needle
    - Estrogen receptor (ER), progesterone receptor (PR), and HER-2/neu overexpression testing may be performed on the cores of tissues.
  - Mammographic localization biopsy
    - Mammogram taken in two perpendicular views and with placement of a needle or hook-wire near the lesion that is used as a guide to locate the abnormality
  - Open biopsy
    - Performed under local anesthesia through an incision with the intent to remove the entire lesion, not just a sample
    - Most reliable means of diagnosis
- Laboratory studies
  - Sedimentation rate
    - Persistently elevated
  - Serum alkaline phosphatase
    - Elevated with bone involvement
  - Hypercalcemia
    - Seen in advanced breast cancer
  - Carcinoembryonic antigen (CEA), CA 15-3, CA 27-29
    - May be used as markers for recurrent breast cancer
    - Not helpful in diagnosing early lesions
- Imaging

- Mammography
  - If suspicious lesion is found, patient is reimaged
    - Images reviewed by radiology, breast oncologist, and surgeon
    - If lesion identified on mammogram is considered suspicious, it is graded as follows:
      - 0
      - 1
      - 2
      - 3
      - 4: 25% chance of cancer with biopsy
      - 5: 50% chance of cancer with biopsy
      - 6: cancer identified with biopsy
- For metastases
  - Chest x-ray
    - Pulmonary metastatic disease
  - CT of liver, brain
    - Only if metastasis to these areas are suspected
  - Bone scan
    - More sensitive than skeletal x-rays in detecting metastasis
  - PET scan
    - Less useful than a bone scan in identifying metastatic bone lesions
    - Effective for soft tissue or visceral metastasis
  - PET-CT
    - PET scan combined with CT is effective for detecting soft tissue metastasis
- Ultrasound
  - Used to differentiate cystic from solid lesions
- Ductography
- MRI
- Cytology
  - Nipple discharge or cyst fluid
  - Ductal lavage

Differential Diagnosis

- Fibrocystic disease of the breast
- Fibroadenoma
- Intraductal papilloma
- Lipoma
- Fat necrosis

Management

- Treatment is curative or palliative
- Curative advised for stage I, II, III disease
- Patients with locally advanced (T3, T4) and inflammatory tumors may be cured with multi-modality therapy, but in many, palliative treatment is all that can be expected.

- Palliative treatment is appropriate for stage IV disease and for previously treated patients with distant metastasis or unresectable local cancers.

Nonpharmacologic Treatment

- Surgical resection
  - Breast-conserving therapy
    - NSABP trial showed lumpectomy with axillary dissection followed by postoperative radiation therapy is as effective as modified radical mastectomy for stage I and II breast cancer.
    - Breast-conserving surgery with radiation is preferred for patients with early stage breast cancer.
    - Tumor size is a major consideration in determining if the patient will be well-served with breast conservation surgery.
    - The patient must have a breast size large enough to have minimal deformity with the excision of 4-cm tumor (upper limit for breast conservation surgery).
    - Subareolar tumors are difficult to excise without deformity but are not contraindications for breast-conserving surgery.
    - Clinically detectable multifocality, fixation to the chest wall or skin, and involvement of the nipple or overlying skin are relative contraindications.
    - The patient should be the judge of what is cosmetically acceptable.
  - Mastectomy
    - Modified radical mastectomy removes the entire breast, overlying skin, nipple, and areolar complex in addition to the underlying pectoralis fascia with the axillary lymph nodes.
    - The major advantage is that radiation may not be necessary, but radiation is used when multiple lymph nodes are positive for cancer.
    - The disadvantage is the cosmetic impairment.
    - Radical mastectomy, which involves the above plus removal of the underlying pectoralis muscle, is rarely performed.
    - Axillary node dissection is not indicated for noninfiltrating cancers.
    - Breast reconstruction, immediate or delayed, should be discussed.
  - Management of the contralateral breast
    - Noncarriers of the BRCA mutation are predicted to have a 0.7% annual risk of contralateral breast cancer.
    - Carriers of the BRCA mutation have a 3% annual risk of contralateral breast cancer.
    - Contralateral prophylactic mastectomy (CPM) is a decision made by the patient based on cancer stage, desire for symmetry, comorbidities, family history, and potentially difficult surveillance.
    - Patients with locally advanced disease should be discouraged from contralateral prophylactic mastectomy because potential surgical complications could compromise oncologic treatments.
  - Sentinel lymph node dissection
    - Minimally invasive procedure to stage the axilla in breast cancer patients who have clinically negative nodes
    - Sentinel nodes are the first group of nodes to drain from the breast to the axilla.
    - Typically, 1–3 lymph nodes are removed and tested for nodal metastasis.
    - If cancer is detected in a sentinel lymph node, axillary lymph node dissection is recommended by the American Society of Clinical Oncology.

- Axillary lymph node dissection
  - Complete removal of level I (lateral to the pectoralis minor) and II (nodes beneath the pectoralis minor) lymph nodes
  - Level III (medial to the pectoralis minor) are not removed unless a palpable adenopathy is present or there is suspicion that one is present.
  - Lymphedema occurs in about 25% of patients.
  - Other complications include shoulder dysfunction, wound infection, seroma, nerve damage, numbness, chronic pain, and, rarely, brachial plexus injury.
- Radiotherapy
  - Radiotherapy after partial mastectomy is 5–7 weeks of five daily fractions for a total dose of 5000–6000 cGy.
  - Many radiation oncologists use a boost dose at the cancer location.
  - For local control: Accelerated partial breast irradiation (only the part of the breast from which the tumor was removed) for 1–2 weeks is effective in achieving local control.
  - The American Society of Breast Surgeons Registry Trial showed that the 3-year rate of ipsilateral breast cancer recurrence was 2.15% in 1440 patients treated with brachytherapy with no unexpected adverse events.

Pharmacologic Treatment

- Adjuvant systemic therapy
  - Systemic therapy improves survival and is recommended for most patients with curable breast cancer.
  - The goal of therapy is to kill cancer cells that have left the breast and axillary lymph nodes as micrometastases before they become macrometastases (stage IV cancer).
  - Chemotherapy
    - TAC
      - Taxotere 75 mg/m^2 IV day 1, every 21 days for 6 cycles
      - Adriamycin 50 mg/m^2 IV day 1
      - Cyclophosphamide 500 mg/m^2 IV day 1
    - Conventional regimen
      - Adriamycin 60 mg/m^2 IV day 1 every 21 days for 4 cycles
      - Cyclophosphamide 600 mg/m^2 IV day 1
        - Followed by paclitaxel 175 mg/m^2 IV day 1 every 21 days for 4 cycles
    - Dose-dense
      - Adriamycin 60 mg/m^2 IV day 1 every 14 days for 4 cycles
      - Cyclophosphamide 600 mg/m^2 IV day 1
    - Followed by paclitaxel 175 mg/m^2 IV day 1 every 14 days for 4 cycles
    - Metronomic regimen
      - Adriamycin 20 mg/m^2 IV day 1 every week for 12 cycles
      - Cyclphosphamide 50 mg/m^2 p.o. every day
        - Followed by paclitaxel 80mg/m^2 IV day 1 every week for 12 cycles
  - Targeted therapy
    - HER-2/neu overexpression
      - AC-TH
      - Adriamycin
      - Cyclophosphamide

- Trastuzumab 4 mg/kg IV load, then 2 mg/kg weekly with paclitaxel (80 mg/m^2 every week for 12 weeks), then 6 mg/kg IV every 3 weeks for 40 weeks
  - Endocrine therapy: hormonal therapy
    - Traditional regimen
      - 5 years of the estrogen-receptor antagonist/agonist tamoxifen (remains the standard for premenopausal women)
      - Aromase inhibitors (AI)
        - Letrozole
        - Anastrozole
        - Exemestane
      - Ovarian ablation plus AI or tamoxifen is an alternative.
      - Postmenopausal women with hormone receptor–positive breast cancer should be offered an AI, either initially or after tamoxifen therapy.
  - Bisphosphonates
    - When used with standard local and systemic therapy, the relative risk of cancer recurrence was reduced by 35% to 40% for hormone receptor–positive nonmetastatic breast cancer
- Neoadjuvant therapy
  - Use of chemotherapy or endocrine therapy before resection of the tumor
  - Increases the chance of breast conservation by shrinking the primary tumor in women who would otherwise need mastectomy for local control
  - Survival with neoadjuvant chemotherapy is similar to that with postoperative adjuvant chemotherapy.
- Palliative treatment
  - Radiotherapy
    - Used for primary treatment of locally advanced cancers with metastatic disease to control ulceration and pain, and for treatment of some bone or soft-tissue metastases to prevent fractures
    - Useful for isolated bony metastases, chest wall recurrences, brain metastases, and acute spinal cord compression
  - Biphosphonate therapy
    - Targeted therapy
    - Endocrine therapy for metastatic disease
      - Selective estrogen receptor modulator (SERM)
        - Tamoxifen citrate 20 mg orally daily
        - Toremifene citrate 40 mg orally daily
      - Steroidal estrogen receptor antagonist
        - Fulvestrant 250 mg IM monthly
      - Estrogen
        - Diethylstilbestrol 5 mg orally three times daily
      - Synthetic luteinizing hormone releasing analoge
        - Goserelin 3.6 mg subcutaneously monthly
      - Progestin
      - Megestrol acetate 40 mg orally four times daily

- Aromatase inhibitor (AI)
  - Letrozole 2.5 mg orally daily
  - Anastrozole 1 mg orally daily
  - Exemestane 25 mg orally daily
- HER-2/neu–targeted therapy
  - Trastuzumab plus chemotherapy
    - Lapatinib—oral agent approved for the treatment of trastuzumab-resistant HER-2/neu–positive breast cancer in combination with capecitabine
- Targeting angiogenesis
  - Bevacizumab is a monoclonal antibody directed against vascular endothelial growth factor (VEGF) that stimulates endothelial proliferation and neoangiogenesis in cancer.
- Targeting triple-negative breast cancer
  - Breast cancers without expression of the hormone receptors ER, PR, and HER-2/neu.
  - Poly-ADP ribose-polymerase inhibitors (PARP-i) are new agents showing some effectiveness against triple-negative breast cancer and BRCA mutations.
- Palliative chemotherapy
  - Should be considered if:
    - Visceral metastases are present (liver, brain, pulmonary)
    - Hormonal treatment is unsuccessful
    - The disease has progressed after an initial response to hormonal therapy
    - The tumor is ER negative
  - Combination chemotherapy offers higher response and progression-free survival rates.

Special Considerations

- Special forms of breast cancer
  - Paget's carcinoma
    - Not common—about 1% of all breast cancers
    - Ducts of the nipple epithelium are infiltrated; however, gross nipple changes are often minimal and a tumor mass may not be palpable.
    - Diagnosis is frequently missed.
    - First symptom is often itching or burning of the nipple with superficial erosion or ulceration.
    - Diagnosis made by biopsy
    - When lesion consists of nipple changes only, the incidence of axillary metastasis is < 5%
    - When a breast mass is present, there is an increased chance of axillary metastasis and decreased chances for cure by surgery or other treatment.
  - Inflammatory carcinoma
    - Most malignant form of breast cancer and occurs in < 3% of cases
    - Rapidly growing, sometimes painful mass that enlarges the breast
    - Overlying skin is erythematous, edematous and warm
    - Often no distinct mass because the tumor infiltrates the involved breast diffusely
    - Inflammatory changes are mistaken for an infection—they are caused by carcinomatous invasion of the subdermal lymphatics.

- If a patient being treated for a breast infection does not respond in 1–2 weeks, a biopsy should be performed.
- Diagnosis is made when more than one-third of the skin over the breast is erythematous and the biopsy reveals infiltrating carcinoma with invasion of the subdermal lymphatics.
- Radiation, hormone therapy, and chemotherapy are likely to be the most effective approach.
- Mastectomy when chemotherapy and radiation have produced a clinical remission and no evidence of metastasis
- Breast cancer during pregnancy or lactation
  - Occurs in about 1 in 3,000 pregnancies
  - Diagnosis may be delayed because the physiological changes of pregnancy hide the lesion
  - When the cancer is confined to the breast, the 5-year survival is 30% to 40%.
  - Pregnancy is not a contraindication for surgery or treatment.
    - Therapy should be based on the stage of the disease.
    - Radiation and chemotherapy may be given during pregnancy.
    - Overall survival rates have improved because the cancer is being detected earlier.
- Bilateral breast cancer
  - Occurs in < 5% of cases
  - There is a 20% to 25% incidence of later reoccurrence of cancer in the second breast.
  - Is seen more often in familial breast cancer, women < 50 years of age, and when the tumor is lobular.
  - The incidence of a second breast cancer increases with the length of time the patient is alive after the first cancer—about 1% to 2% per year.
- Noninvasive cancer
  - May occur within the ducts or lobules
  - LCIS is thought to be a premalignant lesion or a risk factor for breast cancer, but it may behave like DCIS.
    - The invasive potential is being considered.
  - DCIS tends to be unilateral; most often progresses to invasive cancer if untreated
    - In about 40% to 60% of women who have DCIS treated with biopsy alone, invasive cancer develops in the same breast.
    - Treatment is controversial.
      - May be treated with wide excision with or without radiation therapy or with total mastectomy
      - Lumpectomy may be used for patients with small lesions.
      - Current standard of care offers chemoprevention, which is effective in preventing invasive breast cancer in LCIS and DCIS that has been completely excised, or surgical excision of the area in question, or bilateral total mastectomy.
  - Axillary metastasis usually only occurs with an occult invasive cancer.

When to Consult, Refer, or Hospitalize

- Consult general surgery, gynecology for biopsy, surgical intervention, or both as needed.
- Oncology consult when chemotherapy or radiation therapy required
- Admit for surgical resection—mastectomy, lumpectomy

Follow-up

Expected Outcomes
- 5-year survival rates correlate with tumor stage
  - 99% to 100% with stage 0
  - 85% with stage 1
  - 60% to 70% for stage II
  - 30% to 55% for stage III
  - 5% to 10% for stage IV
- Patients should be followed long-term.
- Local and distant recurrences occur most frequently in the first 2–5 years
- During the first 2 years, patients should be monitored every 6 months with mammogram of the affected breast, then annually.
- BSE should be performed monthly with special attention to the contralateral breast.
- Even in disease-free patients, pregnancy is not recommended.
- Hormone replacement therapy is rarely used after breast cancer even in disease-free patients.
- The incidence of local recurrence depends on the tumor size, presence and number of involved nodes, histologic type of tumor, skin edema, or skin or fascia fixation with the primary tumor and the type of definitive surgery and local irradiation.
  - Local recurrence on the chest wall after total mastectomy and axillary dissection occurs in up to 8% of patients.
  - When axillary nodes are not involved, local recurrence rate is < 5% but it can be as high as 25% when there is heavy involvement.

Complications
- Local recurrence
- Psychological issues
- Upper extremity edema
- Cognitive decline ("chemo brain")
- Weight management problems
- Bone loss
- Fatigue

PROSTATE CANCER

Description

- The prostate lies below the bladder and surrounds the prostatic urethra. It is encased by a capsule and is separated from the rectum by a layer of fascia.
- Most prostate cancers are adenocarcinomas.
- Most begin in the periphery.
- The Gleason score is used to classify the histologic characteristics of prostate cancer.
  - The classification is determined by the glandular architecture within the tumor.
    - Grade 1: a near normal pattern

  - Grade 2–4: low grade
  - Grade 5–7: moderate grade
  - Grade 8–10: high grade
- The sum of the most predominant grade and the second most common histologic pattern determines the Gleason score.
- A score of 6 or higher indicates a likelihood of progressing to advanced cancer.

Etiology

- Inherited predisposition
- Exact etiology unknown

Incidence and Demographics

- Prostate cancer is the second leading cause of cancer death in the United States among men and is the most commonly diagnosed cancer in American males.
- An estimated 1 in 10 men will develop prostate cancer in their lifetime.
- On autopsy, men in their 80s show hyperplastic changes > 90% of the time and malignant changes > 70% of the time.
- Cancer is more common, aggressive, and progressive in Black males.
- Blacks tend to have a higher-grade stage of disease at diagnosis.

Risk Factors

- High-fat diet
- Family history
- Tobacco use
- Black race
- High chromium intake
- Advanced age

Prevention and Screening

- American Cancer Society
  - Prostate-specific antigen (PSA) and digital rectal examination (DRE) on an annual basis for men over age 50 with an anticipated survival of > 10 years up to age 76 years
  - Black men with a family history of prostate cancer should start screening at age 45.
- American Urologic Association
  - Same as American Cancer Society
  - They advise the risks and benefits of the performance of the PSA and DRE are not defined
- The National Comprehensive Cancer Network
  - Advises testing at age 40, tailoring additional testing

Assessment

- Staging: The TNM staging system is used
  - Stage T1NC: organ-confined disease
  - Stage T3a: extracapsular extension of the tumor
  - Stage T3b: invasion of the seminal vesicles
  - Stage T4: tumor fixed or invading adjacent structures other than seminal vesicles (bladder neck, external sphincter, rectum, levator muscles, pelvic floor, or a combination of these)
  - Stage NX: regional lymph nodes cannot be assessed
  - Stage N0: no regional lymph node metastasis
  - Stage N1: regional lymph node metastasis
  - Stage MX: distant metastasis cannot be assessed.
  - Stage M0: no distant metastasis
  - Stage M1: distant metastasis
  - Stage M1a: distant metastasis other than regional lymph nodes
  - Stabe M1b: metastasis to bone
  - Stage M1c: other site(s)
  - Stage pM1c: metastasis to more than 1 site

History
- Weight loss
- Pain
- Hematuria
- Urinary retention
- Urinary incontinence
- Ureteral or bladder outlet obstruction
- Spinal cord compression

Physical Examination
- Obliteration of the lateral sulcus or seminal vesical involvement found during a rectal examination
- Carcinomas are typically hard, nodular, and irregular.
- Lower extremity edema, bony tenderness (metastatic disease)
- Dysfunction of external anal sphincter tone with spinal cord compression

Diagnostic Studies
- Complete blood count
- Complete chemistry panel
- Serum prostate-specific antigen (PSA)
  - PSA level does not always correspond to disease progression.
- Free to total PSA ratio
- Acid phosphatase
- Bone scan
  - Limited to patients with a Gleason score of < 7 and PSA < 20 ng/ml
- Patients with a Gleason score > 6 may be candidates for a bone scan with or without a suspicious PSA score.
- Indicated in patients with symptoms of bony metastasis

- Activity in the bone may not be seen for 5 years after micrometastasis; therefore, a negative bone scan does not always rule out distant metastasis.
- Chest x-ray
- Abdominal/pelvic CT scan
- Abdominal/pelvic MRI
- ProstaScint scan
- Imaging may be enhanced by addition of single-photon emission CT (SPECT) imaging or CT scan

Differential Diagnosis

- Paget's disease of the bone
- Lymphoma
- Spinal cord compression from another cause

Management

Nonpharmacologic Treatment
- Low-fat diet
- The management depends on three factors:
  - Overall life expectancy of the patient, which is determined by age and comorbidities
  - The characteristics of the tumor and its projected aggressiveness and behavior
  - Preferences of the patient with regard to potential complications of therapy, adverse effects, efficacy, and quality of life issues
- Localized disease
  - Standard treatments include surgery, radiation therapy, or observation (watchful waiting, active surveillance)
    - Surgery
      - General criteria
        - Patient < 75 years of age
        - Few comorbidities with life expectancy > 10 years
        - Gleason score of < 7
        - PSA level < 20 ng/ml
      - The goal is disease-free survival.
      - Early localized disease (T1–2N0M0)
        - Radical prostatectomy
          - Removal of prostate and seminal vesicles
        - Pelvic lymphadenectomy
    - Radiation therapy
      - External beam
      - Radioactive sources implanted in the gland
      - Combination of the two
    - Active surveillance
      - Monitoring of the illness at fixed intervals with DRE, PSA, and repeat biopsies without therapeutic intervention until the tumor progresses
      - Progression may be based on PSA changes, local tumor growth, the development of symptoms or metastatic disease

- For patients with a rising PSA
  - Often the rise in PSA after surgery or radiation indicates subclinical metastatic disease
  - The need for treatment depends on the estimated probability that the patient will show evidence of metastatic disease on a scan and when.
  - Immediate therapy is not always required; however, treatment is advised when PSA doubles in 12 months or less.
  - After radical prostatectomy the PSA should be < 0.2 ng/ml and after radiation therapy, < 0.5 ng/ml.
- Cryosurgery
  - Liquid nitrogen is inserted into the prostate with ultrasound guidance.
  - The freezing process results in tissue destruction.
  - The range of positive biopsy rate after cryoablation is 7% to 23%

Pharmacologic Treatment
- Advanced disease
  - Systemic therapy has been aimed at androgen suppression and chemotherapy.
    - Androgen suppression
      - Diethylstibestrol 1–3 mg p.o. daily
      - Luteinizing hormone–releasing hormone (LHRH)
        - Leuprolide
        - Goserelin
          - Monthly or 3-month depot injection
      - Ketoconazole
        - 400 mg p.o. 3 times daily
      - Aminoglutethimide 250 mg p.o. 4 times daily
      - Corticosteroids
        - Prednisone 20–40 mg p.o. daily
      - Orchiectomy
      - Antiandrogens
        - Flutamide 250 mg p.o. 3 times daily
        - Bicalutamide 50 mg p.o. daily
    - Biophosphonates
      - To prevent osteoporosis
      - Decrease bone pain from metastasis
      - Reduce bone-related events
    - Chemotherapy
      - Docetaxel

Special Considerations

- Prostate cancer is most often asymptomatic

When to Consult, Refer, or Hospitalize

- Urology for initial work-up, then radiation, medical oncology, or both as required
- Neurosurgery for spinal cord compression
- Orthopedics for treatment of pathological fractures

Follow-up

Expected Outcomes
- Cancer of the Prostate Risk Assessment (CAPRA)
  - Uses serum PSA, Gleason grade, clinical stage, percent positive biopsies, and patient age in a point system to determine risk and reoccurrence in 3–5 years
    - CAPRA scores: 3-year and 5-year recurrence-free survival rates
      - 0–1: 91% (3-year), 85% (5-year)
      - 2: 89% (3-year), 81% (5-year)
      - 3: 81% (3-year), 66% (5-year)
      - 4: 81% (3-year), 59% (5-year)
      - 5: 69% (3-year), 60% (5-year)
      - 6: 54% (3-year), 32% (5-year)
      - 7+: 24% (3-year), 8% (5-year)

Complications
- Spinal cord compression
- Pathological bone fractures
- Urinary retention or obstruction
- Hematuria

BLADDER CANCER

Description
- The urinary tract is lined with transitional cell epithelium from the renal pelvis to the ureter, urinary bladder, and the proximal two-thirds of the urethra.
- Cancers can occur in any area; 90% develop in the urothelium, a 3- to 7-cell mucosal layer within the muscular bladder.
- 98% of primary bladder cancers are epithelial cancers—90% being urothelial cell carcinomas.
- Adenocarcinomas and squamous cell carcinomas are much less common and account for 2% and 7% (respectively) of bladder cancers in the United States.

Etiology

- Up to 50% of bladder cancers in men and 30% in women may be linked to smoking.
  - Smoking increases the risk of bladder cancer almost fivefold.
- See Risk Factors.

Incidence and Demographics

- Bladder cancer is the 4th most common cancer in men and the 13th in women.
- The incidence is three times higher in men than women and twofold higher in Whites versus Blacks.
- Median age at diagnosis is 65.

Risk Factors

- Cigarette smoking
- Exposure to industrial dyes and solvents
  - Aniline
- Medications
  - Phenacetin
  - Chlornaphazine
  - Cyclophosphamide exposure (chronic)
- Exposure to *Schistosoma haematobium*
  - Parasite found in developing countries
- Vesical calculi
- Prolonged indwelling catheter use
- Chronic bladder infections
- External beam radiation

Prevention and Screening

- Smoking cessation
  - Those who quit smoking have a gradual decline in risk.
- Avoid exposure to suspicious toxins
- Avoid parasite exposure
- Screening for hematuria in asymptomatic patients

Assessment

History
- Hematuria
- Voiding symptoms
  - Urinary frequency, urgency, or both
  - Dysuria
  - Incontinence

- Abdominal pain
- Flank pain
- Bone pain and tenderness
- Weight loss

Physical Examination
- Abdominal mass palpated on bimanual examination
- Hepatomegaly or palpable lymphadenopathy with metastatic disease

Diagnostic Studies
- Abdominal CT scan
- Bladder biopsy during cystoscopy
- Intravenous pyelogram
- Urinalysis
- Urine cytology
- Complete blood count
  - Anemia
- Complete metabolic panel
  - Azotemia

Differential Diagnosis

- Simple ulcers of the bladder
- Endometriosis of the bladder
- Chronic hemorrhagic cystitis
- Granulomatous cystitis
- Tuberculous or syphilitic tumor granulation in the bladder

Management

- Staging: TNM system
  - Stage 0: Noninvasive tumors only in the bladder lining
  - Stage I: Tumor is through the bladder lining but does not reach muscle layer.
  - Stage II: Tumor is in the muscle layer.
  - Stage III: Tumor is past muscle layer into surrounding tissue of the bladder.
  - Stage IV: Tumor has spread to lymph nodes or distant sites (metastasis).

Nonpharmacologic Treatment
- Stage 0 and I
  - Surgery—transurethral resection
    - Diagnostic
    - Allows for staging
- Stage II and III
  - Surgery—radical cystectomy
    - Removal of bladder, prostate, seminal vesicles, surrounding fat and peritoneal attachments in men; the uterus, cervix, urethra, anterior vaginal vault, and typically the ovaries in women

· Bilateral pelvic lymph node dissection
· Urinary diversion
- Ileal conduit
- Continent urinary reservoir
- Orthotopic neobladder
- Surgery with partial cystectomy followed by radiation, chemotherapy, or both
- Stage IV
  - Surgery is not indicated.

Pharmacologic Treatment
- Chemotherapy
  - Stage 0–I
    · Chemotherapy is given via a urethral catheter.
    - Doxorubicin
    - Mitomycin-C
    - Thiotepa
  - Stage II and III
    · Carboplatin
    · Cisplatin
    · Cyclophosphamide
    · Docetaxel
    · Doxorubicin
    · Gemcitabine
    · Ifosfamide
    · Methotrexate
    · Paclitaxel
    · Vinblastine

Special Considerations

- Instruct patient to seek medical care for hematuria, painful urination
- Provide smoking cessation counseling

When to Consult, Refer, or Hospitalize

- Urology consult
- Oncology, surgical consult as warranted

Follow-up

Expected Outcomes
- The frequency of reoccurrence depends on the grade
- At initial presentation, 50% to 80% of bladder cancers are stage I, with survival of 81%.
- 5-year survival with stage II or III disease is 50% to 75% after radical cystectomy.
- Long-term survival with metastatic disease is rare.

Complications
- Anemia
- Hydronephrosis
- Urethral stricture
- Urinary incontinence
- Metastatic disease

OVARIAN CANCER

Description

- Most ovarian cancers (> 90%) are epithelial tumors, with the remainder being several different histologic types.
- Ovarian cancer can metastasize via local extension, lymphatic invasion, intraperitoneal implantation, hematogenous dissemination, and transdiaphragmatic passage.
- Malignant cells tend to implant in sites of stasis along the peritoneal fluid circulation.
- Intraperitoneal dissemination is the most common characteristic of ovarian cancer.
- Hematogenous spread is uncommon early in the disease process and more common with advanced disease.

Etiology

- Exact etiology is unknown.
- One theory is that ovarian cancer is related to ovulation, and when the cycle is suppressed, the risk is decreased.
- May develop from an abnormal repair process on the surface of the ovary, which is ruptured and repaired during each ovulatory cycle

Incidence and Demographics

- The American Cancer Society estimates 1 in 70 women will develop ovarian cancer in their lifetime.
- It is the ninth most common cancer in women and causes 5% of cancer deaths—more than any other gynecological cancer.
- From 2001 to 2005, the incidence declined at a rate of 2.4% annually, and the death rate has been stable since 1998.

Risk Factors

- Ovarian cancer affects females.
- Genetic predisposition or family history
  - Families in which multiple members have ovarian cancer are defined as having hereditary ovarian cancer.
  - Breast and ovarian cancer syndrome
    · Associated with early onset of breast or ovarian cancer
    · Autosomal dominant transmission
    · May be inherited from either parent
    · Most related to BRCA1 gene mutation but some are related to BRCA2 mutations (BRCA1 are tumor suppressor genes that inhibit cell growth)
  - Lynch II syndrome
    · Also known as hereditary nonpolyposis colorectal cancer (HNPCC)
    · These patients and families have a high risk for developing colorectal, endometrial, stomach, small bowel, breast, pancreatic, and ovarian cancers
    · Caused by mutation in the mismatch repair genes
- A history of breast cancer increases the chances of developing ovarian cancer.
- Advancing age—uncommon under the age of 40
  - Incidence increases after the age of 40, with most cases being diagnosed in the seventh decade of life.

Prevention and Screening

- Pregnancy and the use of oral contraceptives decrease the risk of ovarian cancer.
- There is no approved screening method for the general population.
- Screening with transvaginal ultrasonography and CA-125 tumor marker measurement is recommended for women at high risk.
- Prophylactic bilateral salpingo-oophorectomy for women with BRCA1 or BRCA2 mutations by the age of 40 or when childbearing is complete
  - Surgical prophylaxis decreases the risk by about 90%.
  - Not all cases can be prevented because some women are at risk for developing primary peritoneal carcinomas.

Assessment

- Ovarian cancer is staged using the International Federation of Gynecology and Obstetrics (FIGO) staging system.
  - Stage I: Growth limited to the ovaries
  - Stage II: Growth involving one or both ovaries with pelvic extension
  - Stage III: Tumor involving one or both ovaries, with peritoneal implants outside the pelvis, positive retroperitoneal or inguinal nodes, or both.
  - Stage IV: Distant metastases; pleural effusion must have a positive cytology; parenchymal liver metastases indicates stage IV disease

History
- Symptoms may be nonspecific
- Abdominal or pelvic pain
- Vaginal bleeding
- Bloating
- Abdominal distention
- Irregular menses
- Change in bowel habits

Physical Examination
- May not be evident early in the disease process
- Ovarian or pelvic mass
- Pleural effusion
- Abdominal mass or bowel obstruction

Diagnostic Studies
- Complete blood count
- Complete metabolic panel
- CA-125 assay (cancer antigen)
  - May be normal in up to 50% of women with ovarian cancer

Differential Diagnosis

- Adnexal tumors
- Ascites
- Irritable bowel syndrome
- Pancreatic cancer
- Peritoneal cancer
- Rectal cancer
- Gastric adenocarcinoma
- Appendiceal tumors

Management

Nonpharmacologic Treatment
- Surgical care
  - Standard of care includes surgical exploration for primary staging and debulking of the tumor
  - Surgical staging
    - If the disease is confined to the pelvis, then comprehensive surgical staging is needed
    - Staging procedure
      - Peritoneal cytology
      - Multiple peritoneal biopsies
      - Omentectomy
      - Pelvic and para-aortic lymph node sampling

- Debulking (cytoreduction surgery)
    - Should be performed at the time of initial laparotomy
    - The volume of residual disease at the completion of surgery is a reliable prognostic factor.
    - Prognosis after cytoreductive surgery in advanced ovarian cancer
        - Classified in three groups
            - Good risk
                - Microscopic disease outside the pelvis or macroscopic disease less than 2 cm outside the pelvis
            - Intermediate risk
                - Macroscopic disease less than 2 cm outside the pelvis only after surgery
            - Poor risk
                - Macroscopic disease more than 2 cm after surgery or disease outside the peritoneal cavity

Pharmacologic Treatment

- Chemotherapy
    - Standard postoperative chemotherapy is a combination of carboplatin and paclitaxel
    - Neoadjuvant chemotherapy
        - Patients with advanced ovarian cancer who are not candidates for debulking surgery may be treated initially with 2 to 3 cycles of conventional chemotherapy and re-evaluated for cytoreduction.

Special Considerations

- Ovarian tumors are common and most are benign.
- The wide range and types of ovarian cancer are the result of the complexity of ovarian embryology and the differences in tissue origin.

When to Consult, Refer, or Hospitalize

- Gynecologic oncologist when ovarian cancer is suspected

Follow-up

Expected Outcomes

- The prognosis of ovarian cancer is poor and is related to the stage at diagnosis.
- The five-year survival rates according to stage:
    - Stage I: 73%
    - Stage II: 45%
    - Stage III: 21%
    - Stage IV: less than 5%

Complications

- Ascites
- Bowel obstruction
- Pleural effusion
- Bladder obstruction
- Malnutrition
- Edema
- Anemia

CERVICAL CANCER

Description

- A cancer that forms in the tissues of the cervix (organ that connects the uterus and vagina).
- A usually slow-growing cancer that may not have symptoms but can be diagnosed with a Papanicolaou (Pap) test

Etiology

- Almost always caused by human papillomavirus (HPV) infection
- There are more than 100 types of HPV—about 40 are sexually transmitted.
- HPV-16 and HPV-18 cause 70% of cervical cancer.

Incidence and Demographics

- In 2010, there were 12,200 new cases of cervical cancers, with 4,210 deaths.
- Incidence is higher in geographical areas where screening is limited.
- Cervical cancer ranks 14th in frequency of cancer in the United States, but it is the 3rd most common worldwide.
- Since precancerous lesions found by a Pap smear can be treated and cured before cancer develops, the incidence and death rates are relatively low.

Risk Factors

- More common in middle-aged and older women and in Hispanic, Black, and Native American women
- Early onset of sexual activity
- Multiple sexual partners
- Promiscuous male partners
- History of STDs
- Being HIV-positive

Prevention and Screening

- HPV and DNA testing in conjunction with cervical cytology for routine cervical screening of women aged 30 years of age or older
- Pap tests have a relatively high percent of false negatives and are often repeated annually to maximize effectiveness.
- If the results of a Pap and DNA test are negative, a false negative is less likely; therefore, the screening may be extended to every 3 years.
- Vaccines for prevention
  - Gardasil
  - Cervarix
  - Highly effective in preventing persistent infections with HPV types 16 and 18—the two high-risk HPV types associated with the majority of cervical cancers
- Limit sexual partners and avoid sexual activity at an early age
- Use of barrier protection

Assessment

History
- Abnormal Pap test
- Vaginal bleeding—usually postcoital
- Vaginal discomfort
- Malodorous discharge
- Dysuria
- With invasion of bladder or rectum directly
  - Constipation
  - Hematuria
  - Fistula
  - Ureteral obstruction
- With pelvic wall involvement
  - Leg edema, leg pain, or both
  - Hydonephrosis

Physical Examination
- Early in the course the physical examination may be normal.
- With disease progression
  - Cervix may become abnormal in appearance.
    - Gross erosion
    - Ulcer
    - Presence of a mass
  - Rectal exam
    - External mass or gross blood from tumor erosion
  - Bimanual exam
    - Pelvic metastasis
    - Presence of a mass
  - Leg edema
  - Hepatomegaly with liver involvement

- Two staging systems
  - FIGO and TNM
  - TX (No FIGO stage): primary tumor cannot be assessed.
  - T0 (No FIGO stage): no evidence of primary tumor
  - Tis (FIGO 0): cercinoma in situ
  - T1 (FIGO I): ccrvical cancer confined to the uterus
  - T1a (FIGO IA): invasive carcinoma diagnosed by microscopy
  - T1a1 (FIGO IA1): stromal invasion $\geq$ 3 mm in depth and $\leq$ 7 mm in width
  - T1a2 (FIGO IA2): stromal invasion > 3 mm but not > 5 mm with a width of $\leq$ 7 mm
  - T1b (FIGO IB): visible lesion confined to the cervix or microscopic lesion > than IA2
  - T1b1 (FIGO IB1): visible lesion $\geq$ 4 mm
  - FIGO IB2: visible lesion > 4 mm
  - T2 (FIGO II): carcinoma invades tissue beyond the uterus but not as far as the pelvic wall or lower third of the vagina
  - T2a (FIGO IIA): tumor without parametrial invasion
  - T2b (FIGO IIB): tumor with parametrial invasion
  - T3 (FIGO III): extends to pelvic wall, involves the lower third of the vagina, or both
  - T3a (FIGO IIIA): involves the lower third of the vagina, does not extend into the pelvic wall
    - T3b (FIGO IIIB): extends to pelvic wall
    - (FIGO IV): extends beyond the true pelvis or has involved the bladder mucosa or rectal mucosa
    - T4 (FIGO IVA): spread to adjacent organs
    - M1 (FIGO IVB): distant metastasis
    - NX: regional lymph nodes cannot be assessed
    - N0: no regional lymph node metastasis
    - N1: regional lymph node metastasis

Diagnostic Studies
- Pap test
- Complete blood count
- Complete chemistry panel
- Colposcopy for direct endometrial biopsy
- Imaging for staging purposes
  - Chest x-ray
    - To rule out pulmonary metastasis
  - CT of the abdomen and pelvis
    - To rule out metastasis to the liver, lymph nodes, presence of hydronephrosis or hydroureter
  - PET scan
    - For stage IB2 or higher
- Procedures
  - For bulky primary tumor
    - Cystoscopy
    - Proctoscopy
      - To rule out bladder or colon invasion

Differential Diagnosis

- Cervicitis
- Endometrial carcinoma
- Pelvic inflammatory disease
- Uterine cancer
- Vaginitis
- Vaginal cancer

Management

Nonpharmacologic Treatment
- Varies with stage of the cancer
- Early in the course, treatment of choice is surgery
- Stage 0
  - Loop electrosurgical excision procedure (LEEP)
  - Laser therapy
  - Conization
  - Cryotherapy
- Stage IA
  - Surgery
    - Total hysterectomy
    - Radical hysterectomy
    - Conization
    - Pelvic radiation
      - For IA with negative lymph nodes and high risk factors
        - Large primary tumor
        - Deep stromal invasion
        - Lymphovascular space invasion
- Stage IB or IIA
  - Combined external beam radiation with brachytherapy or radical hysterectomy with bilateral pelvic lymphadenectomy
  - Radical trachelectomy with pelvic lymph node dissection
    - Fertility preservation with IA2 disease and IBI disease with lesions ≤ 2 cm

Pharmacologic Treatment
- Stage IIB–IVA
  - Cisplatin based chemotherapy in combination with radiation
- Stage IVB or recurrent cancer
  - Chemotherapy
    - Cisplatin
    - Combined cisplatin and topotecan

Special Considerations

- Proper nutrition is an important adjunct to treatment.
- Use of nutritional supplements is encouraged.
- Megace may be prescribed to promote improved appetite.
- Routine Pap screening must be encouraged.

When to Consult, Refer, or Hospitalize

- When diagnosis made, may need gynecologic oncologist, radiation oncologist, and medical oncologist
- Hospitalization for extensive surgical procedures, chemotherapeutic infusions, or both

Follow-up

Expected Outcomes
- 5-year survival for stage I is 90%, stage II is 60%–80%, stage III is 50%, and stage IV is < 30%.
- Survival outcomes are markedly affected by the extent of the disease at the time of discovery.

Complications
- Invasion of the bladder, rectum, or both
- Pelvic wall involvement
- Pulmonary metastasis
- Radiation
  - Diarrhea
  - Abdominal cramping
  - Rectal discomfort
  - Bleeding
  - Cystourethritis
  - Late complications 1–4 years after treatment
    - Rectal or vaginal stenosis
    - Small bowel obstruction
    - Malabsorption syndromes
    - Chronic cystitis
- Surgical complications
  - Urinary dysfunction
  - Foreshortened vagina
  - Ureterovaginal fistula
  - Bleeding
  - Infection
  - Bowel obstruction
  - Rectovaginal fistula

LYMPHOID CANCER

LEUKEMIAS

Description

- The leukemias are a collection of disorders that produce a variety of bone marrow and white blood cell abnormalities that may be quickly fatal or may remain asymptomatic for years.
- Types include:
  - Malignant proliferation of immature lymphocytes (acute lymphocytic leukemia—ALL) or myeloid cells (acute myeloid leukemia—AML—or acute nonlymphocytic leukemia—ANLL)
  - Proliferation of mature-appearing neoplastic lymphocytes (chronic lymphocytic leukemia—CLL) or immature granulocytes (chronic myeloid leukemia—CML)
  - Rarely: proliferation of mature B cells with prominent projections (hairy cell leukemia)

Etiology

Unknown malignancy that affects the bone marrow and other organs; may be the result of exposure to chemicals, ionizing radiation, or both; genetic factors (chromosomal abnormalities); viral agents

- Commonly see elevated WBC, abnormal WBCs on blood smear, bone marrow failure, and involvement of other organs

Incidence and Demographics

- ALL: most common childhood malignancy with peak incidence at 4 years of age, most common in Whites and boys, higher incidence in industrialized countries; adult ALL approximately 100 cases/year in United States
- AML or ANLL: 50% of cases under age 50
- CLL: most common form of adult leukemia in Western countries, occurring during middle age and in older adults
- CML: Middle age
- Hairy cell leukemia: rare, disease of old age

Risk Factors

- Several immunodeficiency states have an associated risk for lymphoma and leukemia in children (Wiskott-Aldrich, X-linked agammaglobulinemia, severe combined immune deficiency, and ataxia telangiectasia)
- Chemical exposure, radiation exposure, or both
- Chromosomal abnormalities
- Cigarette smoking
- Likelihood of some types increases with age

Prevention and Screening

- Currently there is no standard screening process to detect early stages of leukemia.
- There is no way to prevent leukemia, but people can make lifestyle changes to lower their risk.
- Educate patients to report new onset of symptoms early.
- Patients with family history of leukemia should have regular physical examinations.
- Patients who have been treated with chemotherapy for other types of cancers should have regular physical examinations.
- Avoid exposure to chemicals such as benzene.
- Quit smoking or don't start.

Assessment

History
- General: fever, malaise, weakness, bruising, bleeding, weight loss
- ALL: joint pain, limping, anorexia, infection
- AML: sternal tenderness
- CLL: might be asymptomatic; dyspnea on exertion
- CML: might be asymptomatic; night sweats, blurred vision, anorexia, respiratory distress, sternal tenderness

Physical Examination
- Lymphadenopathy, confirmation of symptoms
- ALL: generalized lymphadenopathy, hepatosplenomegaly, petechiae, and purpura
- AML: mouth sores, occasional lymphadenopathy
- CLL: Hepatosplenomegaly, lymphadenopathy, sustained absolute lymphocytosis, bone marrow and lymphocytes
- CML: splenomegaly, priapism, Philadelphia chromosome in bone marrow

Diagnostic Studies
- CBC with differential and platelets, peripheral smear, chemistries, reticulocyte count, bone marrow aspiration
- Laboratory results: decreased RBC, neutrophils, platelets, reticulocyte count; elevated LDH and uric acid

- Consider chest x-ray, ultrasound or CT scan, coagulation profile
- ALL: peripheral blood lymphoblasts
- CLL: sustained absolute lymphocytosis, in the peripheral blood and bone marrow
- CML: Philadelphia chromosome in bone marrow

Differential Diagnosis

- Aplastic anemia
- Viral diseases
- Mononucleosis
- Pertussis
- Paroxysmal nocturnal hemoglobinuria
- Gaucher's disease
- Myelodysplasia syndromes

Management

Nonpharmacologic Treatment
- Good diet, compliance with treatment, management of side effects and chronic effects of diagnosis
- Avoid activities that might cause injury; avoid medications that affect platelets (e.g., aspirin)
- Bone marrow transplantation
- CML: splenecetomy

Pharmacologic Treatment
- ALL
  - Treatment divided into three phases
    · Remission induction
      - Combination chemotherapy
    · CNS prophylaxis
      - Intrathecal or high-dose systemic chemotherapy, or both
      - Cranial radiation therapy
    · Remission maintenance
    · Average treatment length: 1.5–3 years
    · Gleevec
    · Adriamycin
    · Purinethol
    · Sprycel
    · Arranon
    · Trexall
    · Oncaspar
    · Clolar
    · Vumon

- AML/ANLL
  - Treatment divided into two phases
    · Remission induction
      - Combination chemotherapy
      - CNS therapy only when symptoms present
    · Post-remission
      - No maintenance therapy
  - Oncovin
  - Cerbidine
  - Tarabine PFS
  - Mylotarg
  - Cytosar-U
  - Vincasar PFS
  - Arsenic trixode
- CLL
  - Stage 0
    · No treatment indicated
- Stage I, II, III, or IV
    · Observation in asymptomatic patients
    · Rituximab
    · Ofatumomab
    · Oral alkylating agengts
    · Fludarabine
    · Bendamustine
- CML
  - Targeted therapy with tyrosine kinase inhibitors
  - High-dose therapy followed by allogeneic bone marrow transplant or stem cell transplant
  - Biological therapy with or without chemotherapy
    · Interferon alpha
  - Hydroxyurea
  - Chemotherapy, infection prevention medications
  - Hospitalization required for induction of chemotherapy
  - Interferon

Special Considerations

- Patients with leukemia are prone to other infections.

When to Consult, Refer, or Hospitalize

- Refer to hematologist upon suspicion of diagnosis; patient will be followed by hematologist throughout therapy

Follow-up

Expected Outcomes
- ALL: remission rate is very good
- AML: remission rate is 60% to 80%
- CLL: depends on stage at diagnosis; median survival about 9 years
- CML: usually is transformed into the acute phase within 2 years, then poor survival rate
- Patients who have undergone stem cell transplantation have a 10-year survival rate of 70%

Complications
- Infections, bleeding; side effects of chemotherapy, radiation, or both; relapses

LYMPHOMA

NON-HODGKIN'S LYMPHOMA

Lymphomas are divided into two large groups of neoplasms: Hodgkin's (HL) and non-Hodgkin's lymphoma (NHL).

Description

- NHL tumors originate from the lymphoid tissue—mainly of the lymph nodes
- NHL is a progressive clonal expansion of B cells or T (natural killer—NK) cells
- Most of the NHLs are of B cell origin (about 85%); the rest originate with T/NK cells.
- The tumors are characterized by the following:
  - Level of differentiation
  - The size of the cell of origin
  - The rate of proliferation
  - The histologic pattern of growth
- Lymphomas are low-grade (slow to develop), intermediate, or high-grade (incurable or aggressive)

Etiology

- Chromosomal translocations and molecular rearrangements
- Viruses
  - Epstein-Barr
  - Human T-cell leukemia virus type 1
  - Hepatitis C virus
  - Kaposi sarcoma-associated herpesvirus

- Environmental factors
  - Chemicals
  - Wood preservatives
  - Dusts
  - Hair dye
  - Chemotherapy
  - Radiation exposure
- Congenital immunodeficiency states
  - Severe combined immunodeficiency states
  - Wiskott-Aldrich syndrome
- Acquired immunodeficiency states
  - Immunosuppression
- Chronic inflammation seen with autoimmune disorders
  - Sjögren's syndrome
  - Hashimoto thryoiditis
  - Promotes development of mucosa-associated lymphoid tissue (MALT) and predisposes the patient to subsequent lymphomas
- *Helicobacter pylori* infection implicated in primary GI lymphomas

Incidence and Demographics

- Since the early 1970's, the incidence rates of NHL have almost doubled
  - May be the result of earlier detection
- Incidence varies with race; Whites have a higher risk than Blacks and Asians
- The median age for all subtypes of NHL is older than 50 years, except for patients with high-grade lymphoblastic and small noncleaved lymphomas, which are the most common types observed in children and young adults.
- The incidence is slightly higher in men than women.

Risk Factors

- See Etiology

Prevention and Screening

- Avoidance of carcinogenic environmental factors
- People who are at higher risk should have regular medical examinations
- Knowledge of symptoms—enlarged lymph node that does not resolve in a few weeks (although spontaneous regression of lymph nodes can occur in low-grade lymphoma)
- No preventative or screening protocols for lymphoma

Assessment

- Ann Arbor staging system is used most often for patients with NHL
  - Stage I
    - Single lymph node region
    - Localized involvement of a single extralymphatic organ or site
  - Stage II
    - Involves two or more lymph nodes on the same side of the diaphragm
    - Localized involvement of a single associated extralymphatic organ
  - Stage III
    - Involves lymph node regions on both sides of the diaphragm
    - May also have localized involvement of an extralymphatic organ or site
  - Stage IV
    - Disseminated or multifocal involvement of one or more extralymphatic sites, with or without associated lymph node involvement
    - Isolated extralymphatic organ involvement with distant nodal involvement
  - Subscript letters designate extralymphatic organs
    - L: lung
    - H: liver
    - P: pleura
    - O: bone
    - M: bone marrow
    - D: skin
  - Stages I–IV can be amended by A or B designations.
    - A disease
      - No systemic symptoms
    - B disease
      - Unexplained weight loss > 10% of body weight in the previous 6 months
      - Unexplained fever
      - Night sweats

History
- The Working Formulation classification groups the subtypes of non-Hodgkin's lymphoma by clinical behavior.
  - Low grade
    - Painless adenopathy, slowly progressive
    - Spontaneous regression may occur and can be confused with an infectious process.
    - Extranodal involvement and B symptoms (temperature > 38° C, night sweats, weight loss > 10% from baseline in 6 months) are not common at presentation but are seen with advanced, malignant transformation (low-grade to an intermediate or high-grade lymphoma).
    - Bone marrow is often involved.
    - Fatigue
    - Weakness
  - Intermediate and high grade
    - Adenopathy
    - More than one-third present with extranodal involvement.
      - GI tract
      - Skin

- Bone marrow
- Sinuses
- GU tract
- Thyroid
- CNS symptoms
- B symptoms are common.
- Lymphoblastic lymphoma
  - Anterior superior mediastinal mass
  - Superior vena cava syndrome
  - Leptomeningeal disease with cranial nerve palsies
- Burkitt's lymphoma
  - Large abdominal mass
  - Bowel obstruction
- Obstructive hydronephrosis
- Primary CNS lymphomas are of B cell origin
  - Commonly seen in immunodeficient patients

Physical Examination
- Low grade
  - Peripheral adenopathy
  - Splenomegaly
  - Hepatomegaly
- Intermediate and high grade
  - Rapidly growing and bulky lymphadenopathy
  - Splenomegaly
  - Hepatomegaly
  - Large abdominal mass
  - Testicular mass
  - Skin lesions
    - Mycosis fungoides
  - Mediastinal mass

Diagnostic Studies
- Laboratory
  - CBC
    - Counts may be in the reference range in early stage of the disease
    - Anemia
    - Thrombocytopenia
    - Leukopenia
    - Pancytopenia
    - Lymphocytosis
    - Thrombocytosis
  - Chemistry panel
    - Elevated lactate dehydrogenase
      - Poor prognostic factor
    - Abnormal liver function studies
      - The result of hepatic involvement
      - Hypermetabolic tumor growth

- Hypercalcemia
  - Adult T cell lymphoma-leukemia
- Beta2-microglobulin may be elevated—poor prognosis
- HIV serology
- Imaging studies
  - CT scan of neck, chest, abdomen, and pelvis
  - Chest x-ray
  - Bone scan for patients with bone pain
  - Positron emission tomography (PET)
    - May be used for staging
  - Ultrasound of opposite testis in male patients with primary testicular lesion
  - MRI of the brain when CNS lesions are suspected
- Procedures
  - Tissue biopsy for definitive diagnosis of most accessible lymph nodes
  - Bone marrow biopsy—used for staging purposes
  - Biopsy of extranodal sites—for example the GI tract
  - Lumbar puncture
    - Diffuse aggressive NHL with bone marrow, epidural, testicular, paranasal sinus, nasopharyngeal involvement, or patient with two or more extranodal sites
    - High-grade lymphoblastic lymphoma
    - High-grade, small, noncleaved cell lymphomas
    - HIV-related lymphoma
    - Primary CNS lymphoma
    - Patients with neurological signs and symptoms

Differential Diagnosis

- Infectious monoculeosis
- Solid tumor malignancies
- Benign lymph node infiltration
- Reactive follicular hyperplasia because of infection
- Other hematologic malignancies

Management

Nonpharmacologic Treatment
- Indolent stage I and contiguous stage II
  - Radiotherapy
- Indolent noncontiguous stage II, III, and IV NHL
  - Monoclonal antibodies
  - Asymptomatic, older patients—careful observation
  - Bone marrow transplant
- High-risk lymphoma
  - Stem cell transplant
- The role of surgery in the treatment of NHL is limited.
  - Selected situations

- · If the disease is localized or if risk of perforation, obstruction, or massive bleeding is present, for example, with GI lymphoma
- · Orchiectomy is part of the initial management of testicular lymphoma.

Pharmacologic Treatment
- Indolent noncontiguous stage II, III, and IV NHL
  - Chlorambucil
  - Cyclophosphamide
  - Prednisone
  - Combination chemotherapy
    - · CHOP
      - Cyclophosphamide
      - Hydroxydaunomycin
      - Oncovin-vincristine
      - Prednisone
  - Rituximab used in combination with CHOP
- Aggressive NHL
  - Stage I and contiguous stage II (nonbulky or < 10 cm)
    - · Combination chemotherapy
      - Three cycles of CHOP
      - Radiation therapy
  - Stage II, III, and IV NHL
    - · 40% to 50% are cured with standard therapy.
    - · 35% to 40% will respond and then relapse.
    - · Combined chemotherapy
      - CHOP
      - Rituximab with CHOP
- Recurrent indolent NHL
  - · Combination chemotherapy
  - · Stem cell transplant
  - · Chlorambucil
  - · Bendamustine
- Recurrent aggressive adult NHL
  - High-dose chemotherapy plus stem cell transplantation
- T cell lymphomas
  - CHOP
  - CHOP plus etoposide, gemcitabine
  - Pralatrexate
  - Monoclonal antibodies
- MALT of the stomach
  - Combination antibiotics directed against *H. pylori*
- CNS
  - High-dose IV methotrexate with rituximab
- Treatment of T cell lymphomas
  - Two subgroups
    - · Cutaneous
    - · Systemic T cell

- Combination therapy
  - CHOP
  - CHOP plus etoposide, gemcitabine
  - Single therapy—pralatrexate
  - Monoclonal antibodies—alemtuzumab
  - Immunotoxin—denileukin diftitox
  - Histone deacetylase inhibitors

Special Considerations

- Patients who are neutropenic, thrombocytopenic, or both should take precautions.
  - Avoid exposure to communicable or infectious diseases.
  - Avoid eating raw fruits and vegetables.
  - Use a soft toothbrush.
  - Do not use a razor for shaving.

When to Consult, Refer, or Hospitalize

- A hematologist-oncologist should be consulted.
- Consult a radiation oncologist for treatment of localized or limited-stage low-grade lymphoma or for palliative radiation therapy.
- Consult an infectious disease specialist for patients with neutropenic fever not responding to broad spectrum antibiotics.
- Surgical consultation for lymph node biopsy, palliative procedures, or placement of a venous access device
- Hospitalization may be required for complications of the lymphoma or the treatment of high-grade lymphomas.

Follow-up

Expected Outcomes
- The median survival rate of patients with indolent lymphoma is 10–15 years.
  - These diseases will become refractory to chemotherapeutic agents.
    - This usually occurs at the time of progression to a more aggressive form of lymphoma.
- The International Prognostic Index is used to categorize patients with intermediate-grade lymphoma
  - Factors that affect prognosis
    - Age > 60 years
    - Elevated serum LDH
    - Stage III or IV disease
    - Poor performance status
  - Patients with no or one risk factor have high complete response rates to standard immunochemotherapy (80%), and most responses are long lasting (80%).
  - Patients with two risk factors have a 70% complete response rate, 70% long lasting

- Patients with higher-risk disease have lower response rates and poor survival with standard treatment regimen; alternative regimens are needed.
- For relapse after initial chemotherapy, the prognosis depends on whether the lymphoma is still responsive to chemotherapy.
  - Autologous stem cell transplant offers a 50% chance of long-term remission.

Complications
- Disease-related
  - Cytopenias
  - Bleeding from thrombocytopenia, DIC, or vascular invasion
  - Infection
  - Pericardial effusion
  - Dysrhythmias
  - Pleural effusion or lung parenchymal lesions
  - Superior vena cava syndrome
  - Spinal cord compression
  - Neurological problems from primary CNS lymphoma or lymphomatous meningitis
  - GI obstruction, perforation, bleeding
  - Pain
  - Leukocytosis
- Chemotherapy or treatment-related complications
  - Cytopenias
  - Nausea or vomiting
  - Infection
  - Fatigue
  - Neuropathy
  - Dehydration
  - Cardiac toxicity
  - Catheter-related sepsis
  - Catheter-related thrombosis
  - Secondary malignancies
  - Tumor lysis syndrome
  - Atherosclerosis

HODGKIN'S LYMPHOMA (DISEASE)

Description

- A potentially curable malignant lymphoma defined in terms of its microscopic appearance and the expression of cell surface markers
- Exists in five subtypes
  - Four of these are classic Hodgkin's lymphoma (disease)
    - Nodular sclerosis Hodgkin's disease (NSHD)
    - Mixed cellularity Hodgkin's disease (MCHD)
    - Lymphocyte-depleted Hodgkin's disease (LDHD)
    - Lymphocyte-rich Hodgkin's disease (LRHD)

- The fifth type has unique clinical features and a specific treatment strategy.
  - Nodular lymphocyte predominant (NLPHD)
- In classic Hodgkin's lymphoma, the neoplastic cell is the Reed-Sternberg cell.
  - Reed-Sternberg cells express the CD30 and CD15 antigens.
  - Most Reed-Sternberg cells are of B cell origin.
  - 1% to 2% of Hodgkin's lymphomas have Reed-Sternberg cells that originate from T cells
- Nodular sclerosis accounts for about 60% to 80% of cases.
- Mixed cellularity about 15% to 30% of cases.
- Lymphocyte-depleted lymphoma is < 1% of cases.
- Nodular lymphocyte predominant causes about 5% of cases.
  - Reed-Sternberg cells are absent or infrequent in this type of Hodgkin's lymphoma.
  - Lymphocytic and histocytic (L&H) cells or "popcorn cells" are seen within the background of inflammatory cells—usually benign lymphocytes.
  - L&H cells are negative for CD15 and CD30 but positive for CD19 and CD20 antigens.
- The spread of lymphoma occurs via the lymphatics, hematmogenous routes, and direct extension.

Etiology

- Cause unknown
- Infectious agents may be implicated in the etiology of Hodgkin's lymphoma.
  - Epstein-Barr virus (EBV)
  - Up to 50% of Hodgkin's lymphoma cases have tumor cells that are EBV-positive.
  - Incidence of EBV-positive cells is higher with MCHD (60% to 70%) than with NSHD.
  - Almost 100% of HIV-associated Hodgkin's lymphoma cases are EBV-positive.
- Higher incidence with HIV infection
- Genetic predisposition
  - 1% of patients with Hodgkin's lymphoma have a family history of the disease.
  - Siblings of an affected individual have a three- to sevenfold increased risk for developing Hodgkin's lymphoma.
  - Risk is higher in monozygotic twins.
  - Human leukocyte antigen (HLA)—DP alleles are more common in Hodgkin's lymphoma.

Incidence and Demographics

- Incidence in the United States is slightly higher for males than females per 100,000 people.
  - Males: 3.1
  - Females: 2.6
- Overall incidence is slightly higher in White males.
- Peaks in young adults aged 15–34 years of age and again in individuals > 55 years of age
- Young adults typically have NSHD; young children and older adults have the MCHD subtype more often.

Risk Factors

- See Etiology

Prevention and Screening

- Individuals should be educated regarding behavior that will reduce the risk of cancer.
- Patients should be advised of the risk of infection post-splenectomy and the importance of calling their physician if a fever develops.

Assessment

- The Ann Arbor classification is used most often to stage Hodgkin's lymphoma
  - Stage I
    - Single lymph node area or single extranodal site
  - Stage II
    - Two or more lymph node areas on the same side of the diaphragm
  - Stage III
    - Lymph node areas on both sides of the diaphragm
  - Stage IV
    - Disseminated or multiple involvement of the extranodal organs
    - Involvement of the liver or bone marrow
    - The spleen is considered a lymph node area.
  - A or B designations indicate the presence of B symptoms
    - B: B symptoms are present
    - A: B symptoms are absent
    - X: presence of bulky disease

History
- Asymptomatic lymphadenopathy—above the diaphragm in 80% of patients
- Constitutional symptoms
- Intermittent fever in about 35% of patients
- Chest pain
- Cough
- Shortness of breath
- Pruritis
- Alcohol-induced pain at sites of nodal disease is specific for Hodgkin's lymphoma.
- Back or bone pain (rare)

Physical Examination
- Palpable painless lymphadenopathy in the cervical area (60% to 80%), axilla (6% to 20%), and iguinal area (6% to 20%)
- Involvement of the Waldeyer ring, occipital, or epitrochlear areas
- Splenomegaly
- Hepatomegaly
- Superior vena cava syndrome
- CNS symptoms
  - Paraneoplastic syndromes
  - Cerebellar degeneration
  - Guillain-Barré syndrome
  - Multifocal leudoencephalopathy

Diagnostic Studies
- Erythrocyte sedimentation rate—general marker of inflammation
- Lactate dehydrogenase
  - Elevation may correlate with the bulk of disease.
- Complete blood count
  - Anemia
  - Lymphopenia
  - Neutrophilia
  - Eosinophilia
- Serum creatinine
  - Hodgkin's lymphoma has a rare association with nephrotic syndrome.
- Alkaline phosphatase
  - May be elevated with bone or liver involvement
- HIV testing
- Serum levels of cytokines
  - Interleukin-6 and -10, and soluble CD25 (IL-2 receptor) correlate with tumor burden, systemic symptoms, and prognosis.
- CT of the chest, abdomen, and pelvis
- PET scan used for initial staging
- Procedures
  - If pleural effusion is present: thoracentesis and cytology of fluid
  - May be an exudate, transudate, or chylous
  - Lumbar puncture and MRI for CNS signs or symptoms
  - Excisional lymph node biopsy
  - Bone marrow biopsy
  - Staging laparatomy

Differential Diagnosis

- Cytomegalovirus
- Infectious mononucelosis
- Lung cancer
- Non-Hodgkin's lymphoma
- Sarcoidosis
- Serum sickness
- Syphillis
- SLE
- Tuberculosis
- HIV infection

Management

Pharmacologic and Nonpharmacologic Treatment
- Combined therapy—radiation and chemotherapy are the preferred choice for most patients
- The goal of therapy is induce a complete remission.
  - Complete remission
    - Disappearance of all evidence of disease

- Partial remission
  - Regression of measurable disease and no new sites
- Radiation
  - The dose of radiation is tailored to the clinical situation.
- Chemotherapy
  - MOPP
    - Mechlorethamine
    - Vincristine
    - Procarbazine
    - Prednisone
  - ABVD
    - Adriamycin
    - Bleomycin
    - Vinblastine
    - Dacarbazine
  - Stanford V
    - Doxorubicin
    - Vinblastine
    - Mustard
    - Bleomycin
    - Vincristine
    - Etoposide
    - Prednisone
  - BEACOPP
    - Bleomycin
    - Etoposide
    - Doxorubicin
    - Cyclophosphamide
    - Vincristine
    - Procarbazine
    - Prednisone

Special Considerations

- See non-Hodgkin's lymphoma.
- Patients with refractory or relapsed Hodgkin's lymphoma should be referred to centers capable of high-dose chemotherapy with hematopoietic stem cell support.
- Patients should be educated regarding the psychosocial problems associated with surviving Hodkin's lymphoma.
  - Involve social workers, psychologists, and psychiatrists as needed.

When to Consult, Refer, or Hospitalize

- Hematologist-oncologist
- Radiation oncologist
- Social worker

Follow-up

Expected Outcomes

- The International Prognostic Factors Project (IPFP) score for advanced Hodgkin's lymphoma
    - The following were determined to contribute to an increased risk for Hodgkin's lymphoma progression despite therapy.
        - Serum albumin < 4 g/dL
        - Hemoglobin < 10.5 g/dL
        - Male gender
        - Stage IV disease
        - Age > 45 years
        - WBC > 15,000/mm^3
        - Lymphocyte count < 600/mm^3 or < 8% of the total WBC count
    - The International Prognostic Score (IPS) is the number of these features present at diagnosis and correlates with the rate of freedom from disease progression and overall survival.
        - 0–1 factors: 90% overall survival
        - 4 or more factors: overall survival rate about 59%
        - A limitation of the score is the inability to identify the highest risk subgroup of patients.
- Most relapses occur in the first 3 years.
- Follow-up visits are recommended every 2–4 months for the first 1–2 years and every 3–6 months for the next 3–5 years.
- Follow-up examinations include:
    - History and physical
    - CBC, chemistry panel—LDH, ESR, glucose, and lipid panel
    - Thyroid stimulating hormone annually if the patient had radiation therapy to the neck
    - Chest x-ray or CT scan of the chest every 2–3 years, especially if the disease originally occurred below the diaphragm
    - PET scans for surveillance after complete remission is not encouraged because of the possibility of a false positive.
    - Spiral CT of the chest annually starting 5 years after therapy to screen for lung cancer
    - Female patients with radiation therapy to the chest should be screened annually with mammography starting at age 40 or 5–8 years after the radiation therapy.

Complications

- Cardiac disease
    - Mantle radiotherapy increases the risk of coronary artery disease, chronic pericarditis, pancarditis, valvular heart disease, and conduction defects.
- Pulmonary disease
    - ABVD regimen associated with dose-related pulmonary toxicity—interstitial pneumonitis or fibrosis
    - Mantle irradiation may cause dyspnea on exertion, declining pulmonary function parameters
- Secondary cancers
    - Myelodysplastic syndromes, acute leukemia
    - Breast cancer
    - Solid tumors
        - Lung cancer

- Infertility
- Infections
- Hypothryoidism
- Lhermitte syndrome—an electric shock sensation that radiates along the back and legs upon flexion of the neck that occurs in about 15% of patients after mantle irradiation
- Psychosocial issues
  - Increased fatigue
  - Anxiety
  - Depression
  - Employment problems
  - Sexual dysfunction

MELANOMA

Description

- Malignant melanoma is a neoplasm of melanocytes or cells that develop from melanocytes.
- Melanomas may develop in or near a preexisting lesion or in healthy skin.
  - Melanoma de novo is a cancer that arises from healthy skin.
- Two growth phases
  - Radial
    - Malignant cells grow in a radial pattern in the epidermis.
  - Vertical
    - Most melanomas progress to a vertical growth phase—the malignant cells invade the dermis and are then able to metastasize.
- Five forms of melanoma
  - Superficial spreading
  - Nodular
  - Lentigo maligna
  - Acral lentiginous
  - Mucosal lentiginous
  - Other sites
    - Eyes
    - Mucosa
    - GI tract
    - GU tract
    - Leptomeninges
    - Lymph nodes only—metastatic melanoma with unknown primary sites
- Usually present in two extremes
  - Small skin lesion easily curable by surgical resection
  - Metastatic disease with limited therapeutic options and poor prognosis with a median survival of 6–9 months

Etiology

- Exposure to ultraviolet radiation (UVR)
  - Ultraviolet A and ultraviolet B are potentially carcinogenic.
  - There is not a direct relationship between the development of melanoma and the amount of UVR exposure.
- Chemicals
- Viruses

Incidence and Demographics

- Accounts for 5% of skin cancers
- Responsible for three times as many deaths per year than nonmelanona cancer
- The incidence increases 5% to 7% yearly, second only to lung cancer.
- Affects young and middle-aged people; ≥ 70% of people are under 70 years of age
  - Most common cancer in women 25–29 years of age
- More common in Whites, and those with blond or red hair are more susceptible
  - Whites with dark skin have a much lower risk.
  - Whites who live in Hawaii and the Southwestern United States have the highest incidence.
- The incidence in Blacks is 1/20 that in Whites.
- Melanoma is slightly more common in men than in women.
  - Fifth most common malignancy in men and sixth most common in women
- More common in white collar workers than in those who work outdoors
- Lifetime risk of developing melanoma is 1 in 75.

Risk Factors

- Acute, intermittent, blistering sunburns—particularly areas not usually exposed
  - Lentigo maligna melanoma is the exception to this.
- Changing characteristics of a mole
- > 50 nevi 2 mm or greater in diameter
- One family member with melanoma
- Previous history of melanoma
- Sporadic dysplastic nevi
- Congenital nevus
- Immunosuppression
- Sun sensitivity
- Freckling

Prevention and Screening

- Avoidance of sun exposure
  - Wear protective clothing.
  - Avoid peak sun hours.
  - Avoid tanning booths.

- Use sunscreen with a protection factor of at least 15 (however, no evidence that sunscreen reduces the incidence of melanoma, and some studies have shown that sunscreen use increases the duration of sun exposure and sunburn).
- Annual skin examinations for individuals with a familial melanoma

Assessment

- See staging

History
- Family history
  - Melanoma, other skin caner
  - Irregular, prominent moles
  - Pancreatic cancer
  - Astrocytoma
- Personal history of melanoma
- Frequent sun exposure
- Any change in moles

Physical Examination
- Staging
  - TNM classification
    - T1
      - ≤ 1 mm
      - T1a
        - Without ulceration and mitoses < 1/mm^2
      - T1b
        - With ulceration or mitoses ≥ 1/mm^2
      - T2
      - 1.01–2.00
      - T2a
        - Without ulceration
      - T2b
        - With ulceration
    - T3
      - 2.01–4.00
      - T3a
        - Without ulceration
      - T3b
        - With ulceration
    - T4
      - > 4.00
      - T4a
        - Without ulceration
      - T4b
        - With ulceration
    - N0
      - No nodal involvement

- N1
  - 1 metastatic node
  - N1a
    - Micrometastasis
      - Diagnosed after sentinel node biopsy
  - N1b
    - Macrometastatis
      - Clinically detectable nodes confirmed pathologically
- N2
  - 2–3 metastatic nodes
  - N2a
    - Micrometastasis
  - N2b
    - Macrometastasis
  - N2c
    - In-transit metastases or satellites without metastatic nodes
- N3
  - 4+ metastatic nodes
  - Matted nodes
  - In-transit metastases or satellites with metastatic nodes
- M0
  - No distant metastases
- M1a
  - Distant skin, subcutaneous, or nodal metastases
  - Serum LDH normal
- M1b
  - Lung metastases
  - Serum LDH normal
- M1c
  - All visceral metastases
    - Serum LDH normal
  - Any distant metastases
    - Serum LDH elevated
- Staging by the American Joint Committee on Cancer (AJCC)
  - Stage 0
    - Tis, N0, M0
  - Stage I
    - T1a, N0, M0
    - T2a, N0, M0
  - Stage II
    - T2b, N0, M0
    - T3a, N0, M0
    - T3b, N0, M0
    - T4a, N0, M0
    - T4b, N0, M0
  - Stage III
    - Any T, N 1–3, M0
  - Stage IV
    - Any T, any N, any M

- Must perform a total body skin examination when suspecting melanoma
  - Done on initial examination and on all subsequent examinations
  - Serial photography
- ABCD for differentiating early melanoma from benign nevi
  - A
    - Asymmetry
  - B
    - Border irregularity
  - C
    - Color
      - Very dark black or blue with variation in color
  - D
    - Diameter
      - Mole < 6 mm in diameter usually benign
- Examine all lymph node groups if patient diagnosed with melanoma

Diagnostic Studies
- Complete blood count
- Complete chemistry panel
  - Elevated alkaline phosphatase may indicate metastatic bone or liver disease.
  - Elevated aspartate aminotranserase or alanine aminotransferase may indicate metastatic disease in the liver.
  - Lactate dehydrogenase (LDH) is elevated in malignancies.
    - Not specific to melanoma but is used in the diagnosis and follow-up care
    - Markedly elevated LDH at diagnosis or follow-up may indicate distant metastases—especially in lung or liver.
    - Elevated LDH is a predictive factor for poor prognosis.
- Chest x-ray
  - Used as a baseline for future comparisons
- CT or MRI of the brain
  - Obtain in a patient with known distant metastases, if high-dose interleukin-2 is being considered for treatment, or both
  - Used in patients without metastatic disease if symptoms are present
- CT of the chest
  - Used in staging work-up in stage IV disease to detect metastatic lesions
  - Used in stage I, II, or III disease if clinically indicated
- CT of the abdomen
  - Used when evaluating a patient with stage III melanoma, or locally recurrent or in-transit disease
  - A negative scan may used for future comparisons
- PET scan
  - Used for staging patients with known node disease, or in-transit or satellite lesions
  - Greater sensitivity compared to conventional radiographic studies
  - Used to evaluate response to therapy
  - Not indicated in early disease
- Biopsy
  - Complete excisional biopsy preferred
  - Should include 1–2 mm margin of healthy skin, all layers of skin, and some subcutaneous fat

- If suspected lesion is large or in a cosmetically sensitive area, an incisional or punch biopsy may be used.
  - Biopsy should be taken from the most abnormal area.
    - Shave biopsies are contraindicated

Differential Diagnosis

- Basal cell carcinoma
- Lentigo maligna melanoma
- Mycosis fungoides
- Squamous cell carcinoma
- Blue nevus
- Pigmented spindle cell tumor
- Sebaceous carcinoma

Management

Nonpharmacologic Treatment
- Stage 0 disease
  - Excision with minimal, microscopically free margins
- Stage I
  - Lesions ≤ 2 mm may be treated with radial excision margins of 1 cm.
- Stage II
  - Melanomas with a thickness of 2–4 mm, excision with surgical margins of ≤ 2 cm
  - Lymphatic mapping and sentinel lymph node biopsy to assess for the presence of occult metastasis in regional lymph nodes
- Stage III
  - Wide local excision of the primary tumor with 1–3 cm margins, depending on tumor thickness and location
  - Skin grafts may be needed to close the defect.

Pharmacologic Treatment
- Stage III
  - In addition to above surgical excision
  - High-dose interferon alpha-2b
  - Low-dose interferon
    - No consistent evidence that low-dose interferon improves relapse-free survival (RFS) or overall survival (OS)
  - Unresectable disease
    - These patients are recruited into stage IV clinical trials
- Stage IV
  - Palliative local therapy
    - Reginal lymphadenectomy
    - Local resection of metastases to the lung, GI tract, bone, or brain
    - Palliative radiation may help alleviate symptoms
      - Melanoma is a relatively radiation-resistant cancer by nature.
      - Use for metastases to the brain, bone, and spinal cord

- Systemic therapy
  - Melanoma is refractory to most standard systemic therapies.
  - Two approved treatments
    - Dacarbazine (DTIC)
    - Interleukin-2 (IL-2)
    - Have not demonstrated impact on OS
- Chemotherapy
  - DTIC
  - Nitrosureas
  - Carmustine
  - Lomustine
    - Response rate is about 10% to 20%
    - Short-lived responses—3–6 months
- Immunotherapy
  - IL-2
    - Response is in the 10% to 20% range
    - 5% of patients may experience complete remission.
    - Addition of lymphokine-activated killer cells and tumor-infiltrating lymphocytes has been attempted to improve outcomes
  - Ipilimumab
    - May be used alone or with glycoprotein 100
- Signal transduction inhibitors
  - Sorafenib
  - BRAF inhibitors
    - Use in patients with the BRAF V600E mutation

Special Considerations

- The melanoma risk assessment tool (MRAT) may be used by healthcare providers to estimate risk of developing melanoma
  - It should not be used with patients who already have a diagnosis of melanoma, melanoma-in-situ, nonmelanoma skin cancer, or a family history of melanoma.
  - Risks are estimated for non-Hispanic Whites only.
  - The risk calculator may be found at http://dceg2.cancer.gov/melanomarisktool_prvw
- Clinical trials continue to examine treatment modalities for prolonged survival in patients with stage III and IV melanoma.
- Patients with melanoma have an increased risk of developing a new melanoma, and those with basal or squamous cell skin cancers have a risk of developing another skin cancer of any type.
- Factors predicting a response to treatment include the following:
  - Soft tissue disease or small number of visceral metastases
  - Age < 65 years
  - No prior chemotherapy
  - Normal hepatic and renal function
  - Normal CBC
  - Absence of CNS metastases

When to Consult, Refer, or Hospitalize

- When a suspicious lesion is identified, the patient should be referred to a dermatologist or surgical oncologist for an excisional biopsy.
- When the diagnosis of melanoma is made, an oncology referral should be made
- Hospitalize for complications or treatment for stage III and IV disease.

Follow-up

Expected Outcomes
- The follow-up schedule is influenced by the risk of recurrence, stage of primary lesion, family history, presence of dysplastic nevi, patient anxiety
- Stage 0
  - Annual examination for life
  - Monthly skin self-examination
  - Radiologic testing for specific signs and symptoms only
- Stage I (Ia–Iia)
  - See stage 0
  - History and physical examination (with emphasis on nodes and skin) every 3–12 months for 5 years, then annually as clinically indicated
  - Routine radiologic testing is not recommended.
- Stage II (IIb–IV)
  - See stage 0
  - History and physical examination (with emphasis on nodes and skin) every 3–6 months for 2 years, then every 3–12 months for 3 years, then annually as indicated
  - Consider chest x-ray, CT, PET scan, or a combination every 6–12 months
  - Consider brain MRI annually
  - Routine radiologic testing not recommended past 5 years
- Prognosis
  - Depends on the stage of the disease
    - 5-year survival rate
      - Stage I: > 90%
      - Stage II: 45% to 77%
      - Stage III: 27% to 70%
      - Stage IV: < 20%

Complications
- Damage to deep tissue
- Metastasis
- Fatigue
- Hair loss
- Nausea
- Pain

REFERENCES

Alberio, L. (2008). Heparin-induced thrombocytopenia: Some working hypotheses on pathogenesis, diagnostic strategies and treatment. *Current Opinion in Hematology, 15,* 456–464.

American Joint Commission on Cancer (AJCC). (2009). *Final version of 2009 AJCC melanoma staging and classification.* Retrieved from http://jco.ascopubs.org/content/27/36/6199.full.

Andreoli, T. E. (Ed.). (2007). *Cecil essentials of medicine* (7th ed.). Philadelphia: W. B. Saunders Elsevier.

Ban-Hoefen, M., & Francis, C. (2009). Heparin induced thrombocytopenia and thrombosis in a tertiary care hospital. *Thrombosis Research, 124*(2), 189–192.

Barkley, Jr., T., & Myers, C. (2008). *Practice guidelines for acute care nurse practitioners* (2nd ed.). Philadelphia: Elsevier.

Becker, J., & Wira, C. (2009). Disseminated intravascular coagulation in emergency medicine. *E-Medicine.* Last updated September 10, 2009. Retrieved from www.emedicine.medscape.com

Beers, M. H., Porter, R. S., Jones, T. V., Kaplan, J. L., & Berkwits, M. (2006). *The Merck manual of diagnosis and therapy* (18th ed.). Whitehouse Station, NJ: Merck Research Laboratories.

Beghe, C., Wilson, A., & Ershler, W. B. (2004). Prevalence and outcomes of anemia in geriatrics: A systematic review of the literature. *American Journal of Medicine, 116*(Suppl 7A), 3S–10S.

Blunt, E. (2009). *Family Nurse Practitioner: Nursing Review and Resource Manual.* Silver Spring, MD: American Nurses Credentialing Center.

Dambro, M. R. (2006). *The 5 minute clinical consult.* St. Louis, MO: Lippincott Williams & Wilkins.

Dodd, J., Dare, M., & Middleton, P. (2004). Treatment for women with postpartum iron deficiency anemia. *Cochrane Database of Systematic Reviews, 18*(4), CD004222. Retrieved from http://mrw.interscience.wiley.com/cochrane/clsysrev/articles/CD004222/frame.html

Fauci, A. S., Braunwald E., Kaspar, D. L., Hauser, S. L., Longon, D. L., Jameson, J. L., et al. (Eds). (2007). *Harrison's principles of internal medicine* (17th ed.). New York: McGraw-Hill.

Ferri, F. F. (2008). *Ferri's clinical advisor 2008* (11th ed.). St. Louis, MO: Elsevier Mosby.

Foster, C., Mistry, N. F., Peddi, P. F., & Sharma, S. (2010). *The Washington manual of medical therapeutics* (33rd ed.). Philadelphia: Wolters Kluwer/Lippincott Williams & Wilkins.

Frank, J. E. (2005). Diagnosis and management of G6PD deficiency. *American Family Physician, 72,* 1277–1282. Retrieved from http://www.aafp.org/afp/20051001/1277.html

Gando, S., Saitoh, D., Ogura, H., Mayumi, T., Koseki, K., Ikeda, T., … Japanese Association for Acute Medicine Dissemenated Intravascular Coagulation (JAAM DIC) Study Group. (2008). Natural history of disseminated intravascular coagulation diagnosed based on the newly established diagnostic criteria for critically ill patients: Results of a multicenter, prospective survey. *Critical Care Medicine, 36*(1), 145–150.

Goolsby, M. J., & Grubbs, L. (2006). *Advanced assessment: Interpreting findings and formulating differential diagnoses.* Philadelphia: F. A. Davis.

Hebbar, A. K., Gibson, M. V., & D'Epiro, P. (2006). Recognizing and managing anemia of chronic disease. *Patient Care for the Nurse Practitioner, 40*(11), 36–40.

Hoffman, P. C. (2006). Immune hemolytic anemias. *Hematology: American Society of Hematology Education Program, 13*(8). Retrieved from http://asheducationbook.hematologylibrary.org/cgi/content/full/2006/1/13

Hurley, G. (2007). Anemia: Overview and management. *Primary Health Care, 17*(6), 25–30.

Kelton, J., Hursting, M., Heddle, N., & Lewis, B. (2008). Predictors of clinical outcome in patients with heparin-induced thrombocytopenia treated with direct thrombin inhibition. *Blood Coagulation and Fibrinolysis, 19,* 471–475.

Killip, S., Bennet, J. M., & Chambers, M. D. (2007). Iron deficiency anemia. *American Family Physician, 75*(5), 619–621, 671–678, 756.

Kleigman, R. M., Marcdante, K J., Jensen, H. B., & Behrman, R. E. (2006). *Nelson essentials of pediatrics* (5th ed.). Philadelphia: Elsevier Saunders.

Kulkarni, P., & Cortez, J. (2007). Anemia. *Clinical Pediatrics, 46*(5), 462–465.

Kumar, V. (2007). Pernicious anemia. *Medical Laboratory Observer, 39*(2), 28, 30–31.

McPhee, S. J., Papdakis, M. A., & Tierney, L. M. (Eds.). (2008). *Current medical diagnosis and treatment* (47th ed.). New York: Lange Medical Books/McGraw-Hill.

McPhee, S. J., Papadakis, M. A., & Tierney, L. M. (2011). *Current medical diagnosis & treatment* (50th ed.). New York: Lange Medical Book/McGraw Hill.

Murray, C. K., Chinevere, T. D., Grant, E., Johnson, G. A. Duelm, F., & Hospenthal, D. L. (2006). Prevalence of glucose 6-phosphate dehydrogenase deficiency in Army personnel. *Military Medicine, 171*(9), 905–907.

Napolitano, L., Warkentin, T., Al Mahameed, A., & Nasraway, S. (2006). Heparin-induced thrombocytopenia in the critical care setting: Diagnosis and management. *Critical Care Medicine, 34*(12), 2898–2911.

Novak, B. (2007). The benefits of folic acid. *Nurse Prescribing, 5*(5), 215–220.

Rakel, R. E., & Bope, E. T. (2006). *Conn's current therapy.* Philadelphia: Saunders Elsevier.

Rund, D., & Rachmilewitz, E. (2005). Medical progress: β-thalassemia. *New England Journal of Medicine, 353*(11), 1135–1146, 1193–1196.

Stockman, J., & Lohr, J. (2001). *Essence of office pediatrics.* Philadelphia: W. B. Saunders.

Warkentin, T., Greinacher, A., Koster, A., & Lincoff, M. (2008). Treatment and prevention of heparin-induced thrombocytopenia: American college of chest physicians evidence-based clinical practice guidelines (8th ed.). *Chest, 133*(6), 340s–380s.

Warkentin, T., Maurer, B., & Aster, R. (2007). Heparin-induced thrombocytopenia associated with fondaparinux. *New England Journal of Medicine, 356*(25), 2653–2655.

Made in the USA
Lexington, KY
23 August 2014